# Introduction to Occupational Therapy

# Introduction to Occupational Therapy

**5th Edition**

**Jane Clifford O'Brien, PhD, OTR/L, FAOTA**

Professor
Occupational Therapy Department
Westbrook College of Health Professions
University of New England
Portland, Maine

*Author Emerita:*

**Susan M. Hussey, MS, OT/L**

Professor and Coordinator
Sacramento City College
Science and Allied Health Division
Sacramento, California

ELSEVIER

# ELSEVIER

3251 Riverport Lane
St. Louis, Missouri 63043

INTRODUCTION TO OCCUPATIONAL THERAPY, FIFTH EDITION

ISBN: 978-0-323-44448-4

**Library of Congress Cataloging-in-Publication Data**
Names: O'Brien, Jane Clifford, author. | Hussey, Susan M., author.
Title: Introduction to occupational therapy / Jane Clifford O'Brien, Susan M.
    Hussey.
Description: Fifth edition. | St. Louis, Missouri : Elsevier Inc., [2018] |
    Includes bibliographical references and index.
Identifiers: LCCN 2016039974 | ISBN 9780323444484
Subjects: | MESH: Occupational Therapy
Classification: LCC RM735.4 | NLM WB 555 | DDC 615.8/515--dc23 LC record available at https://lccn.loc.gov/2016039974

*Executive Content Strategist:* Kellie White
*Content Development Specialist:* Kathleen Nahm
*Content Development Manager:* Luke Held
*Publishing Services Manager:* Hemamalini Rajendrababu
*Project Manager:* Janish Ashwin Paul
*Design Direction:* Margaret Reid

Printed in United States of America
Last digit is the print number: 9  8  7  6  5  4  3  2  1

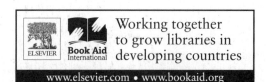

*In memory of Dr. Gary Kielhofner, Dr. Jane Case-Smith, and Dr. Maralynne Mitcham, whose life's work and dedication to the occupational therapy profession made a difference in the lives of persons with disabilities and their families. They inspired and mentored occupational therapy practitioners around the world and in so doing improved the quality of life for those in need of occupational therapy services.*

*In memory of my nephew, 1st Lt. Keith Heidtman, September 2, 1982–May 28, 2007, and the men and women of 2nd Squadron, 6th Cavalry Regiment of the 25th Infantry Division.*

# Reviewers

**Patty Coker-Bolt, Ph.D., OTR/L, FAOTA**
Associate Professor
Division of Occupational Therapy
Medical University of South Carolina
Charleston, South Carolina

**Mary Elizabeth Patnaude, MS, OTR/L**
Assistant Clinical Professor
Occupational Therapy
University of New England
Portland, Maine

# Preface

In the 1980s when I was teaching in the occupational therapy assistant (OTA) program at Palm Beach Junior College, there was no introductory occupational therapy (OT) textbook. When a Mosby representative asked which book I used for my intro class, I responded that I had never found an appropriate introductory text. So I had compiled my own syllabus to include what I thought was needed, using selected readings from other OT books and the *American Journal of Occupational Therapy*. The representative looked over my outline and suggested I forward a copy along with a book proposal for an introductory text. My proposal was accepted; within a year I completed writing the book while testing chapters and exercises on my students. In 1989 the first edition was published under the title *Occupational Therapy: Introductory Concepts*. For the second edition we changed to the present title.

The profession saw many changes prior to and during the 1980s. In its earliest years OT grew from a concern for the humane treatment of all people who were somehow impaired—first those in psychiatric institutions, then later those service members returning from World War I with severe injuries. Crafts were the primary modality and psychiatric hospitals the primary employer. As the treatment of physical disabilities gained prominence, crafts were still featured while new functional modalities emerged.

By the mid-1980s a tension arose within American Occupational Therapy Association (AOTA) between the "soft" and "hard" approaches as the field expanded and grew to encompass new practice areas such as sensory integration, hand therapy, and developmental disabilities/delays. Some occupational therapists were going into private practice, and schools began employing rehabilitation therapists as disabled children were mainstreamed within public schools. Professionalism had become the buzzword, and for many. Fortunately, there were many who believed occupational therapy should incorporate both the holism of its history and contemporary professionalism. I was among them; when I had the opportunity to write the profession's introductory book, I deliberately chose a less formal style and began with a picture essay of people in a spectrum of OT settings to provide a visual overview of the field. I am pleased that has continued throughout all the editions.

I quote from the original text in which I describe the uniqueness of occupational therapy within the broader health field:

An occupational therapist is a facilitator of the patient/client struggle toward independence—of however much or little that person is capable. The occupational therapy profession functions from a mindset that is different from technical specialties. The concern for the whole person is expected in every individual intervention plan. The practitioner is not the repository of some "cure" but the link in assisting a person in finding his or her own abilities or capacities. The professional philosophical base emphasizes that health involves body, mind and spirit in total integration. Dysfunction in any part affects the whole person. If a person loses the ability to walk it is not only his or her legs that are deficient, the entire being is profoundly affected.

I am encouraged that many areas of health care are returning to holism as an essential element of healing. I am also gratified that this text now is in its fifth edition and continues to play an important role in shaping the understanding of the profession for each new generation of OT professionals.

**Barbara Sabonis-Chafee**
(Original author of *Occupational Therapy: Introductory Concepts* and *Introduction to Occupational Therapy*)

This textbook is written for those studying occupational therapy at either the professional level (occupational therapist) or the technical level (occupational therapy assistant) or for those who are exploring the profession to determine whether this is the field for them. *Introduction to Occupational Therapy* gives readers a solid overview of the important concepts of occupational therapy. This edition incorporates the *Occupational Therapy Practice Framework* and the basics of evidence-based practice. Numerous case studies are presented throughout to illustrate the concepts.

The text is divided into four sections. The first section introduces the reader to the field of occupational therapy by providing the history and philosophy of occupational therapy, current issues, future trends in the profession, and a look at OT practice around the globe. Section 2 focuses on the OT practitioner, educational requirements to practice, roles and responsibilities of practitioners, ethical and legal dimensions of practice, and the professional organizations. Section 3 concentrates on the practice of occupational therapy by describing the *Occupational Therapy Practice Framework*, life span changes as related to practice, settings and models of health-care delivery, and service management functions. Section 4 describes the process of occupational therapy. It begins with an overview of the processes involved in evaluation, intervention, and outcomes measurement, followed by a review of models of practice and frames of reference to design intervention. The section concludes with chapters describing the special skills required by OT practitioners, including selecting therapeutic activities and intervention modalities, establishing therapeutic relationships, and developing therapeutic reasoning.

This edition of *Introduction to Occupational Therapy* has been organized to make learning easy for the reader. Each chapter begins with a testimonial written by an occupational therapist or an occupational therapy assistant about his or her experiences in occupational therapy. Each chapter includes objectives outlining the main points and key terms, which are typeset in boldface throughout the text. Case examples are interwoven throughout the chapters, and a summary at the end of each chapter provides a synopsis of the material covered. Learning activities and review questions provide ways to apply the information and concepts covered in the chapter.

Instructors and students may supplement textbook reading with materials available on the Evolve website, which includes separate instructor and student sites that contain the following:

Instructor Resources:
- Test-bank questions
- PowerPoint presentations
- Instructor's Manual: teaching strategies, suggested classroom activities, critical thinking activities, answers to review questions, and additional resources

Student Resources:
- Crossword puzzles
- Fill-in-the blank review questions for each chapter
- Answers to review questions in the textbook
- Sample test-bank questions

Instructors may use test-bank questions to stimulate learning or test knowledge and application of material. PowerPoint presentations of each chapter provide an outline of key content. The Instructor's Manual provides materials to reinforce textbook readings. The teaching strategies and suggested activities (classroom and critical thinking) can be easily incorporated into classes. Many of the strategies and activities require that students present to the class as a way to reinforce learning and facilitate active learning. The review questions at the end of each chapter serve as guides for class discussion. Additional resources enhance content and classroom presentations.

Students may use crossword puzzles, fill-in-the-blank review questions, review questions, and sample test-bank questions to study the material and solidify their knowledge of key concepts.

# Acknowledgments

A special thanks to my family—Mike, Scott, Alison, and Molly—whose support, laughter, play, creativity, and interesting stories energize me every day. I would like to acknowledge Dr. Anita Bundy, Dr. Anne Fisher, Dr. Renee Taylor, Dr. Nancy Carson, Dr. Patti Coker-Bolt and MaryBeth Patnaude for their support, mentoring, guidance, and friendship throughout my career. I would like to recognize my colleagues and students from the University of New England and thank them for allowing me to take photos of them and their families. The American Occupational Therapy Association provided various materials for this book. A special thanks to Susan Hussey and Barbara Sabonis-Chaffee for their work on earlier editions of this text. Thank you to all those at Elsevier, including Kathleen Nahm, Kellie White, Luke Held, Hemamalini Rajendrababu, Janish Paul, and Margeret Reid for their support, guidance, gentle reminders, and professionalism. It is always a joy to work with them.

Finally, I would like to welcome those who read this book and decide to enter this exciting and fulfilling profession. We look forward to your contributions to a profession that makes a difference in people's lives.

**JOB**

# Contents

# SECTION I

# Occupational Therapy: *The Profession*

# 1

# Introductory Questions

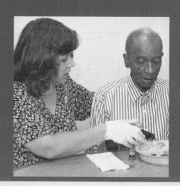

## OBJECTIVES

*After reading this chapter, the reader will be able to do the following:*

- Understand the basic terminology used in occupational therapy.
- Describe the nature and scope of the practice of occupational therapy.
- Identify personality characteristics fitting for a career in occupational therapy.

- Describe levels of occupational therapy personnel.
- Identify types of activities used in occupational therapy intervention.

## KEY TERMS

activity
client
contrived activities
function
goal
independence
media

occupation
occupation-centered activities
occupational performance
occupational therapist
occupational therapy
occupational therapy assistant
occupational therapy practitioner

patient
preparatory activities
purposeful activity
tasks
therapy

*My family is filled with teachers. My grandfather was a teacher. My mother and brother were both teachers, and three of my cousins and an aunt are teachers as well. So why did I become an occupational therapist? As a teenager I was drawn to the idea of helping others. My grandmother was a nurse, and I thought I might like to work as my grandmother did. A medical careers class in high school provided a volunteer opportunity as a candy striper in the West Haven Veterans Administration (VA) hospital. One day a scheduling glitch required my volunteering hours to occur with occupational therapy instead of nursing. Serendipity. At that time, like many people who are not occupational therapists, I had never heard of occupational therapy.*

*My day of volunteering in occupational therapy at the VA hospital included helping wounded or ill veterans engage in a variety of woodworking and other craft-type projects. With my limited understanding of what I was observing that day, I thought that if I were an occupational therapist, I would be paid to do arts and crafts. Amazing! I enjoyed arts and crafts immensely and couldn't think of a better job. I had a lot to learn about occupational therapy though,*

*and as my career turned out, I used crafts very little in my eventual practice.*

*I fell in love with occupational therapy (OT) and have never once regretted my decision. Occupational therapists have a unique way of viewing human behavior. We believe that we strongly influence our own state of health and well-being by what we choose to do and how we use our time. We also believe, as a core tenet of the profession, in the balance between work, self-care, and play/leisure to support and promote health. That concept was one of the first things I learned in OT school, and this idea resonated with me. I always had a variety of hobbies, and I understood as a new OT student that those hobbies were good for me and helped me maintain my sanity as well as my physical health. I feel so fortunate that I have been able to work my entire life in a career that I believe in and relate to, and that this career has afforded me opportunities to help others and make a difference. What more could you ask from a career?*

**HEATHER MILLER KUHANECK, PHD, OTR/L, FAOTA**
**Associate Professor**
**Sacred Heart University**
**Fairfield, Connecticut**

This chapter provides an overview of the occupational therapy (OT) profession, beginning with answers to questions that someone new to the profession may ask. Compare your current knowledge with new insights that may arise while reflecting on the answers to these questions.

## What Is Occupational Therapy?

The *Merriam-Webster's Online Collegiate Dictionary* provides definitions for words that help one to understand OT:[6]

**Occupation:** Activity in which one engages

**Therapy:** Treatment of a physical or mental illness

**Goal:** End toward which effort is directed

**Activity:** State of doing things that requires movement or energy (being active)

**Independence:** State of being self-reliant, not requiring or relying on something else or others

**Occupational therapy:** Therapy based on engagement in meaningful activities of daily life (such as self-care skills, education, work, or social interaction), especially to enable or encourage participation in such activities despite impairments or limitations in physical or mental functioning[6]

OT is a practice that uses goal-directed activity to promote engagement in those things that people find meaningful (i.e., occupations). The *Occupational Therapy Practice Framework: Domain and Process*, from the American OT Association (AOTA) (2014), provides more specificity to the definitions just provided:[4]

**Occupation:** Daily life activities in which people engage, including activities of daily living (ADLs), instrumental activities of daily living, sleep and rest, education, work, play, leisure, and social participation.[4] Occupations are those meaningful activities that give one a sense of identity.

**Occupational performance:** The ability to carry out activities of daily life and one's occupations that result from the interaction among the client, the context, and the activity.[4]

**Purposeful activity:** An activity used during intervention that is goal-directed and typically involves an end product.[5]

AOTA defines OT for professionals and consumers as a profession that uses therapeutic activities to help persons engage in meaningful activities.[3]

## Are There Different Levels of the Occupational Therapy Practitioner?

**Occupational therapy practitioner** refers to two different levels of clinicians: an **occupational therapist** or an **occupational therapy assistant** (OTA). The occupational therapist has more extensive education and training in theory, evaluation, and research than the OTA, who works under the supervision of an occupational therapist. Often, the occupational therapist is referred to as performing at the "professional" level of practice, whereas the OTA performs at the "technical" level. As of 2007, occupational therapists must successfully graduate with a master's degree; OTAs must successfully complete a 2-year associate's degree program. Herein, OT practitioner refers to those within the field at either level. These two roles are discussed in greater depth in Chapters 6 and 7.

## What Does an Occupational Therapy Practitioner Do?

OT practitioners work with clients of all ages and diagnoses. The goal of OT intervention is to increase the ability of the client to participate in everyday activities, including feeding, dressing, bathing, hygiene, self-care, play or leisure, work, education, instrumental activities of daily living, sleep and rest, and social participation. The OT practitioner interacts with a client to assess existing performance, set therapeutic goals, develop a plan, and implement intervention to enable the client to **function** in his or her world. OT practitioners may advocate for clients, make or modify equipment, and/or provide hands-on experiences to help people reengage in life. The OT practitioner records progress and communicates intervention specifics to others (e.g., professionals, families, insurance agencies). The OT practitioner does not simply do something to or for the client; rather, the OT practitioner guides the person to actively participate in intervention. Therefore it is important for the OT practitioner to establish rapport (a relationship of mutual trust) with the client. The therapeutic relationship has value and plays a key role in the intervention process. Section III provides a detailed description of the practice of OT.

## Do Occupational Therapy Practitioners Help People Get Jobs?

Although the term *occupation* commonly refers to jobs in which individuals get paid, it also encompasses the many things people do that are meaningful to them. OT practitioners help clients engage in **occupations** (e.g., activities that have meaning and give people identity). For example, being a mother is an occupation for many clients. This occupation requires that a person complete many activities and tasks. Mothers shop for food and cook meals. Cooking is an **activity** associated with the occupation of being a mother. Cooking may be performed at a much different level for the mother who finds meaning and identity in cooking for her family. **Tasks** refer to the basic units of action (e.g., mixing the batter is a task associated with cooking). See Box 1.1 for examples.

OT practitioners analyze clients' occupations so that they may help clients return to occupations they value. The following example illustrates the distinction between these terms. Gardening is an occupation for Beth; she loves spending time picking out plants, designing layouts, and caring for the garden. She attends many gardening events

| • BOX 1.1 | Examples Describing Key Terms | |
|---|---|---|
| **Occupation** | **Activity** | **Task** |
| Sports team member | Working out in gym or pool | Kicking feet while swimming laps |
| Chef | Preparing a sandwich | Cutting vegetables |
| Mother | Getting children ready for bed | Reading a story to children |
| Student | Going to class | Writing a paper |

with friends who have similar interests. However, she does not necessarily enjoy weeding on hot summer days and finds this to be a chore. Therefore weeding is an activity. She understands the importance of weeding but does not find it essential to her identity. It simply is something she must do within her occupation of gardening. The tasks involved in weeding involve grasping and pulling. Conversely, Jackie does not find gardening enjoyable at all. However, she wants her home to look nice, and, consequently, she plants flowers for this reason. For Jackie, gardening is an activity; her occupation is a homeowner.

## Why Refer to Both "Patient" and "Client"?

OT services are provided to people in many different settings. Professionals use different terms to refer to those served based on the setting. For example, in a hospital or rehabilitation setting, professionals typically use the term *patient,* but they use the term **client** when working in a mental health facility or community center. Individuals receiving services may also be referred to as *residents, participants, consumers, students,* or by their names, according to the setting's policies. In this text, the term *client* is used and is meant to include all settings.

## Are There Personality Characteristics Best Suited for a Career Choice in Occupational Therapy?

OT practitioners have differing interests, personalities, and backgrounds. However, all practitioners possess a desire to help others; they genuinely like people, and they are able to relate to both individuals and small groups. OT practitioners appreciate diversity and value people's ability to change. Generally, OT practitioners are creative thinkers who enjoy hands-on work and are skilled problem solvers. As with any member of the health-care professions, those interested in OT demonstrate the ability to handle their own personal problems and feelings before trying to help others. To support improved engagement in occupation, the OT

practitioner empathizes with clients yet expects and requires effort from them. Because OT practitioners must educate and instruct clients and caregivers, an interest in teaching is also desirable. Practitioners use creative problem solving; they need the ability to find new ways of doing things and flexibility in approaching situations. OT is a lifelong profession; therefore, commitment and dedication are important. As in other professions, the OT practitioner is never finished with education and must always invest in growing with the field and continually maintaining competency.

## What Does an Occupational Therapy Educational Program Cover?

Because of the broad scope of the profession, the knowledge base for students in OT represents several scientific areas, including biological and behavioral sciences, sociology, anthropology, and medicine.[1] The student gains an understanding of typical human development and pathological conditions that affect development and function. With these sciences as a foundation, the student learns the theory and processes related to OT. Educational programs focus on developing students' attitude and awareness so that they are sensitive to the various needs of those seeking intervention. OT education is aimed not only at developing specific skills, but also seeks to develop the student's way of thinking. A problem-solving approach that relies on critical thinking is necessary to evaluate function, analyze activities, and design interventions that facilitate engagement in occupations.

Educational programs teach students how to carefully analyze and evaluate current research. Using the best possible research evidence to assess and intervene is termed evidence-based practice. This is an essential part of any educational program.

Programs provide specific skills training for those techniques most widely used in the profession, although students continue to learn techniques once engaged in clinical practice. All educational programs include a clinical training phase (referred to as *fieldwork*). The student's clinical experiences allow them to integrate the elements of theory and practice. Upon completion of the educational and fieldwork programs, students take a national registry examination, and they are thus prepared to practice in an entry-level position.

## What Is the Main Emphasis of Occupational Therapy Curricula?

Both the occupational therapist (professional) and OTA (technical) educational programs are accredited by the Accreditation Council for Occupational Therapy Education (ACOTE), which is a part of AOTA. Programs are designed to conform to a series of guidelines, called *standards.*[1,2] The course of study features general theory, skills training, and the foundation for therapeutic reasoning. OT curricula have a strong science base and include a focus on human development across the life span.[1,2] Curricula promote professionalism and engagement in occupation through a holistic approach to practice (including the psychological, neurological, and musculoskeletal aspects of occupations). OT education is designed to teach the student problem-solving techniques and skills and prepare students for lifelong learning.

## Who Are the People Served, and What Kinds of Problems or Disabilities Are Addressed by Occupational Therapy?

The mandate of the OT profession is to help clients engage in occupations. The recipients of therapy include people who have problems that interfere with their ability to engage in everyday activities. Clients present with a range of problems, including genetic, neurological, orthopedic, musculoskeletal, immunological, and cardiac dysfunctions, in addition to developmental, psychological, social, behavioral, or emotional disorders. OT practitioners help clients who have functional disabilities by increasing their abilities to do the everyday things they wish to do.

OT practitioners serve all ages (infants to older adults) and clients with physical, cognitive, psychological, and/or psychosocial impairments, which may be the result of an accident or trauma, disease, conflict or stress, social deprivation, genetics, or congenital anomalies (birth defects). For example, an OT practitioner working with children may treat a 2-pound newborn infant in a hospital neonatal unit, a preschool child in an early intervention program, or a child who has cerebral palsy and attends public school. An OT practitioner may work with an adolescent in a drug treatment center or an adolescent in a rehabilitation center who has cognitive limitations as a result of a brain injury. A client may have experienced physical limitations from spinal cord injury after an automobile accident and need to learn to adjust to living with a disability. OT practitioners may teach a homemaker who has had a stroke, resulting in the lack of use of one side of her body, how to manage her home and care for her family again. A client who experiences disability or trauma must learn to establish and embrace his or her new identity. OT practitioners may help with this aspect of disability. A client with a psychological diagnosis, such as schizophrenia, may need help from an OT practitioner to learn skills such as shopping, keeping a checkbook, and using public transportation, or to regain everyday tasks that many take for granted. An OT practitioner might make a splint for a client with a hand injury, work with an older adult in a skilled nursing facility to prepare lunch again, or develop ways to compensate for memory loss. An OT practitioner may also work in a program that helps an individual learn to use assistive technology and train for a new job after an injury. The common goal of all OT interventions is to improve the person's ability to participate in daily living. (See the photographic essay at the end of this chapter.)

## How Are These Services Delivered and in What Kinds of Settings?

OT personnel work in hospitals, clinics, schools, homes, community settings, and even prisons. Some practitioners consult or work in the workplace or in specialty settings (e.g., assistive technology centers). OT practitioners may work in inpatient settings (i.e., clients stay in the setting overnight) or outpatient settings (i.e., clients sleep at home and attend during the day). Acute care settings provide care immediately after trauma and typically involve short hospital stays. Rehabilitation settings provide longer care and intensive therapy from a variety of professionals. Frequently, OT practitioners consult with other team members, who may include physicians, physical therapists, speech therapists, social workers, nutritionists, case managers, nurses, educators, and family members.

OT practitioners evaluate a client's abilities and areas of weakness to develop an intervention plan, which is based on the client's interests, motivations, and goals. Intervention services may be provided in individual or group sessions, depending on the specific needs of the clients. Typically, OT practitioners provide home programs for clients and their families so that therapy goals may be addressed even when the client is not receiving direct service. Further discussion of the intervention process may be found in Section IV.

## What Kinds of Activities Are Used by the Occupational Therapy Practitioner During Intervention?

OT practitioners use purposeful activity (e.g., activities that are meaningful to clients) to help clients regain skills and abilities or compensate for changes in abilities so that they may engage in occupations. Adaptations or modifications may be used to change the way a certain activity is performed so that the client can be successful. For example, clients may use a spoon with a built-up handle to compensate for a weak hand grasp. The goal of therapy sessions is to help clients do the things they wish to do again. Thus OT practitioners analyze the desired occupations and determine the skills and abilities necessary for successful performance.

Intervention may begin with **preparatory activities,** which help get the client ready for the purposeful activity.[4,5] Such things as range of motion (e.g., moving the limbs through a range), exercise, strengthening, or stretching are considered preparatory activities. **Contrived activities** are made-up activities that may include some of the same skills required for the occupation.[5] These activities are used to help simulate the actual activity and may help get the client ready. For example, a client may work on tying shoes by using a doll to simulate this activity before actually tying her own shoes. Or a client may practice the components required to spread jelly before actually preparing a sandwich for lunch. **Purposeful activities** are generally meaningful to the client but may be one task of the occupation.[5] For example, making a sandwich is only part of making lunch. Purposeful activities have an end product and involve allowing the client to have choice. Fisher advocates that OT practitioners facilitate **occupation-centered activities.**[5] In fact, clients retain skills better and are more motivated when performing the actual occupation.[5] Occupation-centered activities are performed in the natural setting (physical, social, and temporal). For example, preparing lunch at home at noon using one's own kitchen supplies is occupation-centered therapy.

OT practitioners develop goals for each client, based upon the client's strengths (abilities) and challenges (weaknesses). The practitioner selects activities using a variety of therapeutic **media,** the objects and materials the practitioner uses to facilitate change. Media may include games, toys, activities, dressing or self-care activities, work activities, arts, crafts, computers, industrial activities, sports, music and dance, role-playing and theater, yoga, gardening, homemaking activities, magic, pet care, and creative writing. Activities may also include the use of assistive technology, aquatics, animal-assisted therapy, ergonomics, yoga, Tai Chi, dance, and community integration. OT practitioners use their creativity and problem-solving skills to design therapy to meet the needs of the client.

## Occupational Therapy Intervention Across the Life Span: A Photographic Essay

The following photographic essay illustrates (see Figs. 1.1 to 1.10) the wonderful diversity of OT intervention across the lifespan.

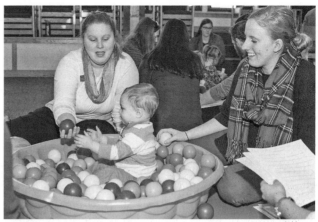

• **Fig. 1.2** An occupational therapy practitioner uses sensory integration treatment to provide a variety of sensory experiences. Immersion in a pool of balls presents challenges to a child with a sensory disorder.

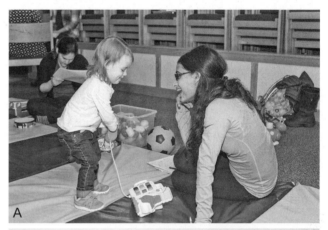

A

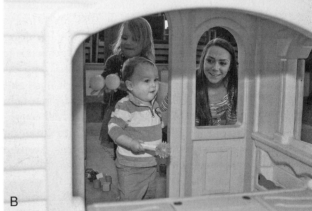

B

• **Fig. 1.3A and Fig. 1.3B** Occupational therapy practitioners working in early intervention or school settings engage children in play.

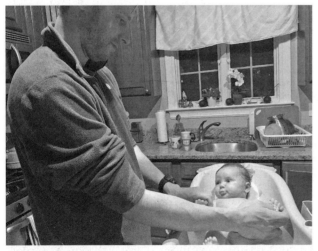

• **Fig. 1.1** Occupational therapy practitioners coach families on the application of calming techniques (such as a warm bath) for infants.

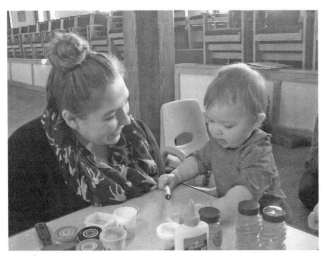

• **Fig. 1.4** An occupational therapy practitioner encourages a young girl to practice using her hands while playing.

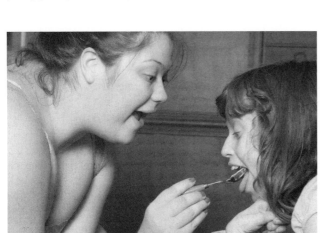

• **Fig. 1.5** The practitioner provides special feeding techniques to help the young girl develop skills to chew and swallow food. (Istockphoto.com)

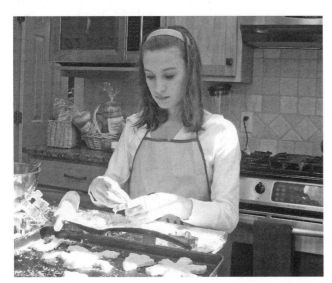

• **Fig. 1.6** Occupational therapy practitioners design activities (such as baking cookies) to enable teens to develop a sense of identity. Occupational therapy practitioners may help teens develop self-confidence through success in a variety of activities.

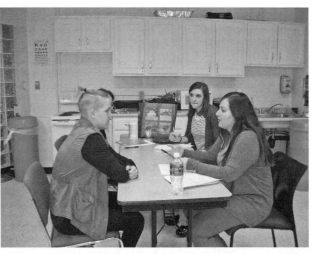

• **Fig. 1.7** Occupational therapy practitioners lead self-help groups for teens to identify support systems and to help teens explore and develop coping and performance skills in a variety of areas.

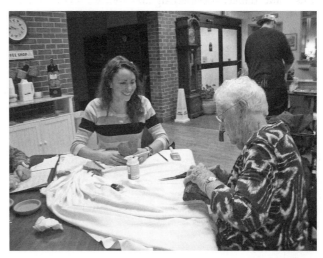

• **Fig. 1.8** The occupational therapy practitioner shows a woman, who has arthritis that causes difficulty in holding objects, how to complete a simple craft project while protecting her hands. Practitioners help adults adjust to physical and psychological challenges.

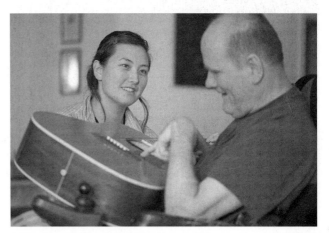

• **Fig. 1.9** An occupational therapy practitioner engages an adult, who had a stroke, in playing his guitar. The occupational therapy practitioner is enabling this man to return to an activity that is meaningful and gives him a sense of self. © iStockphoto.com

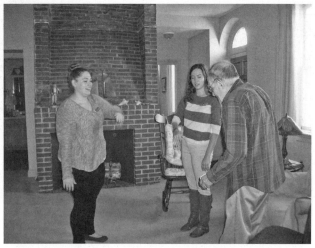

• **Fig. 1.10** Occupational therapy practitioners lead an older man in a physical activity to help with the man's ability to complete daily living tasks, such as walking his dog, walking to the coffee shop, and getting around his apartment.

## Summary

A person pursuing a career in OT must be ready to seek solutions to help clients engage in everyday living. OT practitioners work with diverse clients who have varying abilities, limitations, and desires. Creative persons who have an interest in science and health care and who like working with clients of all ages and abilities will find the career of OT rewarding.

## Learning Activities

1. Ask students to write down three questions they have about the occupational therapy profession prior to reading the text.
2. Require students visit the American Occupational Therapy Association (AOTA) website to learn more about occupational therapy practice.
3. Require students explore the resources and publications available by searching the AOTA website.
4. Illustrate the nature of occupational therapy practice by requesting that students perform their morning routine with only one hand. Discuss how an OT practitioner might help.
5. Select four students, and have each demonstrate preparatory, contrived, purposeful, or occupation-centered activities. Discuss the concepts with the class. For example:
   **Preparatory:** Ask the student to slowly touch each finger with his or her thumb repetitively (to increase coordination and range of motion).
   **Contrived:** Wrap paper around small objects and ask the student to use only one hand to unwrap the object.
   **Purposeful:** Require the student unwrap theraputty surrounding a small object (to increase grip strength and coordination).
   **Occupation-based:** Provide the student with a container full of small wrapped chocolates. Allow the student to enjoy a chocolate snack. Share the chocolates with classmates.
   Discuss the psychological and motor benefits of each activity. Which activity was most motivating? When would you use each? Which was most fun or least fun?
6. Ask students to present a brief overview of the occupational therapy curricula at their educational program.

## Review Questions

1. What is OT?
2. What type of education is required to become an occupational therapist or OTA?
3. What types of things do OT practitioners do?
4. In what kinds of settings do OT practitioners work?
5. What are the differences among preparatory, contrived, purposeful, and occupation-based activities?

## References

1. Accreditation Council for Occupational Therapy Education. *Accreditation Standards for a Master's-Degree Level Educational Program for the Occupational Therapist.* Bethesda, MD: American Occupational Therapy Association; 2008.
2. Accreditation Council for Occupational Therapy Education. *Accreditation Standards for an Educational Program for the Occupational Therapy Assistant.* Bethesda, MD: American Occupational Therapy Association; 2008.
3. American Occupational Therapy Association. *Definition of Occupational Therapy Practice for the AOTA Model Practice Act*; 2011. Retrieved from http://www.aota.org/-/media/Corporate/ Files/Advocacy/State/Resources/PracticeAct/Model%20 Definition%20of%20OT%20Practice%20%20Adopted%20 41411.ashx.
4. American Occupational Therapy Association. Occupational therapy practice framework: domain and process (3rd ed.). *Am J Occup Ther.* 2014;68(suppl. 1):S1–S48. http://dx.doi. org/10.5014/ajot.2014.682006.
5. Fisher AG. Uniting practice and theory in an occupational framework. *Am J Occup Ther.* 1998;52(7):509–521.
6. Merriam-Webster. *Merriam-Webster's Online Collegiate Dictionary.* Springfield, MA: Merriam-Webster; 2015. Retrieved from: www. merriam-webster.com/dictionary/.

# 2

# Looking Back: A History of Occupational Therapy

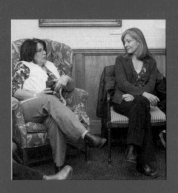

## OBJECTIVES

*After reading this chapter, the reader will be able to do the following:*

- Identify major social influences that gave rise to the field of occupational therapy.
- Name individuals who were involved in the advancement of occupational therapy.
- Recognize how societal influences shaped the field of occupational therapy.
- Describe the concepts that have persisted throughout the history of occupational therapy.
- Describe the influence of historical concepts on the current practice of occupational therapy.
- Identify and describe key pieces of federal legislation that have influenced the practice of occupational therapy.

## KEY TERMS

| | | |
|---|---|---|
| Affordable Care Act | habit training | reductionistic |
| American Occupational Therapy Association (AOTA) | Handicapped Infants and Toddlers Act | Rehabilitation Act of 1973 |
| | Herbert Hall | rehabilitation movement |
| Americans with Disabilities Act of 1990 | holistic | Social Security Amendments |
| arts and crafts movement | Individuals with Disabilities Education Act (IDEA) | Soldier's Rehabilitation Act |
| Balanced Budget Act of 1997 (BBA) | | Susan Cox Johnson |
| Benjamin Rush | Medicare | Susan Tracy |
| Centennial Vision | Meyer Adolf | Technology-Related Assistance for Individuals with Disabilities Act of 1988 |
| Civilian Vocational Rehabilitation Act | moral treatment | |
| deinstitutionalization | National Society for the Promotion of Occupational Therapy | Thomas Kidner |
| Education for All Handicapped Children Act of 1975 | ObamaCare | vision |
| | Philippe Pinel | William Rush Dunton Jr. |
| Eleanor Clarke Slagle | Prospective Payment System (PPS) | William Tuke |
| Gary Kielhofner | reconstruction aides | World War I |
| George Edward Barton | | |

e Visit *www.evolve.elsevier.com* to access the Evolve student resources that accompany your book.

My path to occupational therapy (OT) came through a likely inspiration, my mother, and a less likely one, two physical therapists. As I was recovering from a disastrous end to an alpine ski race with an anterior cruciate ligament (ACL) tear (not my first), I spent some quality time with physical therapists. My physical therapists were top notch, my rehab progressed well, and I was soon back on my two feet again. However, a huge hole was left by my inability to alpine ski race, a role transition that was not addressed through my physical rehabilitation. I was inspired to pursue OT by my mother, a special educator, who suggested OT as a career path. I did what any good high school student does and logged some shadow hours. I shadowed in more than one setting, thank goodness, because I could not have imagined making a career out of the first two. However, it was not long before I caught the OT bug.

*Since the age of 16, I knew I wanted to be an occupational therapist, although initially I wanted to work with clients following neurological injuries and thought I would invent and innovate new assistive devices and aids. Luckily, I learned to adapt and be flexible, a critical part of life, because through fieldwork I found that the hospital setting did not seem to be a good fit.*

*I am grateful every day that I chose the field of OT. I have worked in the field of pediatrics in public school systems, private clinics, and acute care. I have also worked with adults in acute care. Now I am an educator. I often joke about how I am the poster child for embracing OT and career transitions. I knew as a student that I was a lifelong learner, but how wonderful it is to be living that out in my profession. I am still as interested in OT today as I was when I decided to become an occupational therapist. I have loved all of the twists and turns on my career path, and each and every client and family I have encountered has left me a changed and better health-care provider. I have come a long way from not liking hospitals during my fieldwork experience and being the student unable to "stomach" the burn movie in OT school. My last job was at a level 1 trauma center, working with children and adults in the trauma/burn unit. You never know where your OT journey will take you. My advice is to be open to new experiences.*

*I was drawn to becoming an educator because I had the good fortune of working with student programs or OT students at all of my employing organizations. I was impressed by the level of passion and knowledge shown by the students. These experiences inspired me to further my own education to ensure that my practice as an occupational therapist was evidence based and current. Working in academia provides me an opportunity to collaborate with aspiring OT practitioners, thus blending theory and practice. Just as my clients and their families inspired me in practice, I am inspired by the students each day.*

**ELIZABETH CRAMPSEY, MS, OTR/L, BCPR**
**Assistant Clinical Professor**
**Coordinator, Community Therapy Center**
**University of New England**
**Portland, Maine**

Dr. Robert Bing, an occupational therapist and educator, advises, "We exist in the present, yet are future oriented. To make sense of the present or future, we must have knowledge about and an appreciation of the past."[7]

To understand the occupational therapy (OT) profession today, it is necessary to examine the past and understand how the profession originated and developed. The history of OT can be traced with two threads that are intertwined. The social, political, and cultural thread identifies the many currents of human events that influenced the development of OT over time. This includes legislative history that has influenced the delivery of health-care services in general and OT services in particular. The second thread represents the people of the OT profession and how they influenced the direction of the profession. This chapter provides an overview of the social, political, and cultural events that influenced OT and introduces key individuals who developed and shaped today's profession.

## 18th and 19th Centuries

The late 1700s and early 1800s can be distinguished by an awakening of a social consciousness, an awareness that social structures lead to vast inequities. People began to believe that a measure of life's goodness should be available to all people. Evidence of this awakening is found in the novels of Charles Dickens and in the founding of various welfare organizations. This new sense of social conscience gave rise to the Civil War, which eliminated slavery in America, a previously accepted practice that extended back through all of human history. Such social conscience is one thread in the course of human history.

This awakening brought many previously ignored and cruel practices to light, one of which was the treatment of those with mental disorders. Thought to be possessed by the devil, the "insane" were feared by society; locked away like criminals; and often chained, abused, and ignored. The concept of moral treatment developed from this focus on the group of suffering humanity.

### Moral Treatment

**Moral treatment** was grounded in the philosophy that all people, even the most challenged, are entitled to consideration and human compassion. The moral treatment movement sought ways to make the existence of those confined more bearable. One of the ways identified was involvement in purposeful activity.

Two men from different parts of the world are credited with conceiving the moral treatment movement: **Philippe Pinel** and **William Tuke**.[6] Philippe Pinel, a physician in France, introduced "work treatment" for the "insane" in the late 1700s. He used activities to divert the patients' minds away from their emotional disturbances and toward improving their skills.[8] He used physical exercise, work, music, and literature in his treatment. In addition, he introduced farming as an important element of institutional life.[6] Pinel believed that each patient must be critically observed and analyzed, then treatment should commence.[8]

The Society of Friends, also known as Quakers, had a great influence in England. William Tuke, an English Quaker and wealthy merchant, became aware of the terrible conditions in an asylum in York, England, and he suggested establishing the York Retreat.[6] Tuke and Thomas Fowler, the appointed visiting physician, believed that moral treatment methods were preferable to using restraint and drugs. The environment at the York Retreat was like that of a family in which the patients were approached with kindness and consideration.[6,8]

After the publication of Pinel's work in 1801 and Tuke's work in 1813 on the use of moral treatment, many hospitals in both Europe and the United States implemented reforms.[6] In the United States, **Benjamin Rush,** a Quaker, was the first physician to institute moral treatment practices.

Participants in the moral treatment movement followed a structured daily routine and engaged in simple work tasks that promoted better health. Organizing activities for the patients brought order and purpose to unstructured confinement. For these persons, whose day-to-day functioning fell outside the bounds of socially acceptable behavior, there was an individualized routine of personal caretaking and productive involvement in activities.

Although use of the term *moral treatment* began to fade by the mid-1800s, many of the concepts initiated by this movement continued. The practice of OT eventually emerged from this humanitarian concern for each human being and from the use of structured activity that simulated a more normal life for asylum inmates.

## The Early 20th Century and the Beginning of the Occupational Therapy Profession

Changes in science, technology, medicine, and industry toward the end of the 19th century and into the beginning of the 20th century, including new modes of communication and transportation, accelerated the pace of everyday life. Machines were first used in the production of goods; Henry Ford developed the moving assembly line for the production of automobiles in 1913.

In reaction to the expanding use of tools and machines, a contingency of proponents of the arts and crafts developed. John Ruskin and William Morris led the **arts and crafts movement** in England (Fig. 2.1). Proponents of the arts and crafts movement in both England and America were opposed to the production of items by machine, believing that this alienated people from nature and their own creativity. They sought to restore the ties between beautiful work and the worker by returning to high standards of design and craftsmanship not found in mass-produced items. They believed that using one's hands to make items connected people to their work, physically and mentally, and thus was healthier.[24,8] Arts and crafts societies were created to allow people to experience the pleasure of making practical and beautiful items for everyday use. These societies had a long-lasting effect on communities.

At the turn of the 20th century, some members of society became concerned for those who were taken from the mainstream of life by injury or illness and thereafter expected to sit on the sidelines. Until this time, a person with a disability either "got better" or was denied

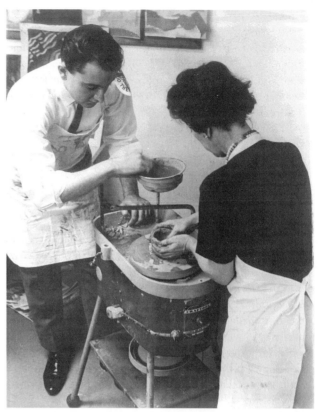

• **Fig. 2.1** Working with clay was part of the arts and craft movement. (Courtesy of the Archive of the American Occupational Therapy Association, Inc.)

competitive involvement in life. The time came to look beyond these two alternatives; there was a need and desire for other options. An awareness that a "handicapped" person is still productive surfaced in sanitariums and hospitals for convalescent individuals. These events influenced the development of the OT profession.

### Founders of the Profession

Several individuals who shared a belief in the benefits of occupation as treatment were influential in the founding of the profession in the United States. These individuals had backgrounds in a variety of disciplines that included psychiatry, medicine, architecture, nursing, arts and crafts, rehabilitation, teaching, and social work. Their backgrounds served to enrich the depth and breadth of the profession of OT.[24] This fledgling form of treatment was called by various names during this period of development, including *ergo-therapy, activity therapy, occupation treatment, moral treatment,* and *the work cure.* The origination of the term *occupation therapy* is ascribed to William Rush Dunton.[12] Later, George Barton recommended that the term be changed to *occupational therapy.*

### Herbert Hall

At the turn of the century, chronic illness and disability, such as tuberculosis, neurasthenia, and industrial accidents, were on the rise as people became victims of urban and industrial life. Adapting the arts and crafts movement for medical purposes was a treatment concept developed by **Herbert Hall,** a physician who graduated from Harvard Medical School (Fig. 2.2). He worked with invalid patients, providing medical supervision of crafts for the purpose of improving their health and financial independence.[24]

In 1904, he established a facility at Marblehead, Massachusetts, where patients with neurasthenia worked on arts and crafts as part of treatment. Neurasthenia, a disorder that was commonly seen in women, caused severe weakness during the performance of work activities. The treatment usually prescribed at the time was total rest. Hall's alternative to the "rest cure" was arts and crafts activities, beginning with participation on a limited basis from bed and gradually increasing the level of activity until the patient went to the workshop, in which she worked on weaving looms, ceramics, and other crafts.[24] He called this approach the "work cure." In 1906, he received a grant of $1000 to study the "treatment of neurasthenia by progressive and graded manual occupation."

Even though Hall was not present at the founding meeting of the National Society for the Promotion of Occupational Therapy (discussed later in the chapter), his work with occupation was widely published and recognized by the other founders. He also took on a leadership role in the early history of the organization by serving as its president from 1920 to 1923.

### George Edward Barton

**George Edward Barton** was a dynamic and resourceful architect who studied in London under William Morris, one of the leaders of Britain's arts and crafts movement (Fig. 2.3). Later, he returned to Boston to incorporate the Boston Society of Arts and Crafts. After personally experiencing a number of disabling conditions—tuberculosis, foot amputation, and paralysis of the left side of his body—Barton was determined to improve the plight of convalescent individuals. In 1914, Barton opened the Consolation House for convalescent patients in Clifton Springs, New York, where occupation, in the form of arts and crafts, was used as a method of treatment.

Barton studied rehabilitation courses available at the time and made contact with people dedicated to reforming the conditions in asylums, many of whom were influenced by the moral treatment movement. Among those whom Barton established contact with were Dr. William R. Dunton Jr., Eleanor Clarke Slagle, Susan Tracy, and Susan Cox Johnson.

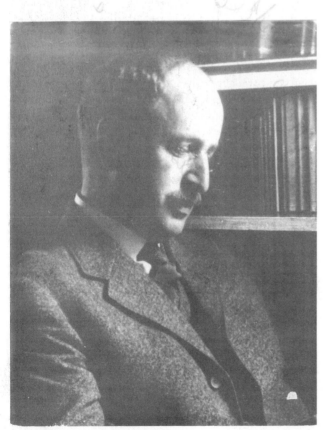

● **Fig. 2.2 Herbert Hall.** (Courtesy of the Archive of the American Occupational Therapy Association, Inc.)

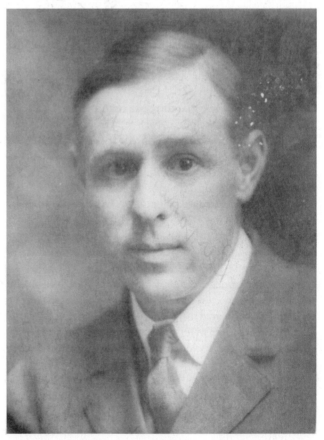

● **Fig. 2.3** George Edward Barton. (Courtesy of the Archive of the American Occupational Therapy Association, Inc.)

## Dr. William Rush Dunton Jr.

**Dr. William Rush Dunton Jr.,** considered the father of occupational therapy, was a psychiatrist who spent his career treating psychiatric patients (Fig. 2.4). In 1891, he was hired as the assistant staff physician at the Sheppard Asylum (later named the Sheppard and Enoch Pratt Hospital) in Towson, Maryland. Having studied the treatment programs of Pinel and Tuke, he was interested in implementing a similar program at the Sheppard Asylum.

In the early 1910s, the hospital introduced a regimen of crafts for its patients. Hospital staff performed necessary medical procedures and provided a structured environment, and the patients were expected to actively participate in their rehabilitation by working in the workshop.[24] Dunton was known for his writings on the value of occupation for treatment. In 1915, he published *Occupational Therapy: A Manual for Nurses*, which describes simple activities that the nurse can use or adapt in the treatment of patients. Dunton served as treasurer and president of the National Society for the Promotion of Occupational Therapy and edited the association's journal for 21 years.

## Eleanor Clarke Slagle

Often referred to as the mother of occupational therapy,[24] **Eleanor Clarke Slagle** began her career as a student in social work (Fig. 2.5). She attended training courses in curative occupations in 1908 at the Chicago School of Civics and Philanthropy, which was affiliated with Hull House and Jane Addams. After this training, she worked at state hospitals in Michigan and New York. In 1912, she was asked by Adolf Meyer to direct a new OT department at the Henry Phipps Psychiatric Clinic of Johns Hopkins Hospital in Baltimore, Maryland. It was at this time that Slagle developed the area of work for which she is most noted, "habit training." **Habit training** is described as a "re-education program designed to overcome disorganized habits, to modify other habits, and to construct new ones, with the goal of restoring and maintaining health."[7,8] Habit training involved all hospital personnel and took place 24 hours a day. Slagle summarized it as a "directed activity, and [it] differs from all other forms of treatment in that it is given in increasing doses as the patient improves."[15]

In 1914 Slagle returned to Chicago, where she lectured at the Chicago School of Civics and Philanthropy and started a workshop for the chronically unemployed.[24] Soon after

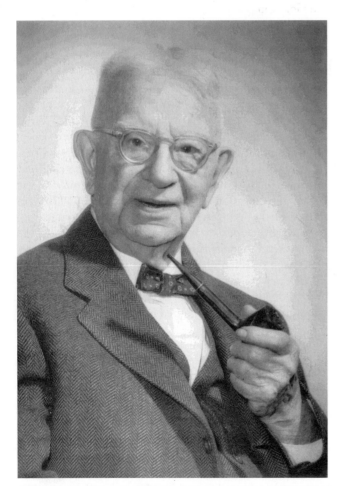

**Fig. 2.4** Dr. William Rush Dunton Jr. (Courtesy of the Archive of the American Occupational Therapy Association, Inc.)

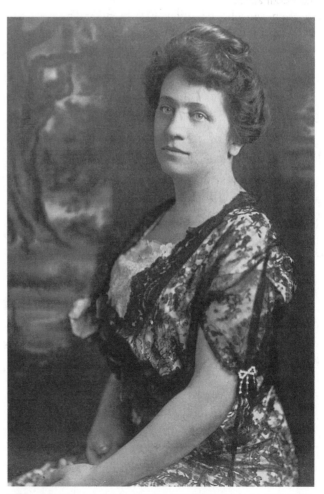

**Fig. 2.5** Eleanor Clarke Slagle. (Courtesy of the Archive of the American Occupational Therapy Association, Inc.)

the move, she organized the first professional school for OT practitioners, the Henry B. Favill School of Occupations.

Slagle's dedication to the profession can be illustrated by the fact that her home was the first unofficial headquarters of the National Society for the Promotion of Occupational Therapy (NSPOT), which later became the American Occupational Therapy Association (AOTA). During her lifetime she held each office within the AOTA and served as executive secretary for 14 years. In 1953 the AOTA established the Eleanor Clarke Slagle Lectureship Award, named in her honor. Today, AOTA awards this prestigious honor to occupational therapists who have made significant contributions to the profession. The recipient provides a lecture to the association members as a way to direct the future of the profession.

### Susan Tracy

**Susan Tracy** was a nursing instructor involved in the arts and crafts movement and in the training of nurses in the use of occupations. She was hired in 1905 to work at the Adams Nervine Asylum, a small mental institution in Jamaica Plain, Massachusetts. While at this institution, she supervised the nursing school, developed the occupations program, and conducted postgraduate courses for nurses.[24] Tracy's *Studies in Invalid Occupations*[30] is the first-known book about OT. In it she describes the selection and practical use of arts and crafts activities for patients. Throughout her career, Tracy was involved in teaching training courses. She believed only nurses were qualified to practice occupations, and she tried to make patient occupations a nursing specialty. Tracy was involved with her work and not able to attend the first meeting of the NSPOT, but she actively served as chair of the Committee of Teaching Methods.

### Susan Cox Johnson

**Susan Cox Johnson** was a designer and arts and crafts teacher from Berkeley, California. She later became the director of occupations at the Montefiore Home and Hospitals in New York. In this position she sought to demonstrate that occupation could be morally uplifting, that it could improve the mental and physical state of patients and inmates in public hospitals, and that these individuals could contribute to their self-support.[18] Following her work in this capacity, she joined the nursing faculty of Columbia University, where she taught OT.[22] She was an advocate for high educational standards and for the training of competent practitioners versus the training of large numbers of practitioners.

### Thomas Kidner

**Thomas Kidner** was a friend of George Barton's and fellow architect and teacher. He was influential in establishing a presence for OT in vocational rehabilitation and tuberculosis treatment (Fig. 2.6). In 1915 he was appointed to the position of vocational secretary of the Canadian Military Hospitals Commission. In this position he was responsible

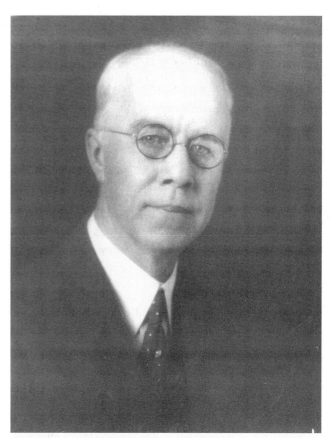

• **Fig. 2.6** Thomas Kidner. (Courtesy of the Archive of the American Occupational Therapy Association, Inc.)

for developing a system of vocational rehabilitation for disabled Canadian veterans who served in World War I. As a Canadian architect, he was recognized for constructing institutions for individuals with physical disabilities. In many of his architectural drawings for these facilities, he included workshops for OT. When the United States passed the Vocational Rehabilitation Act in 1920 (described in the following section), Kidner encouraged occupational therapists to capitalize on this opportunity. He became interested in tuberculosis when he realized that many men disabled in World War I were diagnosed with the disease. He helped promote the movement to hospitalize individuals with tuberculosis and designed hospitals in both Canada and the United States for the treatment of tuberculosis patients.[24]

## National Society for the Promotion of Occupational Therapy

The formal "birth" of the profession of OT can be traced to a specific event. On March 15, 1917, a small group of people from varied backgrounds convened the initial organizational meeting and produced the Certificate of Incorporation of the **National Society for the Promotion of Occupational Therapy** in Clifton Springs, New York (Fig. 2.7). Included in this group were George Barton, William Dunton, Eleanor

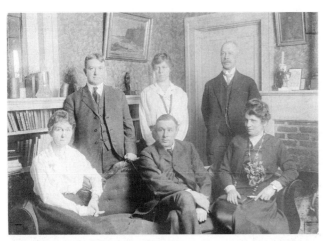

**Fig. 2.7** The National Society for the Promotion of Occupational Therapy in Clifton Springs, New York. (Courtesy of the Archive of the American Occupational Therapy Association, Inc.)

Clark Slagle, Susan Cox Johnson, Thomas Kidner, and Isabel Newton, who attended in the capacity of Barton's secretary (and later became his wife) and was, in fact, made secretary of the new organization. Reportedly, George Barton rejected William Dunton's nomination of Herbert Hall for inclusion at the founding meeting.[18] Susan Tracy could not attend but was made a charter member of the association. The object of the association as set forth in its Constitution was "to study and advance curative occupations for invalids and convalescents; to gather news of progress in OT and to use such knowledge to the common good; to encourage original research, to promote cooperation among OT societies, and with other agencies of rehabilitation."[4]

In September 1917, 26 men and women held the first annual meeting of the organization. Early in these formative years, a set of principles was developed (Box 2.1).

---

**• BOX 2.1 | Dunton's Principles of Occupational Therapy**

- Any activity should have a cure as its objective.
- The activity should be interesting.
- There should be a useful purpose other than to merely gain the patient's attention and interest.
- The activity should preferably lead to an increase in knowledge on the patient's part.
- Activity should be carried on with others, such as a group.
- The occupational therapist should make a careful study of the patient and attempt to meet as many needs as possible through activity.
- Activity should cease before the onset of fatigue.
- Genuine encouragement should be given whenever indicated.
- Work is much to be preferred over idleness, even when the end product of the patient's labor is of poor quality or is useless.

From Dunton, W. R. (1919). *Reconstruction therapy*. Philadelphia, PA: Saunders, p. 320.

---

## Philosophical Base: Holistic Perspective

Another individual's influence helped shape the emerging profession of OT, although he was not present at the first organizational meeting. **Adolf Meyer**, a Swiss physician who immigrated to the United States in 1892 and later became a professor of psychiatry at Johns Hopkins University, expressed a point of view that eventually formed the philosophical base of the profession (Fig. 2.8).

Meyer was committed to a **holistic** perspective and developed the psychobiological approach to mental illness. He advocated that each individual should be seen as a complete and unified whole, not merely a series of parts or problems to be managed. He maintained that involvement in meaningful activity was a distinct human characteristic. Further, he believed that providing an individual with the opportunity to participate in purposeful activity promoted health.

In 1921 at the fifth annual meeting of the NSPOT in Baltimore, Maryland, Meyer delivered the keynote address. The "Philosophy of Occupational Therapy" was later published in the organization's first journal in 1922 and emphasized developing habits to achieve a balance between work, play, rest, and sleep. In his keynote, address he stated that:

*There are many ... rhythms which we must be attuned to: the larger rhythms of night and day, of sleep and waking hours ... and finally the big four—work and play and rest and sleep, which our organism must be able to balance even*

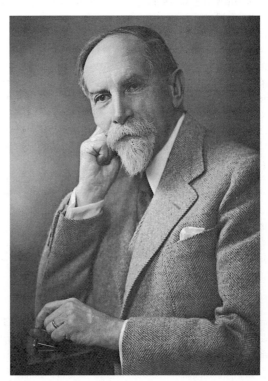

**Fig. 2.8** Adolf Meyer. (Courtesy of the Archive of the American Occupational Therapy Association, Inc.)

*under difficulty. The only way to attain balance in all this is actual doing, actual practice, a program of wholesome living as the basis of wholesome feeling and thinking and fancy and interests.*[20]

Thus, Adolph Meyer provided the foundational philosophical statement for the profession. An examination of political, social, and cultural events that shaped the profession follows.

## World War I

Along with the use of occupations for the "insane" and the early sheltered workshops for convalescent individuals, **World War I** and the creation of **reconstruction aides** served to influence the profession (Fig. 2.9).

In May 1917, 1 month following President Woodrow Wilson's declaration of war, the US military initiated a reconstruction program. The purpose of the program was to rehabilitate soldiers who had been injured in the war so that they could either return to active military duty or be employed in civilian jobs. The program was placed under the direction of orthopedic professionals and included OT aides, physiotherapy aides, and vocational evaluators. In early 1918 the program began on a trial basis at Walter Reed Hospital in Washington, DC, with a group of physiotherapy aides and OT aides who were civilian women with no military ranking.[13] The physiotherapy aides used techniques such as massage and exercise in their therapy, and they worked primarily with orthopedic patients, whereas the OT aides used arts and crafts to treat the mind and the body.[24] The OT aides worked with both orthopedic and psychiatric patients.

Several training programs were implemented, and hundreds of women were trained to be practitioners. The program was also implemented overseas when the first group of reconstruction aides was sent to France to assist in the rehabilitation of US soldiers. Under poor working conditions—no rank, no uniforms, no materials or equipment, no prepared working areas—the reconstruction aides demonstrated to the US Army that involvement in activities had a beneficial effect on hospitalized soldiers suffering from "shell shock."[19] The approach proved to be beneficial to the US Army, and the demand for the aides' services increased throughout the war.

As the need for reconstruction aides increased, so did the need for training. Not only did existing schools and hospitals add training courses, but new schools were created to meet the need. Typically, the programs consisted of instruction in arts and crafts, medical lectures, and hospital etiquette, in addition to practical experience in a hospital or clinic. Although only a high school diploma was required, many of the women accepted into these programs had previous training in social work, teaching, or the arts.[24] Many supporters of OT viewed this as an opportunity to expand the field. Others felt that the training programs were hastily developed in response to the war, and they were concerned about the proficiency of the newly trained practitioners.

The war ended in November 1918, and many of the women who trained to become reconstruction aides left the field. Only a small percentage of the aides were actually occupational therapists. Others eventually became occupational therapists, and some went back to their prior roles (e.g., artist, teacher).[19] Many of the training programs closed. Reconstruction aides showed the validity of activity as therapy and linked OT with physical disabilities.

## Post–World War I Through the 1930s

Rehabilitation remained important after the war. Two pieces of federal legislation provided the impetus for the development or expansion of vocational rehabilitation programs that often included OT practitioners. The Smith–Sears Veterans Rehabilitation Act of 1918, also known as the **Soldier's Rehabilitation Act,** established a program of vocational rehabilitation for soldiers disabled on active duty (Fig. 2.10). When injured soldiers returned home, OT practitioners had a role in helping the soldiers to adjust to their "industrial responsibilities" in civilian life. OT practitioners focused on rehabilitating the soldiers so they could return to productive living.

In 1920 Congress passed the Smith–Fess Act, also known as the **Civilian Vocational Rehabilitation Act** (Public Law [PL] 66-236). This act provided federal funds to states on a 50-50 matching basis to provide vocational rehabilitation services to civilians with physical disabilities. To be eligible for benefits, applicants for the program had to be unable, because of their disability, to engage "successfully" in "gainful employment." Funds were provided for vocational guidance, training, occupational adjustment, prosthetics, and placement services. Passage of the Smith–Hughes Act and the Smith–Sears Act marks the beginning of the federal government's involvement in funding health-care services. The OT profession became valued as a provider of some of these prevocational and rehabilitation services.

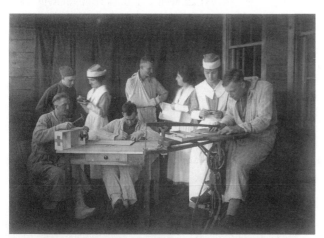

• **Fig. 2.9** Reconstruction aides served soldiers during WWI. (Courtesy of the Archive of the American Occupational Therapy Association, Inc.)

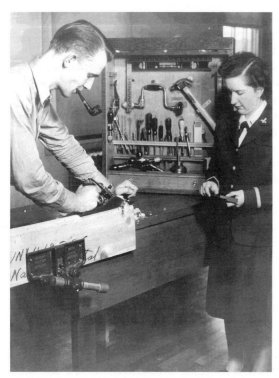

• **Fig. 2.10** Occupational therapists continued to serve soldiers after WWI. (Courtesy of the Archive of the American Occupational Therapy Association, Inc.)

Another important area of growth for OT during this time was in treating and caring for patients with tuberculosis. Thomas Kidner was instrumental in promoting OT services for vocational rehabilitation and tuberculosis treatment, and tuberculosis sanatoriums throughout the United States employed occupational therapists.

The Great Depression, from 1930 to 1939, affected all aspects of society, including the health-care fields. It slowed the development of OT, bringing department closures and reductions of OT staff positions. Schools closed, and membership in the NSPOT decreased. Attention to rehabilitative care, which began with World War I, did not reemerge until World War II brought new and similar needs.

## Progress of the Profession

In 1921 the membership voted to change the name of the National Society for the Promotion of Occupational Therapy to the **American Occupational Therapy Association (AOTA).** The profession continued to grow and evolve under this new name.

### Minimum Standards Adopted for Training

Several of the emergency schools set up to provide training during World War I remained open in the 1920s and attempted to recruit practitioners to the new profession. The training courses varied considerably. Furthermore, the heterogeneous nature of the existing workforce (arts and crafts instructors, reconstruction aides, and some college-educated practitioners) called for the development of a workforce that

was uniform so that OT could advance as a profession.[24] At the time, there were eight OT schools in the United States. The first set of standards for OT training, *Minimum Standards for Courses of Training in Occupational Therapy*, was adopted in 1923 by the membership of AOTA. The standards included prerequisites for admission into training programs, length of courses, and content of courses. The standards stipulated that courses of training for OTs needed to be a minimum of 1 year, with 8 or 9 months of medical and craft training and 3 or 4 months of clinical work in hospitals. Lacking any legal ability to close schools that did not meet the standards, the association endorsed those schools that met the standards. These standards were revised twice by AOTA during the 1920s, with each revision requiring more training.

In 1929 AOTA established a national registry that identified practitioners who had graduated from schools that the association endorsed.[4] The registry began on January 1, 1931. In 1935, the American Medical Association (AMA), at the request of AOTA, assumed responsibility for the inspection and accreditation of OT schools. Five schools were accredited in 1938. This collaboration with the AMA continued until 1994, when it was determined that the profession of OT should be responsible for accrediting and monitoring its own educational programs.

### Growth Through Publication

An emphasis on publication shaped the profession of OT and continued to mold its emerging character. Within 5 years of the organization's founding, AOTA published a journal devoted to the profession. Dunton, who published works on the use of occupation for treatment purposes, served as the editor for the *Archives of Occupational Therapy* from 1922 through 1947. The journal name changed to *Occupational Therapy and Rehabilitation* in 1925 and *American Journal of Occupational Therapy* in 1947.[25] The journal has become known informally as *AJOT* (pronounced *a-jot*). Since 1925, membership in the national organization has included a journal subscription.

The postwar period allowed OT to become closely coupled with medicine and the medical model of education. This led to the beginning of specialization and of a more scientific approach. It set the stage for attempts by physical medicine to control the developing profession of OT. On one hand, the support OT received from physicians was instrumental in the growth of the profession. On the other hand, the profession's unique philosophy based on occupation and a holistic perspective was threatened by the **reductionistic** views of medicine at the time.

## World War II: 1940–1947

World War II created a new demand for more occupational therapists. Because they had not achieved military status during World War I, few occupational therapists were employed in the US Army or in army hospitals when World War II broke out.[29] Initially, the War Department required occupational therapists to be graduates of an accredited school. However, these educational requirements took 18 months to complete, which was too long for the army to wait to get trained occupational therapists.[29] Once again, War Emergency Courses were implemented to quickly train the needed occupational therapists. As a result, the number of employed practitioners increased significantly. AOTA data indicate that in 1945 there were 2177 members.

Beginning in 1945, successful completion of an examination became a requirement for registering as an OT practitioner. The examination was initially in essay format; in 1947, it adopted the format of an objective test.

## Post–World War II: 1950s–1960s

The OT profession changed quickly and in numerous ways after WWII. Overall, there was a continued shift away from a generalist approach to one of specialization in physical rehabilitation.

### New Drugs and Technology

The discovery of neuroleptic drugs (tranquilizers and antipsychotics) in the mid-1950s changed the course of psychiatric treatment. As psychotic behavior yielded to chemical control, it became possible to discharge many people, eventually leading to a national plan to release clients—the national **deinstitutionalization** plan. In anticipation of local care needs, community mental health programs were developed.

New technologies also were developed, such as splinting materials, wheelchairs, and more advanced prosthetics and orthotics. Special training was required for OT practitioners using the new therapeutic material and equipment.

### Rehabilitation Movement

The time from 1942 to 1960 is often called the period of the **rehabilitation movement.**[23] The Veterans Administration (VA) hospitals increased in size and number to handle the casualties of war and continued care of veterans. The VA hospitals, which had employed occupational therapists in psychiatric and tuberculosis units since the administration's beginnings in 1921, developed physical medicine and rehabilitation departments to serve veterans with physical disabilities. After the war, in 1947, the US Army established the Women's Medical Specialist Corps, through which women in the fields of OT, physical therapy, and dietetics, who were classified as civilian employees during the war, were commissioned as officers of the US Army. The Corps later became the Army Medical Specialist Corps to allow both men and women to serve as commissioned officers in the military. The Korean War, which began in 1950, called for the continuation of army hospitals with active OT departments.

Growth in health care was not limited to the VA hospitals. As a result of the polio epidemic and new medical procedures and antibiotics that were saving lives, more individuals were living with disabilities. Facilities and services were needed to meet the needs of individuals with disabilities. The Hill–Burton Act assisted states in determining what hospitals and health-care facilities were needed and provided grants to states to construct these facilities. OT practitioners were hired as one type of rehabilitation professional; their responsibilities included teaching patients activities of daily living, designing orthotic devices, training patients on how to use prosthetics, implementing progressive resistive exercise techniques, introducing muscle reeducation techniques, and evaluating patients' vocational aptitudes and abilities.[23]

### Federally Mandated Health Care

**Medicare** (PL 89-97) was enacted in 1965, and it increased the demand for OT services. Under Medicare guidelines, those who are 65 years of age or older or those who are permanently and totally disabled receive assistance in paying for their health care. Medicare covers OT services in the inpatient setting and provides limited coverage for outpatient services. Initially, this legislation did not provide for services provided by OT practitioners in independent practice settings. In 1988 legislation granted OT practitioners the right to Medicare provider numbers, permitting direct reimbursement for OT services.

### Changes in the Profession

The 1950s and 1960s brought organizational changes to AOTA to improve both the overall function of and the membership representation in the ever-growing and expanding organization. The American Occupational Therapy Foundation (AOTF) was founded in 1965 to promote research in OT through financial support.[4] AOTA and AOTF are discussed further in Chapter 9.

A shift in practice to physical rehabilitation and working with individuals with severe disabilities required practitioners to expand their knowledge. Services that were once based on occupation and arts and crafts changed to a more technical focus, using modalities particular to the area of specialization. OT faculty decreased the emphasis on teaching of arts and crafts and focused on a medical and scientific approach. Leaders of the profession spoke out against specialization and encouraged the profession to return to its roots of occupation. However, the trend toward the reductionistic model and specialization continued throughout the 1960s.

#### New Level of Practitioner: The Occupational Therapy Assistant

With an increasing number of occupational therapists practicing in medical and rehabilitation facilities, there was a shortage of therapists working in psychiatric settings. Aides and technicians working under OT practitioners in psychiatric settings became knowledgeable in the intervention techniques used.

"Supportive personnel knew how to do things, but lacked goal-oriented intervention methods necessary to work without immediate supervision."[6] This led to the development of a new level of practitioner, the occupational therapy assistant (OTA). The first 3-month educational program for OTAs began in 1958 in psychiatry, and a second course for general practice was offered in 1960. Initially, these training programs were based in hospitals. Later, the programs were offered in technical schools and community colleges. The first directory of OTAs was published in 1961 and listed 553 names.[2] Although the introduction of this new level of practitioner was a major milestone for the profession, there was a lack of agreement as to the appropriate roles of the OT practitioner and the OTA.

## 1970s Through 1980s

The period from the 1970s to the 1980s included the introduction of personal computers, a substantial increase in drug and alcohol abuse, and the appearance of a new disease with no known cure, AIDS. The deinstitutionalization plan gained acceptance and was implemented across the United States. Consequently, individuals who previously resided in mental hospitals and facilities for the developmentally delayed were transferred from these institutions to smaller community facilities. Many of the large state institutions closed. Some services were developed in communities to support these individuals, but overall there was a lack of services. As a result, many individuals with chronic mental illness and intellectual deficits (previously referred to as mental retardation) ended up homeless, which remains an issue today.

The US Congress passed several important pieces of legislation for persons with disabilities in the 1970s and 1980s: the Rehabilitation Act of 1973, the Education for All Handicapped Children Act of 1975, the Handicapped Infants and Toddlers Act of 1986, and the Technology-Related Assistance for Individuals with Disabilities Act of 1988.

The **Rehabilitation Act of 1973** came during a time of great social change and unrest. Persons with disabilities, inspired by the civil rights movement of the 1960s, became a new force and exerted significant influence on rehabilitation legislation. The Rehabilitation Act of 1973 established several important principles. First, the act emphasized priority service for persons with the most severe disabilities and mandated that state agencies establish an order of selection that would place the most severely disabled person first for service. Second, under the act, every client accepted for services was mandated to participate in the service-planning process by completing an individualized written rehabilitation program (IWRP) specifying the client's vocational goal and key supporting objectives, such as physical restoration,

counseling, educational preparation, work adjustment, and vocational training. Third, the act called for the development of a set of standards by which the impact of rehabilitation services could be assessed. Fourth, the act emphasized the need for rehabilitation research. Finally, it included civil rights provisions that gave equal opportunity for people with disabilities. It prohibited discrimination in employment or in admissions criteria to academic programs solely on the basis of a disabling condition.

OT practitioners' work with children in schools emerged during this time as another specialty area, aided in part by passage of the **Education for All Handicapped Children Act of 1975** (PL 94-142). This act establishes the right of all children to a free and appropriate education, regardless of handicapping condition. This law includes OT as a related service. Before the passage of PL 94-142, many children with disabilities did not attend school or receive therapy services. This law requires a written individualized education program (IEP) for each student that describes the student's specialized program and measurable goals. The **Handicapped Infants and Toddlers Act** (PL 99-457) was passed in 1986 as an amendment to the Education for All Handicapped Children Act. The amendment extends the provision of PL 94-142 to include children from 3 to 5 years of age and initiates new early intervention programs for children from birth to 3 years of age. OT is considered a primary service. These two laws increased OT services provided to children and the number of OT personnel employed within the school environment.

The **Technology-Related Assistance for Individuals with Disabilities Act of 1988** (PL 100-407) addresses the availability of assistive technology devices and services to individuals with disabilities. Many OT practitioners are involved in providing these services.

These pieces of legislation increased the demand for OT services. However, the 1970s also saw rises in the cost of health care. The 1980s brought about changes in the health-care system in an attempt to contain health-care costs.

### Prospective Payment System

In 1983 President Reagan made a fundamental change to the way in which health-care dollars were dispersed by signing the **Social Security Amendments** into law. Up until this point, hospitals were reimbursed based on the actual cost of services provided. With the implementation of the Medicare **Prospective Payment System (PPS)** created by these amendments, a nationwide schedule was established that delineated what the government would pay for each inpatient stay of a Medicare beneficiary. The level of payment is set by descriptive categories according to the individual's diagnosis, called diagnosis-related groups, or DRGs. With this new system of fixed payment for DRGs, massive changes in hospital organization and care delivery occurred. Most notably, patient length of stay in acute care hospitals was shortened, and there was an increased use of long-term care facilities and home health services.

## Advances at AOTA

AOTA expended great efforts to ensure that OT would be appropriately included in the onslaught of new federal governmental legislation directed at the delivery of health care. Lobbying for the interests of OT became a function of AOTA during the 1970s and 1980s and remains an important aspect of the association's role.

In the 1980s, AOTA moved into its own building, thus signifying a new era that began to yield results from AOTA's long-standing emphasis on research. This decade witnessed a wealth of new books and publications, including a new research journal, the *Occupational Therapy Journal of Research*. There was also growth in the number of educational programs that offered a graduate degree.

In 1986, AOTA separated professional membership and certification procedures by declaring the association no longer responsible for board certification. Instead, on completion of all requirements, an OT practitioner is certified through the National Board for Certification in Occupational Therapy (NBCOT), subject to certification regulations; AOTA membership is separate and voluntary.

## State Regulation of Occupational Therapy

State regulatory legislation became a controversial issue in the 1970s. Individual states began to introduce laws requiring that OT practitioners become licensed to practice. AOTA's Representative Assembly supported state licensing to ensure quality OT services in 1975. (Regulation and licensure are discussed in detail in Chapter 6.)

## A Return to the Roots of the Profession: Occupation

By the 1970s, there was a large contingent of OT practitioners urging the profession to return to its roots in occupation. Occupational therapists such as Mary Reilly, Elizabeth Yerxa, Phil Shannon, and Gail Fidler called upon therapists to reject the practices of reductionism and return to the principles of moral treatment and occupation. Shannon described the "derailment of occupational therapy."[28] He observed that there were two philosophies in conflict with each other. One, based on the philosophy of moral treatment, held a holistic and humanistic view of the individual. The other saw the individual as a "mechanistic creature susceptible to manipulation and control via the application of techniques."[28] He further noted, "If OT persists in this direction, what was once and still is one of the great ideas of 20th-century medicine will be swept away by the tide of technique philosophy."[28]

There was growing realization that something needed to be done. OT was lacking a science unique to occupation, theories of practice, and research that demonstrated the effectiveness of OT. It was during this time that different theories and models for OT started to emerge. One such model is the Model of Human Occupation, described earlier, developed by Kielhofner and his associates.[16] The field of occupational science, a basic science that supports occupational practice, also emerged.[31,32]

## Gary Kielhofner: Return to Occupation

*"Life takes on meaning in the minute-by-minute reality in which we experience ourselves achieving the ordinary things."*
**GARY KIELHOFNER**

**Dr. Gary Kielhofner** (February 15, 1949–September 2, 2010) developed the Model of Human Occupation (MOHO) as a graduate student under the supervision of Dr. Mary Reilly, a professor of OT at the University of Southern California (Fig. 2.11). Over 30 years, Dr. Kielhofner further developed and refined this model.[16,17] Dr. Kielhofner was a prolific scholar who published 19 textbooks and over 150 journal articles. He listened to feedback from students, colleagues, and clinicians to develop a model that would allow OT practitioners at all levels to better address the important issues concerning their clients. In so doing, Dr. Kielhofner provided the profession with evidence to support occupation-based practice and tools (21 assessments) to evaluate clients. MOHO is the most evidence-based model of practice in OT.[14,16,21] At the time of this writing, there were over 400

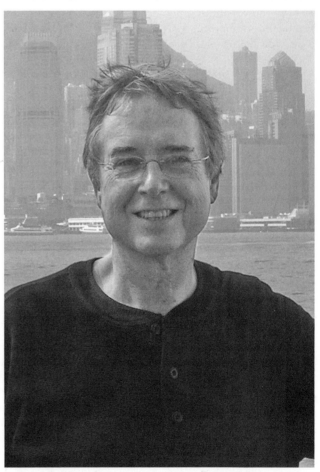

• **Fig. 2.11** Gary Kielhofner, DrPH, OTR/L, FAOTA. (Photo Courtesy Dr. Renee Taylor).

research-based articles published on MOHO. Dr. Kielhofner never lost sight of his goal to make a difference in the lives of those with disabilities. He was a visionary who promoted the field of OT through the quality of his scholarship.

Dr. Kielhofner received his bachelor's degree in psychology from St. Louis University. He earned his master's degree in OT and doctoral degree in public health from the University of Southern California. He held faculty appointments at Boston University, Virginia Commonwealth University, and, most recently, the University of Illinois at Chicago, where he served as a professor and Wade Meyer chair for 30 years. By engaging in participatory research work with the community, Dr. Kielhofner furthered the scholarship of practice model to bridge the gap between practice and academics. The scholarship of practice model helped develop effective programming and research supporting the use of MOHO in practice and making a difference in many clients' lives. Notably, Dr. Kielhofner worked to help persons with HIV/AIDS reengage in meaningful occupations and experience improved quality of life. With colleagues from around the world, he designed programs to help those with mental illness and children and adults with physical disabilities. He was a dynamic leader who encouraged all to achieve. Dr. Kielhofner mentored numerous students, practitioners, and faculty around the world, always encouraging and inspiring others to excel. His creativity, passion, and energy helped move the profession forward to benefit clients. His legacy continues as the profession embodies occupation-based practice.

## Occupational Science

Occupational science was created to examine the knowledge base and research related to occupation. Elizabeth Yerxa founded the first doctoral program in occupational science (at the University of Southern California). Later, Dr. Florence Clark became the chair of the program. Dr. Clark conducted a randomized controlled trial, the results of which were published in the *Journal of American Medical Association*, showing the importance of OT with well elders.[11] Occupational science has generated research that helps scholars and practitioners better understand the uniqueness of occupation to support the profession. The yearly Study for the Science of Occupation (SSO) conference allows practitioners and scholars to network, discuss current research, and advance the field.

## 1990s to the Present

The information age, characterized by technologies such as cell phones, fax machines, personal computer applications, and the networking of computers through the Internet, allows individuals to have immediate access to news and world events at the click of a button. In OT, computer technology also is used as an intervention modality, such as the use of computer software to retrain cognitive skills. Billing and documentation of services are typically done on a computer.

The modern societal climate includes two-income families as the norm. The number of individuals living with disabilities is increasing, as is the number of individuals over 65 years of age. The population in the United States is becoming ever-more culturally diverse, and many individuals and families cannot afford the cost of health care.

One of the most significant pieces of legislation passed during the 1990s is the **Americans with Disabilities Act of 1990** (**ADA**; PL 101-336). The ADA provides civil rights to all individuals with disabilities. It guarantees equal access to and opportunity in employment, transportation, public accommodations, state and local government, and telecommunications for individuals with disabilities. OT personnel provide consultation to private and public agencies to assist them in meeting these guidelines.

The Education for All Handicapped Children Act of 1975 (PL 94-142), was reauthorized and renamed the **Individuals with Disabilities Education Act (IDEA)** in 1991. IDEA requires school districts to educate students with disabilities in the least restrictive environment (LRE). Specifically, IDEA requires states to establish procedures to ensure that students with disabilities are educated, to the maximum extent appropriate, in settings with students without disabilities. IDEA also mandates that the local school district is responsible for providing assistive technology devices and related services as deemed appropriate to the child's education. In 1997, the president signed the Individuals with Disabilities Education Act Amendments of 1997 (PL 105-17; IDEA 97), which further improves the educational opportunities for children with disabilities. The focus of IDEA 97 is on improving educational results for children with disabilities. The law stipulates that the assistive technology needs of children with disabilities must be considered, along with other special factors, by the IEP team in formulating the child's IEP. IDEA 97 also strengthens the role of parents in educational planning and decision making on behalf of their children. IDEA defines OT as a related service that can be provided to a student to enable him or her to participate in and benefit from the educational process. OT practitioners' role in schools increased dramatically as a result of this law. Some practitioners were employed directly by the school system whereas others contracted with schools a a private practice practitioner.

In the medical arena, OT services are restricted by what insurance companies will cover, and managed care continues in efforts to contain spiraling health-care costs. OT practitioners have to continuously adapt to the regulations and reimbursement limitations affecting the health-care environment. Furthermore, health-care practitioners struggle on a daily basis with ethical questions related to the allocation of health-care services.

The intent of the **Balanced Budget Act of 1997 (BBA)** was to reduce Medicare spending, create incentives for the development of managed care plans, encourage enrollment in managed care plans, and limit fee-for-service payment and programs. Under the Medicare Part B outpatient rehabilitation benefit, there is an annual $1500 cap per person receiving OT services and a separate $1500 cap per person for physical therapy and speech–language pathology services combined.

The uncertainty around the BBA forced practitioners to broaden their horizons and look beyond traditional areas of practice. More therapists are working in community-based programs, and the job market is on the upswing. The Bureau of Labor Statistics (BLS)[9] predicts that employment for OT practitioners is projected to increase much faster than the average for all occupations (increase of 27%) through 2024. Employment of OTAs is expected to grow much faster than average (increase of 40% or more) through 2024.[9] The BLS expects the demand for OT practitioners to rise as a result of growth in the number of individuals with disabilities or limited function, the baby-boom generation's movement into middle age (when incidence of heart attacks and stroke increases), and growth in the population aged 75 years and older. All of these populations will require therapy services.[10] To help meet the challenges associated with the costs of providing services to an aging population, the Centers for Disease Control and Prevention (CDC) encourages community organizations and public health agencies to include health promotion among older adults, prevention of disability, maintenance of capacity, and enhancement of quality of life in their scope.[10] These are all areas in which OT can have a role.

## Affordable Care Act (ACA): ObamaCare

The Patient Protection and Affordable Care Act (PPACA), or Affordable Care Act (ACA), also referred to as ObamaCare was signed into law on March 23, 2010. The ACA was created to address the rising cost of healthcare, shortage of healthcare providers, and lack of insurance available to many Americans. The intent of ObamaCare is to lower federal government spending on healthcare by decreasing emergency room visits and increasing preventative care (such as provided to those with health insurance). Americans are allowed to choose their insurance plan (private, through employers, Medicaid, Medicare, or state) but may choose the federal ObamaCare plan.[21a] ObamaCare provides health insurance to all (with no discrimination based on gender or health status). However, those Americans who do not have insurance may be taxed. The ACA caps out of pocket expenses and covers all preventative care. Furthermore, ObamaCare sets clear rules for insurance companies to prevent abuse and fraud.[21a] The ACA also funds scholarships and loan repayment programs for students in health-related professions. It promotes inter-professional collaboration and funds community health centers.[21a] OT practitioners are encouraged to educate themselves on how this law influences occupational therapy services. Specifically, OT practitioners should investigate how much ObamaCare covers for OT services and what type of services are expected. The intent of the law is to cover medical services that increase the client's ability to regain quality of life and avoid emergency room visits, which is congruent with occupational therapy services. Since the law recently passed, it is unclear how this will affect occupational therapy services. AOTA is advocating for the inclusion of occupational therapy services.

## Vision 2025

A **vision** leads the future direction of a profession or organization. The vision is developed with the members and constituents over time, and it clarifies values, creates a future, and focuses the mission. Visioning helps organizations "stretch the horizon," develop a clear picture for the future,[27] and develop goals and objectives. Thus, a vision helps organizations move forward in a clear direction by encouraging all participants to work toward the same goals. In acknowledgment of 2017 being the 100-year anniversary of the OT profession, after much discussion and input from members, constituents, and consumers, AOTA adopted the **Centennial Vision**[1], which reads "We envision that occupational therapy is a powerful, widely recognized, science-driven, and evidence-based profession with a globally connected and diverse workforce meeting society's occupational needs."[1] This vision for the OT profession emphasizes evidence-based practice and the value of the diversity of clients and practitioners. It highlights the work that OT practitioners do to meet society's needs and articulates the need for science to support practice.

The current Vision 2025 builds upon the Centennial vision and states, "Occupational therapy maximizes health, well-being, and quality of life for all people, populations, and communities through effective solutions that facilitate participation in everyday living." [1a] Vision 2025 emphasizes accessible (culturally responsive and customized services); collaborative (working with clients and within systems to produce effective outcomes); effective (evidence-based, client-centered and cost-effective); and leadership (changing policies, environments and complex systems).[1a]

## Occupation

AOTA's Vision 2025 reflects the commitment to return to the roots of the profession: occupation. Practitioners are encouraged to engage in occupation-based practice, focusing on helping clients reengage in occupations, as opposed to focusing on specific component skills. The emphasis on occupation-based practice is prevalent in the OT literature, including the *Occupational Therapy Practice Framework*,[5] standards for accreditation, conference programs, textbooks, and research publications. Educational programs have designed curricula around the uniqueness of occupation. Therefore, the trend to return to occupation remains a focus of research, education, and scholarly work.[5] OT practitioners embrace the uniqueness of the profession by helping persons do what they wish to do. Furthermore, research supports the premise that engagement in the actual occupation is beneficial and leads to increased physical, psychological, and social benefits.[5] Participation in occupations leads to increased motivation, generalization, and improved motor learning.[5]

## Occupational Therapy Entry-Level Education, Continuing Competence, and Recertification

Ongoing issues for the profession include the need to develop scientists in the profession to conduct research, the need to gather and disseminate OT research, the application of evidence-based knowledge in practice, and continuing competency of practitioners.

Following the phase-out of baccalaureate programs in OT in 2007, students must earn a graduate degree to be eligible to take the OT certification exam. This requirement trains OT practitioners who have the knowledge and skills to be competent in today's practice environment and to be consumers of research. As of January 2015, AOTA reported 159 accredited occupational therapist programs and 213 accredited OTA programs.[3]

State licensure laws typically require evidence that the practitioner is keeping current in the field. The Commission on Continuing Competence and Professional Development (CCCPD) was put in place by AOTA to recommend standards for continuing competence and to develop strategies for communicating information to OT practitioners and consumers about issues of continuing competency affecting OT. The NBCOT implemented recertification, which requires the completion of professional development units to maintain certification as an occupational therapist or OTA (see Chapters 6 and 9).

## Occupation-Based Practice

It is an exhilarating time to be practicing in OT. The richness and complexity of occupation and the evidence of its impact on clients are being documented through research. Academic leaders in the profession are creating a science of occupation, developing theories to guide practice, identifying best practices by examining evidence-based practice, and generating research that demonstrates the effectiveness of OT.[26]

AOTA adopted a framework of practice for the profession. The *Occupational Therapy Practice Framework: Domain and Process*[5] delineates language and concepts that describe the focus of the profession. The document is meant to be used by OT practitioners to examine current practice and to consider emerging practice areas. It was also written to assist external audiences, such as third-party payers, in understanding OT's unique focus on supporting function and health and the process by which that is achieved. The framework reflects a return to the roots of the profession because it is centered on the use of occupation to support participation in life (see Chapter 10).

As history demonstrates, OT is a dynamic and ever-evolving profession. Many of the issues that have been identified in the current era will continue to evolve. The profession and practice of OT will remain responsive to societal, cultural, and political needs.

## Summary

By studying the history of OT, we gain knowledge that will enhance current practice. OT grew out of the rising social consciousness of the early 20th century and became a profession in March 1917. It evolved out of moral treatment in psychiatric facilities, rehabilitation in sanitariums, and restoration for soldiers injured in battle. The profession views the use of occupation as a course of treatment. Changes in society have often meant changes in the profession. OT has evolved through merging theory and research while focusing on health and function. As a field of practice, OT's history of a holistic approach and use of occupation provide its distinction from other health-care services.

## Learning Activities

1. Refer to Box 2.1 and Dunton's "Principles of Occupational Therapy." How could you update these principles to reflect current OT practice?
2. Research and write a short paper on the moral treatment movement of the 1800s. Compile short biographies on the founders of occupational therapy after consulting three or four information sources.
3. Search the past volumes of the *American Journal of Occupational Therapy* (and the older *Archives of Occupational Therapy* and *Occupational Therapy and Rehabilitation*, if available). Compile lists of article titles to show the changes in emphasis from decade to decade.
4. Research and write a short paper on any single social influence, legislation, or technical development. Elaborate on how the event affected the practice and profession of occupational therapy.
5. Research AOTA's history and make a wall chart with a timeline that depicts significant events and changes in AOTA since its inception.
6. Read an Eleanor Clarke Slagle lecture and provide a brief discussion of the concepts presented.
7. Research the work and biographies of current leaders in the profession. If possible, send an email to or interview one of these leaders to find out more about the individual and his or her influence on the profession.

## Review Questions

1. What major social influences gave rise to the field of OT?
2. Who are some of the key people involved in the evolution of the OT profession?
3. What key concepts have persisted throughout the history of OT?
4. How has the profession changed over time?
5. What are some key pieces of federal legislation that have influenced the practice of OT?

## References

1. American Occupational Therapy Association. *AOTA's Centennial Vision: Shaping the Future of Occupational Therapy*. http://www.aota.org/-/media/corporate/files/aboutaota/centennial/background/vision1.pdf; 2011.
1a. American Occupational Therapy Association. *Vision 2025*. http://www.aota.org/AboutAOTA/vision-2025.aspx; 2016.
2. American Occupational Therapy Association. *Directory Certified Occupational Therapy Assistants for the Year 1961*. New York, NY: Author; 1961.
3. American Occupational Therapy Association, Division of Academic and Scientific Affairs. *Academic Programs Annual Data Report Academic Year 2014–15*. Bethesda, MD: Author; 2015. Retrieved from, http://www.aota.org/-/media/corporate/files/educationcareers/educators/2014-2015-annual-data-report.pdf.
4. American Occupational Therapy Association. *History of AOTA Accreditation*; 2011, January25. Retrieved from, http://www.aota.org/education-careers/accreditation/overview/history.aspx.
5. American Occupational Therapy Association. Occupational therapy practice framework: domain and process (3rd ed.). *Am J Occup Ther*. 2014;68(Suppl. 1):S1–S48.
6. Bing R. Looking back, living forward: occupational therapy history. In: Sladyk K, Ryan SE, eds. *Ryan's Occupational therapy Assistant: Principles, Practice Issues and Techniques*. 4th ed.Thorofare, NJ: Slack; 2005:366–379.
7. Bing R. Living forward, understanding backward. In: Ryan S, ed. *The Certified Occupational Therapy Assistant: Principles, Concepts, and Techniques*. 2nd ed.Thorofare, NJ: Slack; 1993:3–20.
8. Bing R. Occupational therapy revisited: a paraphrasatic journey (Eleanor Clarke Slagle lecture). *Am J Occup Ther*. 1981;35(8):499–518.
9. Bureau of Labor and Statistics. *Occupational Outlook Handbook—Occupational Therapists*. Retrieved from, http://www.bls.gov/ooh/healthcare/occupational-therapists.htm; 2015.
10. Centers for Disease Control and Prevention. Public health and aging: trends in aging—United States and worldwide. *Morb Mortal Wkly Rep*. 2003;52(6):101–106. Retrieved from, http://www.cdc.gov/mmwr/preview/mmwrhtml/mm5206a2.htm.
11. Clark F, Azen SP, Zemke R, et al. Occupational therapy for independent-living older adults: a randomized controlled trial. *JAMA*. 1997;278:1321–1326.
12. Dunton WR. *Reconstruction Therapy*. Philadelphia, PA: Saunders; 1919.
13. Gutman SA. Influence of the US military and occupational therapy reconstruction aides in World War I on the development of occupational therapy. *Am J Occup Ther*. 1995;49:256–262.
14. Haglund L, Ekbladh E, Thorell LH, Hallberg IL. Practice models in Swedish psychiatric occupational therapy. *Scand J Occup Ther*. 2000;7:107–113.
15. Kidner TJ. Occupational therapy: its development, scope, and possibilities. *Occup Ther Rehabil*. 1931;10:1–11.
16. Kielhofner G. *A Model of Human Occupation*. Baltimore, MD: Williams & Wilkins; 1985.
17. Kielhofner G. *A Model of Human Occupation: Theory and Application*. 4th ed. Baltimore, MD: Lippincott Williams & Wilkins; 2008.
18. Licht S. The founding and founders of the American Occupational Therapy Association. *Am J Occup Ther*. 1967;21:269–277.
19. Low JF. The reconstruction aides. *Am J Occup Ther*. 1992;46:38–43.
20. Meyer A. The philosophy of occupational therapy. *Occup Ther Ment Health*. 1983;2(3):79–83 [Reprint from October 1921].
21. National Board for Certification in Occupational Therapy. A practice analysis study of entry-level occupational therapist registered and certified occupational therapy assistant practice. *Occup Ther J Res: Occupation, Participation, and Health*. 2004;24(Suppl. 1):S1–S31.
21a. ObamaCare: An Independent Site for ACA Advice ObamaCare Facts. http://obamacarefacts.com/obamacare-facts/
22. Peloquin S. Occupational therapy service: individual and collective understandings of the founders (part 2). *Am J Occup Ther*. 1991;45:733–744.
23. Punwar AJ, Peloquin SM. *Occupational Therapy Principles and Practice*. 3rd ed. Baltimore, MD: Lippincott Williams & Wilkins; 2000.
24. Quiroga V. *Occupational Therapy: The First 30 Years 1900 to 1930*. Bethesda, MD: American Occupational Therapy Association; 1995.
25. Reed KL, Sanderson SR. *Concepts of Occupational Therapy*. 4th ed. Philadelphia, PA: Lippincott Williams & Wilkins; 1999.
26. Schwartz KB. Reclaiming our heritage: connecting the founding vision with the Centennial Vision (Eleanor Clarke Slagle lecture). *Am J Occup Ther*. 2009;63:681–690.
27. Scott C, Jaffe D, Tobe G. *Organizational Vision, Values, and Mission: Building the Organization of the Tomorrow*. Menlo Park, CA: Crisp Publishers; 1993.
28. Shannon PD. The derailment of occupational therapy. *Am J Occup Ther*. 1977;31(4):229–234.
29. The Historical Unit, U.S. Army Medical Department. *Medical Department, United States Army Medical Training in World War II*. Washington, DC: Office of the Surgeon General, Department of the Army; 1974. Retrieved from, http://history.amedd.army.mil/booksdocs/wwii/medtrain/default.htm.
30. Tracy SE. *Studies in Invalid Occupation*. Charleston, SC: BiblioBazaar; 2010.
31. Yerxa E. An introduction to occupational science: a foundation for OT in the 21st century. *OT Health Care*. 1989;6(4):3.
32. Yerxa EJ, Clark F, Jackson J, Pierce D, Zemke R. An introduction to occupational science, a foundation for occupational therapy in the 21st century. *Occup Ther Health Care*. 1990;6(4):1–17.

# 3

# Philosophical Principles and Values in Occupational Therapy

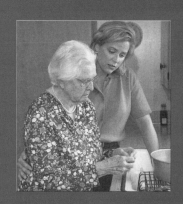

## OBJECTIVES

*After reading this chapter, the reader will be able to do the following:*

- Understand the importance of a profession's philosophical base.
- Describe the general components of a philosophy.
- Describe the philosophy of occupational therapy.
- Articulate occupational therapy's view of humankind.
- Explain the meaning of *occupation* in the context of the profession and understand its role in occupational performance and well-being.

- Name the values of the profession.
- Describe adaptation as used in occupational therapy.
- Distinguish between occupation as a means and occupation as an end.
- Describe the client-centered approach and its relevance to occupational therapy.

## KEY TERMS

active being
activity
adaptation
altruism
axiology
client-centered approach
dignity
epistemology
equality

freedom
holistic approach
humanism
justice
metaphysics
occupation
occupation as a means
occupation as an end
occupational performance

professional philosophy
prudence
quality of life
role
reductionistic
tasks
truthfulness
volition

 Visit *www.evolve.elsevier.com* to access the Evolve student resources that accompany your book.

*Occupational therapy (OT) is by far the most unique of allied health-care professions. The delicate balance of art, science, and human interaction on which the profession is based contributes not only to this uniqueness but also to the obvious effectiveness of OT intervention throughout the life span.*

**GLEN GILLEN, EDD, OTR, FAOTA**
**Assistant Professor in Clinical Occupational Therapy**
**Columbia University**
**New York, New York**

Students in occupational therapy (OT) or occupational therapy assistant (OTA) programs will better understand the profession when they are familiar with its philosophical base. A **professional philosophy** refers to the set of values, beliefs, truths, and principles that guide the education, practice, and scholarship of the profession. OT philosophy defines the nature of the profession, guides the actions of practitioners, and supports the profession's domains. Theories, models of practice, frames of reference, and intervention approaches that guide OT practice are derived from the profession's philosophy. This chapter begins with a general description of philosophy before examining OT philosophy and describing the core concepts of OT practice.

## Understanding Philosophy

Philosophy refers to a set of basic principles or concepts that underlie practice or conduct.[18] The philosophy of a profession can be divided into three areas of concern—metaphysics, epistemology, and axiology—that seek to address questions regarding the values and beliefs of the profession.[15] **Metaphysics** is concerned with the nature of humankind and addresses how humans engage, organize their lives, and find meaning and interact with others. **Epistemology** is related to the nature, origin, and limits of human knowledge and investigates such questions as "How do we know things?" and "How do we know that we know?"[15] **Axiology** is concerned with the study of values. Therefore this area explores questions of desirability and questions of ethics, such as "What are the standards and rules of right conduct?"[15] These questions serve as guidelines to understand the core concepts and philosophical base of the OT profession.

## Philosophical Base of Occupational Therapy

The philosophical base of OT was adopted in 1979 and most recently updated in 2011.[4] (Box 3.1.) It explains the profession's values and beliefs by addressing questions regarding metaphysics, epistemology, and axiology. Fig. 3.1 illustrates the elements that make up the philosophical base of OT. The core values (depicted in the roots of the tree) inform the practice, education, and research of the profession in the areas represented in the branches. The philosophy is further defined in the core concepts (Box 3.2), which are described more fully throughout this chapter.

### What Is Humankind?

The metaphysical component of philosophy examines the question, "What is humankind?" This philosophical question becomes the basis to understanding the OT profession's focus on enhancing a person's ability to engage in life. Specifically, OT practitioners are committed to holistic and humanistic practice.

### *Occupational Therapy Views Humans Holistically*

The US health-care system typically uses a **reductionistic** approach, wherein humankind is reduced to separately functioning body parts. Professionals using a reductionistic approach specialize in specific areas and treat these body functions independently for greater expediency and efficiency; their purpose is to isolate, define, and treat

---

> **• BOX 3.1  The Philosophical Base of Occupational Therapy**
>
> Occupations are activities that bring meaning to the daily lives of individuals, families, and communities and enable them to participate in society. All individuals have an innate need and right to engage in meaningful occupations throughout their lives. Participation in these occupations influences their development, health, and well-being across the lifespan. As such, participation in meaningful occupation is a determinant of health.
>
> Occupations occur within diverse social, physical, cultural, personal, temporal, or virtual contexts. The quality of occupational performance and the experience of each occupation are unique in each situation due to the dynamic relationship between factors intrinsic to the individual, the contexts in which the occupation occurs, and the characteristics of the activity.
>
> The focus and outcome of occupational therapy are individuals' engagement in meaningful occupations that support their participation in life situations…Occupational therapy is based on the belief that occupation may be used for health promotion and wellness, remediation or restoration, health maintenance, disease and injury prevention, and compensation/adaptation. The use of occupation to promote individual, community, and population health is the core of occupational therapy practice, education, research, and advocacy.
>
> From American Occupational Therapy Association. (2011). The philosophical base of occupational therapy. *American Journal of Occupational Therapy*, 65(Suppl. 6), S65.

body functions and to focus on a specific problem. The reductionistic approach has been successful in producing cures and technological developments. However, clients remain frustrated with health-care systems that are inefficient and costly. Therefore many medical practitioners are returning to approaches that allow them to address the body and mind of the client (i.e., the patient-centered approach).[13]

Since its beginning, OT has adhered to a **holistic approach.** The holistic perspective can be traced to Adolf Meyer. In *The Philosophy of Occupational Therapy,* he states, "Our body is not merely so many pounds of flesh and bone figuring as a machine, with an abstract mind or soul added to it. [Rather, it is a live organism acting] in harmony with its own nature and the nature about it."[12] The holistic approach emphasizes the organic and functional relationship between the parts and the whole being. This approach maintains that a person is a whole—an interaction of biological, psychological, sociocultural, and spiritual elements. If any element (or subsystem) is negatively affected, a disruption or disturbance will be reflected throughout the whole.

Belief in a holistic approach is a core concept of the OT profession. This means that evaluations and intervention plans reflect the needs of the whole person. OT practitioners treating only the body (or parts of the body) or only the mind are not following the profession's commitment to holism.[2,9] In such cases, the consumer is denied one of the unique aspects of OT: the holistic approach.

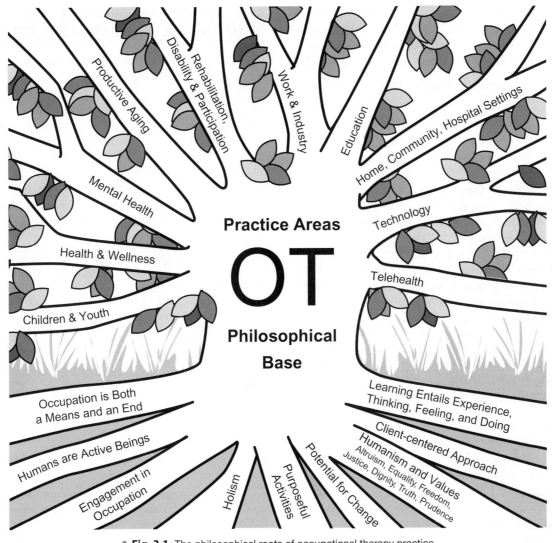

Practice Areas

OT

Philosophical

Base

Productive Aging

Rehabilitation: Disability & Participation

Work & Industry

Education

Home, Community, Hospital Settings

Technology

Telehealth

Mental Health

Health & Wellness

Children & Youth

Occupation is Both a Means and an End

Humans are Active Beings

Engagement in Occupation

Holism

Purposeful Activities

Potential for Change

Learning Entails Experience, Thinking, Feeling, and Doing

Client-centered Approach

Humanism and Values
Altruism, Equality, Freedom, Justice, Dignity, Truth, Prudence

**Fig. 3.1** The philosophical roots of occupational therapy practice.

---

**• BOX 3.2    Core Concepts of Occupational Therapy**

- People are viewed holistically.
- People are active beings for whom occupation is critical to well-being.
- Occupations are classified as: activities of daily living, instrumental activities of daily living, self-care, education, work, play and leisure, sleep and rest, and participation in social activities.
- Learning entails experience, thinking, feeling, and doing.
- The profession views occupation as both a means and an end.
- Every person has the potential for change.
- The client, family, and significant others are active participants throughout the therapeutic process - the client-centered approach.
- Occupational therapy is based on humanism, wherein the values of altruism, equality, freedom, justice, dignity, truth, and prudence are central to the profession.

---

*Occupational Therapy Views People as Active Beings for Whom Occupation Is Critical to Well-Being*

OT views people as **active beings.** People are actively involved in controlling and determining their own behavior and are capable of changing behavior as desired. Furthermore, people are viewed as open systems in which there is continuous interaction between the person and the environment. The person's behaviors influence the physical and social environment; in turn, the person is affected by changes in the environment.

**Occupation** refers to "the ordinary and familiar things that people do every day."[1] It is the term used to "capture the breadth and meaning of 'everyday life activity.'"[1] Occupations are activities that are meaningful to individuals and add to their daily lives. Each person performs certain occupations (e.g., feeding, dressing, bathing, social participation, work, education, sleep and rest, leisure). Occupations fulfill each individual's need for security, belonging, physiological esteem, and self-actualization. OT practitioners believe that engagement and participation in occupations are essential to one's identity and well-being. People have an innate need to engage in meaningful occupation. Engagement in occupation is a determinant of health and well-being.

## Occupational Therapy Classifies Occupations

OT classifies occupations under activities of daily living, instrumental activities of daily living, self-care, education, work, play and leisure, and participation in social activities. OT practitioners explore many aspects of occupations in practice, including (1) the range of occupations and activities that make up people's lives; (2) the skills used by people to perform occupations and activities (performance skills); (3) the habits, routines, and roles that are assumed by individuals in carrying out occupations or activities (performance patterns); (4) the internal or external context, or conditions, in which occupation occurs and influences performance (cultural, personal, physical, social, temporal, and virtual); (5) the demands of the activity that require skill and affect the success of performance; and (6) the factors that reside within the client (e.g., client factors) and influence performance, such as physiological and psychological body functions and anatomical body structures (organs and limbs).[1] These various dimensions of occupation all make up OT's domain of concern and are described in detail in Chapter 10.

At a given time, an individual may be occupied with caring for himself or herself by bathing, dressing, or eating. A person may be occupied with productive tasks, such as paid employment or tasks that are necessary for the care of his or her family. At other times, the individual may be involved in activities that he or she simply finds pleasurable, such as playing cards, watching a movie, or exercising. This is referred to as **occupational performance,** or "the ability to carry out activities of daily life."[1] These activities are categorized in the following occupations:[1]

- Activities of daily living (e.g., feeding, dressing, bathing, toileting, hygiene)
- Instrumental activities of daily living (e.g., meal preparation, budgeting, homemaking, care for pets, care for others)
- Rest and sleep
- Education activities (e.g., going to school, studying, formal or informal)
- Work activities (e.g., activities related to employment and volunteer work)
- Play and leisure activities (e.g., activities that promote pleasure and diversion)
- Social participation (e.g., activities related to interacting with others)

Occupations performed on a daily basis are also influenced by individual occupational roles. Christiansen and Townsend define **role** as "a pattern of behavior that involves certain rights and duties that an individual is expected, trained, and encouraged to perform in a particular social situation."[5] Role has also been defined as "a culturally defined pattern of occupation that reflects particular routines and habits."[16] Expectations of the individual's culture provide

subtle messages about which roles to adopt and when.[5] Occupations occur within a variety of contexts, including social, physical, cultural, personal, temporal, and virtual.[1] The duration of roles varies, depending on the role. For example, it may be a long-term role, such as a parent or spouse, or a short-term role, such as a patient in a hospital. A specific occupation may also be carried out in different roles and contexts, which will influence how that occupation is performed. For example, the activity of reading may be carried out in the role of a parent reading a story to a child at home, in the role of a student reading a textbook in the library, or in the role of a consumer reading food labels in the grocery store. The role in which the activity is being performed gives meaning to it as an occupation.[5]

## How Does a Person Know What He Knows?

Epistemology investigates the nature, origin, and limits of human knowledge.[15] This component of philosophy provides a base for understanding motivation, change, and learning. OT practitioners examine a client's motivations, interests, and values as part of the therapy process. Clients engage in occupations for longer periods of time and with better quality when they are motivated or value the activity. Kielhofner uses the term **volition** to define a client's desire, motivations, and interests.[10] Volition includes a client's motivations and values.

## Learning Entails Experience, Thinking, Feeling, and Doing

OT believes that people learn through experience—thinking, feeling, and doing. This principle is found in many of the early writings of the founding members of the profession.[4,12,15] People are unique in that they have a sense of time—past, present, and future. This enables humans to remember past experiences and use them for present and future knowing. For example, a child who touches a hot stove and burns himself will learn rather rapidly (and painfully) from this experience not to touch a stove again. Past experiences also play a role in what the person finds meaningful. A child who likes the sound of a toy may be motivated to activate it again.

OT emphasizes *doing* as the primary mechanism for learning and relearning various skills. Meyer saw OT's role as "giving *opportunities* rather than prescriptions." He saw a need for "opportunities to work, opportunities to do and to plan and create, and to learn to use material."[12] The philosophical base mentions the use of purposeful activity (occupation) to improve or maintain health. On a broad level, OT practitioners use both the terms *occupation* and *activity* to describe participation in daily life pursuits. However, there are important differences in these terms. Occupations refer to those daily life events that give one meaning and identity.[8] Occupations include one's roles, such as mother, teacher, or athlete. Occupations are made up of many activities. The term **activity** describes a general class of human actions that are goal directed.[8,14] Goal-directed behavior implies that the person is focused on the goal of the activity rather than the processes involved in achieving the goal.[3] AOTA delineates an activity from an occupation as something an individual may participate in to achieve a goal, but activity may not have importance or meaning in the person's life.[1] **Tasks** are considered the basic units of behavior and are the simplest form of an action (i.e., reaching for a ball). OT practitioners engage clients in occupations as a way to improve skills, abilities, and performance so clients can participate in life. The focus and outcome of OT is engagement in meaningful occupations that support participation in life.[4]

### The Profession Views Occupation as Both a Means and an End

Through the therapeutic use of occupation and activity, the client is involved on many levels. Coordination between the person's sensorimotor, cognitive, and psychosocial systems is necessary and elicited when an individual engages in occupations and activities.[3] OT practitioners use occupation and activity as a means to help a client learn a new skill, restore a deficient ability, compensate in the presence of a functional disability, maintain health, or prevent dysfunction.[3] By doing, clients improve performance skills and engage in life activities. OT practitioners value doing and use occupation to facilitate goal achievement and to help clients reengage in daily life. Gillen underscores the importance of using occupation-based intervention activities to achieve effective outcomes in practice.[9] Occupation-based activities allow clients to integrate a variety of skills, movements, and sensations within the natural context. This promotes motor learning and generalization.

In the practice of OT, occupation is seen as both a means and an end. **Occupation as a means** is the use of a specific occupation to bring about a change in the client's performance.[3,7,9,14,17] When occupation is used as a means, it may be equivalent to activity. **Occupation as an end** is the desired outcome or product of intervention (i.e., the performance of activities or tasks that the person deems as important to life), and it is derived from the person's values, experiences, and culture.[17] See Box 3.3 for examples. Occupation may be used for health promotion and wellness, remediation or restoration, health maintenance, disease and injury prevention, compensation, or adaptation.[1]

The therapeutic use of occupation and activity requires that the OT practitioner analyze both of these professional tools from multiple perspectives. Analysis of occupation and activity is a skill specific to OT and is discussed in detail in Chapter 14.

### Every Person Has the Potential for Change

OT practitioners believe that all people have the ability to change. This principle is based on humanistic theory, which centers on valuing the person. People learn to adapt by "doing." The philosophical base of OT defines individual **adaptation** as "a change in function that promotes survival and self-actualization." [2,4] The concept of adaptation can be traced back to Adolph Meyer, who stated that diseases

| • BOX 3.3 | Comparison Between Occupation as a Means and an Ends | |
| --- | --- | --- |
| **Occupation** | **Occupation as a Means** | **Occupation as an End** |
| Meal preparation | Increase fine motor skills by preparing a meal | Make lunch for a family of three |
| Play | Increase posture and balance while playing catch with peer | Play with peer for 30 minutes |
| Dressing | Increase bilateral hand skills through dressing | Dress oneself independently |

in psychiatry are "largely problems of adaptation" and that "psychiatry was among the first disciplines to recognize the need for adaptation and the value of work as a help in the problems of adaptation."[12] Adaptation takes place as part of the normal developmental progression, in the process of adjusting to stress or change.[11]

In OT, occupation and activity are used to promote change. Through occupation and activity, the individual achieves mastery over the environment, which contributes to the individual's feeling of competency.[6] Gail Fidler and Jay Fidler describe the development of competence. They write, "The ability to adapt, to cope with the problems of everyday living, and to fulfill life roles requires a rich reservoir of experiences gathered from direct engagement with both human and nonhuman objects in one's environment." They continue, "It is through such action with feedback from both human and nonhuman objects that an individual comes to know the potential and limitations of self and the environment and achieves a sense of competence and intrinsic worth."[7]

OT practitioners set up intervention so clients are successful and develop a sense of competency. People will repeat activities in which they are successful and gain mastery. The process of adaptation is viewed as coming from within the individual. The client is actively involved in creating the change. The role of the OT practitioner in this process is to arrange the surroundings, materials, and demands of the environment to facilitate a specific adaptive response.[11] Practitioners of OT are optimistic that each and every individual has the potential to grow, adapt, and change.

## What Is Desirable?

Axiology examines values and what is considered just and right in terms of the profession. For OT, the concepts of client-centered care, quality of life, and ethics fall under axiology.

### The Client, Family, and Significant Others Are Active Participants

The profession understands the importance of having the client, family, and significant others as active participants throughout the therapeutic process. The client is actively involved, not only in the modality itself, but also in identifying personal goals and preferences for intervention. This allows the practitioner to understand the individual's idea of what constitutes quality of life. OT professionals believe that **quality of life** is important. What is meaningful and provides satisfaction to an individual is determined by the experience of that individual.[10] Therefore, OT practitioners involve the client, family, and significant others in the OT process to ensure that they are addressing concerns that improve the client's quality of life.

OT seeks to improve the quality of life for any person whose functional ability is impaired or limited. This goal is achieved by helping the client develop greater independence in the performance of any area of occupational behavior. For example, the goal of intervention may be to enable a client to independently brush his or her teeth, manage a checkbook, or become more alert to the body mechanics that help avoid injury on the job. Likewise, the goal of intervention may be to ensure that the client increases strength in the body part needed to perform a necessary task, achieves better coordination for all activities, becomes better able to enjoy life by developing a hobby, or participates more fully in life by developing social skills. The OT practitioner works with the client to identify those occupations that are meaningful and will improve his or her quality of life. Together, the OT practitioner and client focus intervention on maximizing occupational performance in these areas. The **client-centered approach** is central to OT practice because only the client can determine his or her quality of life, and, consequently, he or she must help the practitioner understand his or her experience.[13]

### What Are the Rules of Right Conduct?

As discussed in Chapter 2, the profession of OT emerged from the era of moral treatment, which valued the humanitarian treatment of individuals who were mentally ill. OT is based on **humanism,** a belief that the client should be treated as a person, not an object.

### Occupational Therapy Is Based on Humanism

From this humanistic perspective, values and attitudes central to the profession have evolved. In *Core Values and Attitudes of Occupational Therapy Practice,* the American Occupational Therapy Association (AOTA) identifies the concepts of altruism, equality, freedom, justice, dignity, truth, and prudence as the core values and attitudes of OT.[2]

**Altruism** is the unselfish concern for the welfare of others. OT practitioners demonstrate this commitment to the profession and to the client with caring, dedication, responsiveness, and understanding. **Equality** refers to treating all individuals equally, with an attitude of fairness and impartiality, and respecting each individual's beliefs, values, and lifestyles in day-to-day interactions.[2]

The OT practitioner also values **freedom,** an individual's right to exercise choice and to "demonstrate independence, initiative, and self-direction."[2] Freedom is demonstrated through nurturing, which is very different from controlling or directing. OT practitioners nurture their clients by providing support and encouragement, enabling each client to develop his or her inherent potential. Nurturing encourages the development of independence in the client, rather than retaining all direction and control in the hands of the practitioner.

**Justice** is the need for all OT practitioners to abide by the laws that govern the practice and to respect the legal rights of the client. Through the value of **dignity,** the uniqueness of each individual is emphasized. OT practitioners demonstrate this value through empathy and respect for each person. **Truthfulness** is a value demonstrated through behavior that is accountable, honest, and accurate, and that maintains one's professional competence. **Prudence** is the ability to demonstrate sound judgment, care, and discretion.[2] These values and attitudes are reflected in the *Occupational Therapy Code of Ethics* (see Chapter 8).

## Summary

This has been a brief introduction to the philosophy of OT and its role in shaping the knowledge base and practice of the profession. The philosophical base of a profession represents its core beliefs, values, and principles. The philosophy of the profession addresses questions concerning the nature of humankind, ethical practice, and rules of conduct.

OT practitioners work in a variety of settings with diverse clients. However, all practitioners abide by the philosophical principles of the profession, which include valuing a holistic and humanistic approach, occupation, purposeful activity, adaptation, and quality of life. The common bond between OT practitioners is the importance of occupation and the facilitation of occupational performance. From a holistic perspective, OT views humans as active beings. Occupation is seen as an essential part of human existence, and it refers to all of the daily activities in which people participate. The underlying goal of OT is to increase the individual's independence in any area of occupational performance; thus, the OT practitioner must recognize inhibitors of activity and be able to design client-centered intervention plans. Humans learn by doing, and through the process of adaptation, they develop a mastery of self and competence. Improving a client's quality of life (particularly, increasing a person's independence) is the focus of the services provided by OT practitioners. OT facilitates the adaptive process by providing clients with opportunities to adapt and improve their quality of life.

## Learning Activities

1. Identify your values and beliefs. Do they relate to the values and beliefs of the OT profession?
2. Review Chapter 2 and research other historical OT resources to trace consistencies between the early and current philosophies of the profession.
3. From case-study articles (i.e., in *OT Practice*), gather examples of quality-of-life changes that result from OT intervention.
4. In your own words, write a description of OT.
5. In a small group, identify the various roles within which each person functions. Discuss how your different roles give individual meaning to the activities you perform.
6. List the core beliefs of OT. Interview a practitioner to identify how he or she has embodied the core beliefs and OT philosophy.

## Review Questions

1. What is OT's view of humans?
2. What are the similarities and differences between occupation, activity, and tasks?
3. What is meant by the terms *occupation as a means* and *occupation as an end?*
4. What are the core concepts of OT practice? Provide examples of each.
5. What is the philosophical base of OT?

## References

1. American Occupational Therapy Association. Occupational therapy practice framework: domain and process (3rd ed.). *Am J Occup Ther.* 2014;68(suppl. 1):S1–S48.
2. American Occupational Therapy Association. Core values and attitudes of occupational therapy practice. *Am J Occup Ther.* 1993;47:1085–1086.
3. American Occupational Therapy Association. Position paper: purposeful activity. *Am J Occup Ther.* 1993;47:1081–1082.
4. American Occupational Therapy Association. The philosophical base of occupational therapy. *Am J Occup Ther.* 2011; 65(suppl. 6):S65.
5. Christiansen CH, Townsend EA, eds. *Introduction to Occupation: The Art and Science of Living.* Upper Saddle River, NJ: Prentice Hall; 2004.
6. Fidler GS. From crafts to competence. *Am J Occup Ther.* 1981;35:567–573.
7. Fidler GS, Fidler JW. Doing and becoming: purposeful action and self-actualization. *Am J Occup Ther.* 1978;32:305–310.
8. Fisher A. Uniting practice and theory in an occupational framework (Eleanor Clarke Slagle Lecture). *Am J Occup Ther.* 1998;52:509–521.
9. Gillen G. A fork in the road: an occupational hazard? (Eleanor Clarke Slagle Lecture). *Am J Occup Ther.* 2013;67:641–652.
10. Kielhofner G. *The Model of Human Occupation: Theory and application.* 4th ed. Philadelphia, PA: Lippincott Williams & Wilkins; 2008.
11. King LJ. Toward a science of adaptive responses. *Am J Occup Ther.* 1978;32:14.
12. Meyer A. The philosophy of occupation therapy. *Arch Occup Ther.* 1922;1:1–10 [Reprinted in 1977 in American Journal of Occupational Therapy, 3, 10].
13. Mroz TM, Pitonyak JS, Fogelberg D, Leland NE. Health policy perspectives: client centeredness and health reform: key issues for occupational therapy. *Am J Occup Ther.* 2015;69:1–8.
14. Pierce D. Untangling occupation and activity. *Am J Occup Ther.* 2001;22:138–146.
15. Shannon PD. Philosophy and core values in occupational therapy. In: Sladyk K, Ryan SE, eds. *Ryan's Occupational Therapy Assistant: Principles, Practice Issues, and Techniques.* 4th ed. Thorofare, NJ: Slack; 2005:24–32.
16. Townsend EA, Polatajko HJ. *Enabling Occupation: An Occupational Therapy Perspective.* Ottawa: Canadian Association of Occupational Therapists; 2007.
17. Trombly CA. Occupation: Purposefulness and meaningfulness as therapeutic mechanisms (Eleanor Clark Slagle Lecture). *Am J Occup Ther.* 1995;49:960–972.
18. The Free On-line Dictionary. (n.d.). *Philosophy.* Retrieved from http://dictionary.reference.com/browse/philosophy?s=t.

# 4

# Current Issues and Emerging Practice Areas

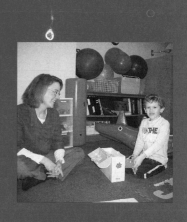

## OBJECTIVES

*After reading this chapter, the reader will be able to do the following:*

- Identify current issues facing the occupational therapy profession.
- Outline the progress toward the Centennial Vision.
- Describe emerging practice areas.

- Discuss the value of evidence-based practice.
- Review the influence of policy on practice.
- Identify the distinct value of occupational therapy.

## KEY TERMS

Affordable Care Act
aging in place
assistive technology
Centennial Vision

distinct value
driver rehabilitation specialists
ergonomics
evidence-based practice

primary care
telehealth vision 2025

e Visit *www.evolve.elsevier.com* to access the Evolve student resources that accompany your book.

---

*It may seem children are heard, but that is not always the case. Not yet. Social and physical participation and inclusion are still things we have to strive for. I started in occupational therapy (OT) in 1974, and I have seen OT grow, become more important, and become a lovely profession. For me, first and foremost, OT is about helping people do everyday things. And the starting point is what people can do, what they are able to do, and what they want to do. That goes for all people, including people with challenges, and especially children. From the start, my heart went out to children with special needs. And that has remained over all these years. The voice of the individual child needs to be involved in the intervention, and the voices of all the children need to be recognized regarding their health and well-being.*

**MARJON TEN VELDEN, MSC, OT**
**Lecturer Occupational Therapy**
**Amsterdam University of Applied Sciences**
**Faculty of Health**
**School of Occupational Therapy**
**Amsterdam, The Netherlands**

The role of the occupational therapy (OT) practitioner has developed significantly since its beginnings in the work of reconstruction aides. OT practitioners provide services to clients of all ages (children to older adults) and diagnoses in such settings as hospitals, schools, rehabilitation clinics, private companies, community agencies, and day-treatment centers. With advances in science and technology, the OT practitioner today provides a wide range of technological and occupation-based services supported by research. The OT practitioner is skilled at problem solving and therapeutic reasoning and adept at interpersonal interactions, also referred to as therapeutic use of self. OT practitioners today are consumers of research, which enables them to provide quality, evidence-based service to clients. They advocate for the rights of clients and participate in the political process to help generate policy to assist those in need. In general, today's OT practitioner is an informed, active professional whose interest in the client helps serve the public, the profession, and the individual. This chapter provides an overview of the profession's progress in addressing the

**Centennial Vision**, examines emerging areas of practice, describes policy issues facing OT, and outlines future issues.

## Vision

A **vision** leads the future direction of a profession or organization. The vision is developed with the members and constituents over time, and it clarifies values, creates a future, and focuses the mission. Visioning helps organizations "stretch the horizon," develop a clear picture for the future, and develop goals and objectives.[21] Thus, a vision helps organizations move forward in a clear direction by encouraging all participants to work toward the same goals.

### Centennial Vision

The year 2017 marks the centennial year of the OT profession. After much discussion and input from members, constituents, and consumers, the American Occupation Therapy Association (AOTA) adopted the Centennial Vision.[2]

AOTA's Centennial Vision statement reads, "We envision that occupational therapy is a powerful, widely recognized, science-driven, and evidence-based profession with a globally connected and diverse workforce meeting society's occupational needs."[2] The vision for the OT profession emphasizes evidence-based practice and the value of the diversity of clients and practitioners. It highlights the work that OT practitioners do to meet society's needs and articulates the need for science to support practice.

### Vision 2025

AOTA's Vision 2015 builds on previous work and states "Occupational therapy maximizes health, well-being, and quality of life for all people, populations, and communities through effective solutions that facilitate participation in everyday living."[2a] This vision emphasizes the profession's role in providing culturally responsive and customized services; working collaboratively with clients and within systems to produce effective outcomes; conducting evidence-based, client-centered, and cost-effective services; and being influential in changing policies, environments, and complex systems.[2a]

## Occupation

AOTA's vision reflects the commitment to return to the roots of the profession: occupation. Practitioners are encouraged to engage in occupation-based practice, focusing on helping clients reengage in occupations, as opposed to focusing on specific component skills. The emphasis on occupation-based practice is prevalent in the OT literature, including the *Occupational Therapy Practice Framework*,[3] standards for accreditation, conference programs, textbooks, and research publications. Educational programs have designed curricula around the uniqueness of occupation. Therefore the trend to return to occupation remains a

focus of research, education, and scholarly work.[2,3,15] OT practitioners embrace the uniqueness of the profession by helping persons do what they wish to do. Furthermore, research supports the premise that engagement in the actual occupation is beneficial and leads to increased physical, psychological, and social benefits.[3,10] Participation in occupations leads to increased motivation, generalization, and improved motor learning.[3,10,15]

## Emerging Areas of Practice

As health care and society's needs change, opportunities and new areas of OT practice emerge. Events such as the aging of baby boomers (those persons born between 1946 and 1964), advancements in technology, and changes in healthcare policy provide OT practitioners with new opportunities. Former AOTA president Carolyn Baum identified six emerging areas of practice:
1. Aging in place
2. Driver assessments and training programs
3. Community health and wellness
4. Needs of children and youth
5. Ergonomics consulting
6. Technology and assistive-device developing and consulting [2]

These areas of practice illustrate the diversity of the profession and the breadth of services that OT practitioners provide. In addition to these areas of practice, OT practitioners continue to provide service in settings such as hospitals, skilled nursing facilities, community agencies, rehabilitation clinics, private clinics, schools, day-care centers, and mental health facilities. OT practitioners provide services to underprivileged populations, including the homeless, migrant workers, and victims of disaster. OT practitioners continue to work with returning veterans; they are examining the current issues these veterans face to better address their unique needs.

### Aging in Place

With advances in medicine and health care, Americans are living longer, and more older adults wish to remain in their homes and live independently (or with minimal support). This trend toward staying in the home is termed **aging in place.** The OT practitioner offers a wide range of services to older individuals to allow them to remain at home and continue to be active in their community; these services include home modification, consultation, community mobility, energy conservation, education, and remediation. Safety in the home includes the ability to manage medications, access emergency numbers, carry through with emergency procedures, show adequate judgment and cognition for daily living (e.g., cooking safety), demonstrate physical safety in the home, and the ability to safely protect oneself from strangers (Figs. 4.1A and 4.1B). Not only does the practitioner evaluate the

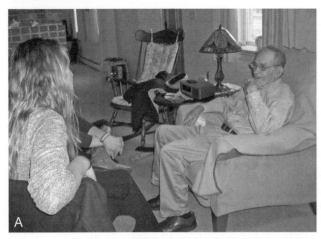
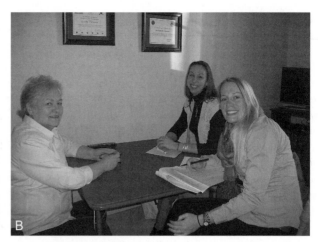

• **Fig. 4.1A and 4.1B** Older adults may require supports to stay in their own homes.

client's skills, abilities, and safety in the home, but the OT practitioner also examines the support systems and resources in place for the client.

Socializing with others is important to the psychological well-being of individuals living at home. The OT practitioner may direct older persons to new social activities or help clients continue a previous activity with modifications or assistance. OT practitioners can be key players in developing creative programs to address the needs of older persons. Clark et al. conducted a large, randomized control trial to examine the effectiveness of OT services on well older adults.[10] The results of this study support OT intervention as a cost-effective service to improve the health and quality of life of older adults. OT practitioners are meeting the needs of older adults by developing expertise in Alzheimers' disease and dementia, low vision, or community mobility and driving.[24]

## Driver Assessments and Training Programs

Safe driving requires many factors (e.g., judgment, reaction time, sequencing, visual perceptual skills). OT practitioners determine a person's ability to drive after a trauma, illness, or decline in function by evaluating cognitive and physical abilities. Intervention is designed to remediate poor abilities or to make adaptations to accommodate for weak or dysfunctional skills. The OT practitioner and a team of providers are responsible for assessing whether the client is capable of driving safely; state laws provide driving licensure regulations. Clients may need special modifications to their vehicles in order to drive (Fig. 4.2).

OT practitioners train individuals in the necessary foundational skills to ensure that drivers are safe. Because OT practitioners are trained to examine clients in a holistic manner, occupational therapists are well suited to succeed as **driver rehabilitation specialists.** Namely, the OT practitioner evaluates and intervenes in physical, social, cognitive, and psychosocial aspects of functioning that affect driving skills. OT practitioners may consult with technology specialists or mechanics on adapting vehicles to help clients with disabilities.

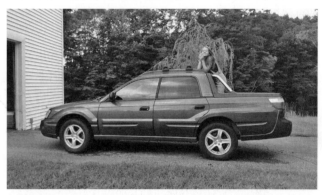

• **Fig. 4.2** Driving is an important occupation for adolescents. This teen is anxious to get her license so she can drive the family car.

## Community Health and Wellness

Because the goal of OT is to help individuals engage in activities of daily living, work, education, leisure, play, and social participation, OT practitioners may develop programs to keep clients and communities healthy. Such programs focus on wellness and prevention of disability, and they help those with disabilities and chronic conditions integrate into the community and contribute to society (e.g., vocational rehabilitation programs).

Advances in health care have enabled individuals to survive many conditions that interfere with functioning. Policymakers and consumers have begun to realize the benefits to helping individuals remain active in their communities. OT practitioners facilitate health and wellness in communities through educational programs and services to individuals and groups. Providing services to the community promotes wellness and quality of life. For example, programs such as Miracle League baseball, adapted skiing or sailing programs, dance and theater, and arts groups can all be adapted so everyone can participate (Figs. 4.3A and 4.3B).

An individual's quality of life is based on many things, including standard of living, finances, freedom, happiness, and access to goods and services. Therefore helping older adults or those with chronic conditions access health care, social groups, transportation, and daily living activities can increase their quality of life. For example, OT practitioners may consult with a group of older persons about the benefits of physical activity or speak to support groups on a variety of topics, including safety at home, driving tips, cooking modifications, and medication management.

OT practitioners may design programs to increase wellness in the community or to address a specific concern, such as childhood obesity. They may work in the community to address the needs of the homeless, migrant workers, or victims of disaster. OT practitioners might also work with communities as consultants to assure accessibility for persons with disabilities (e.g., playgrounds, public buildings). OT practitioners are beginning to play an increasing role in designing preventative programs.  Furthermore, OT practitioners may have an important role in helping clients manage chronic disease.

## Needs of Children and Youth

The needs of children and youth continue to be a growing area for OT practitioners. Childhood obesity is a concern among this population. In fact, *Healthy People 2020* cites childhood obesity in America as one of the leading health issues.[17] Because there are many factors associated with childhood obesity, OT practitioners are well suited to developing programs for children to address health and wellness (Figs. 4.4A and 4.4B).

OT practitioners serve children in early intervention programs that begin as early as birth. Although federal law mandates these programs for the age range of birth to 3 years old, states are responsible for the implementation of services. With limited funding and increased need for services, OT practitioners working in early intervention may need to advocate for the children they serve. There continues to be a need for training and programming in this area.

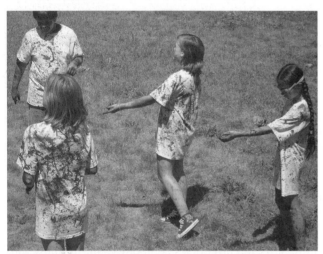

• **Fig. 4.3A** Occupational therapy practitioners provide services to enable children to play with their peers in the community. These children enjoy a party game of tie-dye tag.

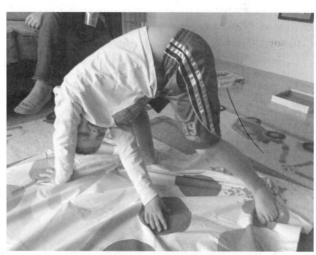

• **Fig. 4.4A** Occupational therapy practitioners may design programs to increase physical activity and nutrition for children and youth. This child plays an active game of Twister.

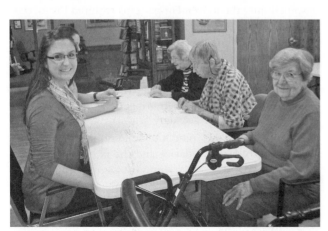

• **Fig. 4.3B** Occupational therapy practitioners provide services to enable older persons to socialize in their communities. Playing board games can be fun for older adults and allows them to socialize.

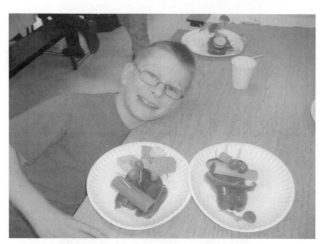

• **Fig. 4.4B** This child learns about healthy snacks by making "Vegetable Aliens."

When children with special needs transition to the public school system, an OT practitioner helps them function in the education environment. OT practitioners provide services within systems with limited funding, despite the vast needs. They may be involved in creating after-school programs or evening social programs for children and youth. Creative solutions are needed to address the needs of children and youth. Current issues regarding mental health needs, bullying, and transitioning to adulthood have increased the scope of services provided to children and youth in school settings.[24]

### Dr. Jane Case-Smith

Dr. Jane Case-Smith (1953–2014) was a dedicated OT professional, educator, and researcher who addressed the needs of children, youth, and their families in her life's work (Fig. 4.5). Dr. Case-Smith served as primary editor for five editions of the *Occupational Therapy for Children and Adolescents.* She advocated that practitioners conduct occupation-based intervention with clear measureable outcomes. Dr. Case-Smith engaged in research to demonstrate the effectiveness of OT intervention with children and youth. Her high-quality work made a difference in the OT profession and supports the **distinct value** of OT. Most recently, she engaged in national studies examining the effectiveness of pediatric constraint-induced movement therapy.[11,12] Dr. Case-Smith completed a systematic review of the work on autism, examined the effectiveness of handwriting programs, and explored sensory-based practice.[8,9,14,20] Dr. Case-Smith promoted OT practice with children and youth, emphasizing the importance of the family. She mentored practitioners, students, and faculty across the

country.[19] Her work influenced the profession and the lives of children and their families. Her colleague, Dr. Andrew Persch, advises OT practitioners and scholars to "pay it forward" in Dr. Case-Smith's honor by engaging in work to promote OT.[19]

### Ergonomics Consulting

**Ergonomics** refers to the study of the problems of people in adjusting to their work environment.[23] Ergonomics consulting involves providing recommendations to individuals and companies on workstation setup to promote safety, efficiency, and comfort to prevent work-related musculoskeletal injury. Examination of seating and positioning, lifting, and other physical requirements falls well within the OT practitioner's expertise. Proper ergonomics may prevent injury to the client, which may result in fewer missed work days and lower costs to the company and client. OT practitioners are addressing issues regarding an aging workforce through ergonomics consulting and evaluation of the worker's habits and routines. OT practitioners use new technology to assist employees.

### Technology and Assistive-Device Developing and Consulting

**Assistive technology,** or adaptive technology, commonly refers to "products, devices or equipment, whether acquired commercially, modified, or customized, that are used to maintain, increase, or improve the functional capabilities of individuals with disabilities."[7] Assistive technology, which includes equipment to assist with communication, computer access, daily living, education and learning, hearing and listening, mobility and transportation, recreation and leisure, seating and position, vision and reading, and prosthetics and orthotics,[7] has improved life for those with disabilities. OT practitioners use technology to help clients function independently in many areas of performance. Because OT practitioners are skilled at analyzing activities, including the movement patterns required for success, many practitioners serve as consultants in the development of devices. Practitioners may be involved in creatiing, developing and evaluating the effectiveness of new technology is for rehabilitation, wounded warrior care, and children and youth. Some practitioners are involved in working with clients who have had hand transplants and may be using bionic limbs.

Frequently, the OT practitioner consults with the team on the type of assistive device and the physical, cognitive, or psychological skills the client possesses to use the device. The OT practitioner is an important member of the team because he or she determines whether the device helps the client perform his or her daily occupations in a reasonable amount of time. The OT practitioner and client determine whether the device is practical and helpful to the client after careful analysis.

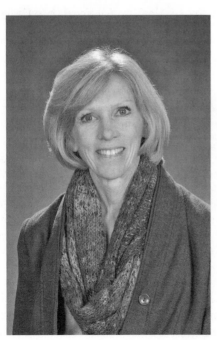

• **Fig. 4.5** Dr. Jane Case-Smith. (Photo courtesy Greg Smith)

## Technology Applications

Computer, phone or tablets provide a variety of opportunities for clients who receive occupational therapy. OT practitioner explore these programs (referred to as Apps) to allow clients to engage in everyday living. For example, a client may benefit from an App that notifies him when to take medication or provides directions. A client may have the bus schedule read to her. This area of technology has many more possibilities.

## Telehealth

Telehealth refers to the use of technology to provide health care services, such as occupational therapy. For example, a practitioner may Skype with a family to review a home program. This may be an effective way to deliver occupational therapy services and practitioners are urged to look at state licensure requirements and reimbursement policies, talk with other therapists, and carefully consider this service delivery model.[7a]

## Educational Trends

Educators consistently evaluate how to teach OT and OTA students to succeed in practice. Educators acknowledge that practitioners entering a diverse workplace with expanding areas of practice need to be lifelong learners and critical consumers of research. Practitioners must be able to support their decisions based on available research. The need to justify intervention and examine evidence requires practitioners who are able to generate and critically analyze research. Basing practice on the best available research evidence is termed **evidence-based practice.** Insurance companies, consumers, and employers require professionals, including OT practitioners, to provide evidence for what they do. Given so many options for spending one's health-care dollar, practitioners must show that therapy is beneficial and cost-effective.

This need to become critical consumers of research prompted the move to a master's level degree as the entry-level requirement for therapists in 2007. This degree reflects the advanced critical analysis and synthesis required of today's practitioners, especially with regard to the ability to analyze research for practice. The associate's degree is still the educational requirement for OTAs. Faculty strive to educate OT students who are critical and innovative thinkers—people who are able to interact therapeutically with clients and peers. Educators hope to bridge the clinical practice and theory gap so that students become practitioners who use current research and sound judgment to benefit their clients. Current issues regarding OT education include the need for faculty, distance learning, and education for those who would like to re-enter the profession.[24]

Because of the demands in health care, trends in interprofessional work, and desire to allow OT practitioners to be primary referral sources, the OT profession is considering changing the entry-level requirement to the clinical doctorate (OTD), with a proposed date of 2025. After discussion and input from members, the Accreditation Council on Occupational Therapy Education (ACOTE) decided that entry-level certification will remain at both the master's and doctoral degree.[1] See Chapter 6 for more information on the levels of education for OT practitioners.

## Policy and Reimbursement

Policy affects health services, including OT. For example, the Prospective Payment System of 1983 resulted in shorter hospital stays, but OT practitioners continued to treat these clients in other settings (such as skilled nursing facilities and home health agencies). Federal laws mandate services, but they require state legislation to determine how the laws will be carried out. OT practitioners must become familiar with policies while they are being developed and advocate for services for those with disabilities. Box 4.1 provides a partial listing of some of the laws that have affected OT services.

OT practitioners advocate for the profession by participating in policymaking. Practitioners may advocate on local, regional, or national levels. The first step toward addressing these challenges is for OT practitioners to be familiar with the scope of practice and the foundations for it. Remaining current on topics by reading professional journals, newsletters, and federal and state news can increase one's awareness of the issues that affect the profession. Practitioners can keep up-to-date on health-care policy through active involvement in the state and national OT associations. See Chapter 9 for more information on professional organizations.

### Patient Protection and Affordable Care Act of 2010

The **Affordable Care Act** of 2010 (ACA) seeks to reduce spending while increasing quality of care.[18] It addresses the need for efficiency by rewarding settings that prevent hospital-acquired conditions (such as falls), prevent hospital readmission, and provide quality care in which patients are satisfied.[13,16,18] Occupational therapists are well suited to play a key role in increasing the efficiency and quality of care because practitioners deliver client-centered care using validated assessments with clear outcomes. OT practitioners are adept at analyzing skills and encouraging clients to move and engage in daily activities, which may prevent hospital-acquired conditions that result in staying in bed.

AOTA is working closely with federal policymakers to ensure that OT is considered an essential health benefit and covered under the ACA.[13,16] However, each state decides the scope and nature of coverage, so OT practitioners must advocate and document outcomes for payment under this act. The importance of research, outcomes, and documenting the effectiveness of OT is key to future funding of these needed services.

> ● BOX 4.1 | **Laws That Have Affected Occupational Therapy Services**
>
> 1. *Section 504 of the Rehabilitation Act of 1973:* "No other-wise qualified handicapped individual in the United States … shall, solely by reason of … handicap, be excluded from participation in, be denied the benefits of, or be subjected to discrimination under any program or activity receiving federal financial assistance."[22] Section 504 provides rights and benefits to persons with disabilities and provides services to children in school systems who may not qualify for services under Individuals with Disabilities Education Act (IDEA). This law requires that programs or activities receiving federal financial assistance provide reasonable accommodations so persons with disabilities may participate.
> 2. *Americans with Disabilities Act (ADA) of 1990:* Provides protection from discrimination on the basis of disability. The ADA upholds and extends the standards for compliance set forth in Section 504 of the Rehabilitation Act of 1973 to employment practices, communication, and all policies, procedures, and practices that affect the treatment of students with disabilities.[22] ADA expanded services to include the workplace and public places. This law required that public places be accessible to those with disabilities. For example, OT professionals work with architects and employers to make work settings accessible to those with disabilities.
> 3. *Individuals with Disabilities Education Act (formerly Public Law 94-142, or the Education for All Handicapped Children Act of 1975):* Requires public schools to make available to all eligible children with disabilities a free, appropriate public education in the least restrictive environment appropriate to their individual needs.[22] OT practitioners working in school systems work under this act. Thus the role of the OT practitioner is to provide intervention that will allow the child to engage in education. Intervention takes place in the least restrictive environment and is appropriate to the child's needs.
> 4. *Balanced Budget Act of 1997:* Set out to contain health-care costs by placing caps on therapy services and resulted in a decrease in OT jobs. Many therapists changed settings during this time or moved on to private practice. Managed care pushed for productivity.[22]
> 5. *Medicare:* This health insurance program is for people 65 years of age or older and those with certain disabilities. It is a federally funded program that provides limits on spending and reimbursement for OT services.
> 6. *Patient Protection and Affordable Care Act of 2010 (ACA; Public Law 111-148):* This law seeks to strengthen existing health insurance access, choice, cost, and coverage. It expanded coverage to uninsured Americans. It includes a package of essential health benefits. Rehabilitative and habilitative services and devices likely include OT services, but this is decided at the state level.[18]

## Role of Occupational Therapy in Primary Care

**Primary care** refers to the provision of integrated, accessible health-care services by clinicians who are accountable for addressing a large majority of personal health-care needs, developing a sustained partnership with patients, and practicing in the context of the family and community.[4,18]

As the ACA becomes recognized, new models of practice are being developed. The goals of these models have the following aims:
1. Improving the individual experience of care,
2. Improving the health of populations, and
3. Reducing the costs of care.[18 (p. S25)]

Consequently, there is incentive to coordinate care and delivery to reduce cost and improve health outcomes. OT is in a prime position to contribute to primary care because it recognizes and addresses the impact of habits and routines on the management of chronic conditions and the development of healthy lifestyles.[18] Occupational therapists can play a role in increasing self-efficacy, reducing disability, improving health status, and decreasing health-care utilization.[5,6,18] Practitioners may provide interventions to promote safety, prevent falls, facilitate driving and community mobility, manage conditions, promote lifestyle modifications, educate on medication management, adapt the environment, and provide family and caregiver support. The ACA offers many opportunities for OT to demonstrate its unique contributions to health care.

## Distinct Value of Occupational Therapy

OT practitioners must advocate and document the value of OT by incorporating interventions that have strong or moderate evidence and allow OTs to provide effective, high-quality, and cost-effective services. Evidence exists to support the effectiveness of occupation-based interventions for client issues such as stroke, autism, mental health, and neurological conditions.[6,9,10,20] A variety of research evidence supports OT's work with driving, school-based practice, and cognition.[5,6,8–10] Use of research evidence and assessment tools (with validity and reliability) to produce occupation-based intervention supports the profession and allows others to see the distinct value of OT. Articulating the importance and uniqueness of OT in an interprofessional team educates others about the role of OT and further strengthens the distinct value of OT. The OT profession has made strides in conducting research to support the value of intervention to clients and their families, and further research will continue to promote the profession and show the value of occupation-based interventions. OT intervention allows clients to engage in those things that they find meaningful and that give them identify. Documenting the power of OT to enhance clients' lives will help the profession gain funding so that the work can continue.

## Summary

The Centennial Vision provides a message of growth and support for the profession.[2] Continued evidence supporting OT practice reinforces the work and ensures that the profession will thrive. The diversity of clients, in addition to the diversity in practitioners, makes the profession exciting and valuable in a changing health-care system. OT practitioners will need to continue to advocate for the profession and be involved in policy and reimbursement issues.

## Learning Activities

1. Review five current *OT Practice* magazines and list the current issues. Present your findings to your classmates.
2. Review the AOTA national conference program to identify current issues.
3. Pick one of the six emerging practice areas. Describe the role of the OT practitioner in the area and how you could develop future programs.
4. Develop a resource list around one of the six emerging practice areas.
5. Examine one health-care policy by discussing the history and intent of the policy. In small groups, describe how the policy has been implemented in practice.
6. Interview an OT practitioner to inquire about how the ACA has influenced documentation and practice.

## Review Questions

1. What are some current issues facing the OT profession?
2. What are the emerging practice areas?
3. What is evidence-based practice?
4. How has policy affected OT practice?
5. What are some current trends in OT education?
6. What is the ACA, and how might it affect OT practice?

## References

1. Accreditation Council for Occupational Therapy Education. *ACOTE's Statement on the Entry-Level Degree for the OT and OTA*; 2015, August. Retrieved from, http://www.aota.org/Education-Careers/Accreditation/acote-entry-level-degress.aspx.
2. American Occupational Therapy Association. *AOTA's Centennial Vision: Shaping the Future of Occupational Therapy*. Retrieved from, http://www.aota.org/-/media/corporate/files/aboutaota/centennial/background/vision1.pdf; 2007.
2a. American Occupational Therapy Association. *Vision 2025*. Retrieved from, http://www.aota.org/AboutAOTA/vision-2025.aspx. 2016.
3. American Occupational Therapy Association. Occupational therapy practice framework: domain and process (3rd ed.). *Am J Occup Ther*. 2014;68(suppl. 1):S1–S48.
4. American Occupational Therapy Association. The role of occupational therapy in primary care. *Am J Occup Ther*. 2014;68(suppl. 3):S25–S33.
5. Arbesman M, Lieberman D, Metzler CA. Health policy perspectives—using evidence to promote the distinct value of occupational therapy. *Am J Occup Ther*. 2014;68:381–385.
6. Arbesman M, Mosley LJ. Systematic review of occupational therapy and mental health promotion, prevention, and intervention for children and youth. *Am J Occup Ther*. 2012;67:277–283.
7. Assistive Technology Act of 1998. (2004 revised). Retrieved from http://www.parentcenterhub.org/repository/ata/#defs.
7a. Cason J. An introduction to telehealth as a service delivery model within occupational therapy. *OT Practice CE Article*. 2012.
8. Case-Smith J, Holland T, White S. Effectiveness of a co-taught handwriting program for first grade students. *Phys Occup Ther Pediatr*. 2014;34:30–43.
9. Case-Smith J, Weaver LL, Fristad MA. A systematic review of sensory processing interventions for children with autism spectrum disorders. *Autism*. 2015;19:133–148.
10. Clark F, Azen SP, Zemke R, et al. Occupational therapy for independent-living older adults: a randomized controlled trial. *JAMA*. 1997;278(16):1321–1326.
11. DeLuca SC, Case-Smith J, Stevenson R, Ramey SL. Constraint-induced movement therapy (CIMT) for young children with cerebral palsy: effects of therapeutic dosage. *J Pediatr Rehabil Med*. 2012;5:133–142.
12. DeLuca SC, Ramey SL, Trucks MR, Wallace DA. Multiple treatment of pediatric constraint-induced movement therapy (PCMIT): a clinical cohort study. *Am J Occup Ther*. 2015;69. Retrieved from 69066180010, http://dx.doi.org/10.5014/ajot.2015.019323.
13. Fisher G, Friesema J. Health policy perspectives—implications of the Affordable Care Act for occupational therapy practitioners providing services to Medicare recipients. *Am J Occup Ther*. 2013;67(5):502–506.
14. Hall L, Case-Smith J. The effect of sound-based intervention on children with sensory processing disorders and visual-motor delays. *Am J Occup Ther*. 2007;61:209–215.
15. Law M, Polatajko H, Baptiste W, et al. Core concepts of occupational therapy. In: Townsend E, ed. *Enabling Occupation: An Occupational Therapy Perspective*. Ottawa, Canada: Canadian Association of Occupational Therapists; 1997:29–56.
16. Metzler C, Tomlinson J, Nanof T, Hitchon J. Health policy perspectives—what is essential in the essential health benefits? And will occupational therapy benefit? *Am J Occup Ther*. 2012;66:389–394.
17. Office of Disease Prevention and Healthy Promotion (ODPHP). (n.d.). *Healthy People 2020*. Retrieved from http://www.healthypeople.gov/2020/leading-health-indicators/2020-lhi-topics/Nutrition-Physical-Activity-and-Obesity/data.
18. Patient Protection and Affordable Care Act. (2010). Pub. L. No. 111–148 3502. 124 Stat. 119, 124. Retrieved from www.healthcare.gove/law/full/index.html.
19. Persch AC. Guest editorial: paying it forward: honoring Jane Case-Smith for commitment to occupational therapy education and research. *Am J Occup Ther*. 2015;69:6906170010. http://dx.doi.org/10.5014/ajot.2015.696004.
20. Schaff RC, Case-Smith J. Sensory interventions for children with autism. *J Comp Eff Res*. 2014;3:225–227.
21. Scott C, Jaffe D, Tobe G. *Organizational vision, values and mission: building the organization of the tomorrow*. Menlo Park, CA: Crisp Publishers; 1993.
22. US Department of Justice, Civil Rights Division, Disability Rights Section. *A Guide to Disability Rights Laws*; 2009, July. Retrieved from, http://www.ada.gov/cguide.htm.
23. Webster's New World College Dictionary. *Ergonomics*. Cleveland, OH: Wiley Publishing, Inc; 2010. Retrieved from, http://www.yourdictionary.com/ergonomics.
24. Yamkovenko, S. (nd). The emerging niche: What's next in your practice area? Retrieved from, http://www.aota.org/Practice?Manage/Niche.aspx.

# 5

# A Global Perspective of Occupational Therapy

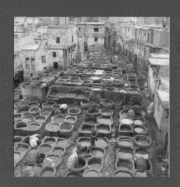

## OBJECTIVES

*After reading this chapter, the reader will be able to do the following:*

- Describe the importance of a global perspective on occupational therapy.
- Identify the influence of culture in occupational performance.
- Describe how to develop cultural competence.

- Understand the importance of interprofessional education and practice.
- Provide examples of occupational therapy practice around the world.
- Define and provide examples of occupational justice.

## KEY TERMS

contexts
cultural competence
cultural sensitivity

culturally responsive care
culture
interprofessional education (IPE)

occupational justice
polytrauma

℮ Visit *www.evolve.elsevier.com* to access the Evolve student resources that accompany your book.

Occupation and the use of occupation to enhance well-being, whether physically or psychologically, is the essence of what drew me to the profession of occupational therapy (OT). Before entry into the field, I worked in a psychiatric hospital on a locked unit for individuals with severe mental health issues. During my tenure on the unit I noticed that several days a week a person would roll in a cart filled with different activities for the clients to engage in. Many of the clients would not leave their rooms except to eat, and even then it was not a certainty that they would come out of their rooms. What I found was that those same individuals would come out and engage with the person and the activities. I was rather awestruck, and I had to know who this person was, what he was doing, and why it made a difference in the lives of our clients. What I found was that he was an occupational therapist, providing meaningful activity and engaging the clients in desired occupations. From that point I was hooked. I had to become an occupational therapist. Throughout my career I have been pursuing keener understanding of what I observed on that locked unit. The Model of Human Occupation has proven

to be a most beneficial aid in my quest for understanding the "why" of what occupational therapists undertake in service provision.

**PATRICIA BOWYER, EDD, MS, OTR, FAOTA**
**Associate Director/Professor/Doctoral Program Coordinator**
**Texas Woman's University–Houston**
**School of Occupational Therapy**
**Texas Medical Center**
**Houston, Texas**

## Introduction

The World Federation of Occupational Therapists (WFOT) and the American Occupational Therapy Association (AOTA) support a globally connected profession that responds to the needs of diverse societies.[2,24] The *Occupational Therapy Practice Framework* cites culture as affecting occupational performance. As such, occupational therapy (OT) professionals consider the customs, beliefs, and expectations of the client's culture.[3] Furthermore, understanding how OT practice is theorized, conducted, and measured in other countries allows professionals to compare and contrast approaches and contemplate best practice, which benefits clients.[12] Even if a practitioner does not travel outside of his or her home country, he or she will encounter clients from different cultures. Being aware and understanding cultural expectations allows the practitioner to develop a therapeutic relationship and prevents missteps that may slow intervention progress.

This chapter explores the global nature of OT by providing an overview of practice around the globe. The chapter begins by describing the importance of understanding culture for OT practitioners. The author provides descriptions of cultural competence and culturally responsive care, along with strategies to strengthen one's knowledge and skills in working with people from a variety of cultures. Educational programs design a variety of experiences to promote cultural awareness, including cultural immersion programs and interprofessional education experiences. The chapter concludes with a discussion of practice around the world.

## Importance of Culture in Understanding Clients in Occupational Therapy

OT practitioners have the privilege of working with clients of all ages and from numerous cultures. **Culture** affects all aspects of OT. It is considered a context and is defined as "customs, beliefs, activity patterns, behavioral standards, and expectations accepted by the society of which the client is a member. The cultural context influences the client's identity and activity choices."[3] Culture is a pattern of behaviors and includes thoughts, communications, actions, customs, beliefs, values, and institutions of a racial, ethnic, religious or social group.[21] One's beliefs influence the types of activities and occupations in which a person engages. Because OT practitioners are concerned with a person's activity choices, they must understand the influence of the culture (Fig. 5.1). Behavioral standards dictated by the culture provide the practitioner with information that is useful when designing intervention. For example, many cultures have standards and expectations regarding mealtime behaviors. The practitioner uses cultural expectations as the marker for success in OT. OT practitioners analyze activities in consideration of the cultural requirements and design intervention that respect the person's cultural values and beliefs.

Although the groups (e.g., racial, ethnic, religious, or social) to which the person belongs may define behavioral and occupational expectations, individuals may behave outside of established norms. Therefore practitioners use general knowledge of cultural groups for baseline information, but spend time learning about the individual's interpretation and behavioral presentation of the group norms. General cultural expectations and standards provide guidelines that help OT practitioners understand clients' motivations, occupational choices, and standards and expectations of behavior. A practitioner can use the overall knowledge of

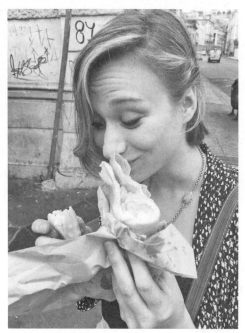

• **Fig. 5.1** Occupational therapy practitioners consider the cultural influences on how people engage in occupations, such as eating.

the specific cultural grouping as a starting point to develop intervention and establish a therapeutic relationship.

## Influence of Culture on Occupational Performance

Culture includes the values, customs, and rituals of a group of individuals. Values are those things that people have interest in or hold meaningful.[3] Rituals are routines or habits that people follow to fulfill roles. Roles are defined by cultures. Cultures define the role expectations, responsibilities, and standards. These influence occupational performance and include the person's actions, skills, and client factors (what is required to perform).

Meg is a 25-year-old student from a middle-class family in New England who is completing her level II fieldwork in a large medical center in the South. Meg has not traveled and is nervous about working with clients from different cultures, although she is excited to learn about and live in a new culture. Meg takes the following steps to develop cultural competence:

- She does research on the cultures she is likely to encounter. She investigates the values of the cultures and beliefs regarding health care, family, work, and leisure. She engages in conversation with students who previously completed fieldwork at the site to find out more tips to better understand the cultures.
- Meg completes a culturally sensitivity assessment to gauge her abilities and skills.
- She reads about various cultures, especially regarding health-care values and beliefs.

- Meg observes her supervisor interacting with people of different cultures and takes notes on specific intervention protocols that may be considered when working with clients from these cultures.
- Meg asks her supervisor to observe her interactions with the clients. She specifically asks for feedback on how she could be more culturally sensitive to clients.
- Meg uses culturally sensitive assessments (e.g., Model of Human Occupation assessment and the Canadian Occupational Performance Measure) because they inform practitioners of how clients engage in their daily lives and can be structured for people from any culture.
- Importantly, Meg engages in self-reflection throughout the process and enjoys learning about and working with clients from different cultures.

## Cultural Competence

**Cultural competence** refers to one's ability to be sensitive to other cultures.[4] Cultural competence requires the practitioner to understand the history and cultural practices of different cultures. In OT practice, consider ethnicity, access to technology, cultural practices, and language spoken.[18] For example, in one program in Peru, individuals greet each other with a kiss on both cheeks; staff, participants, and family members are very warm and welcoming to outsiders. However, unlike what may be the norm in Peru, staff at the site communicate via email.[18]

For OT practitioners providing services in foreign countries, developing cultural competency may first begin by developing understanding of the local and national cultural **contexts** by exploring the literature and discussing the culture with those who are familiar with it. It may be beneficial to study local and national government policy on health, education, and disability; local beliefs around health and the stigma of disability; and cultural norms and expectations.[23] OT personnel (students, faculty, and practitioners) may want to review World Health Organization (WHO) materials.[25] Once in the host country, participants gain cultural sensitivity by visiting community and local cultural attractions (Fig. 5.2). Before recommending interventions that may not be culturally accepted, students and practitioners may benefit from observing local therapists and discussing the intervention strategies they follow.[23]

## Culturally Responsive Care

OT practitioners respond to the attitudes, feelings, and circumstances of groups of people who share a common cultural heritage (racial, national, linguistic, or religious). They use awareness of their cultural group as a starting point. **Cultural sensitivity** refers to the ability to understand the needs and emotions of one's own culture and the cultures of others.[10,11]

Suarez-Balcazar et al.[18] suggested a model for developing cultural sensitivity that includes three key components:

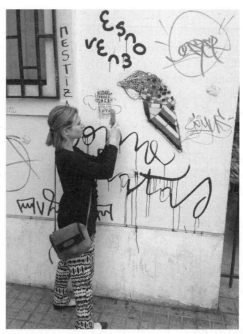

**Fig. 5.2** This college student engages in leisure occupation specific to this Chilean culture (art). The wall is developed each week as people create the piece of art.

*Cognitive (awareness/knowledge):* A desire and curiosity to learn about different cultures paired with an awareness of one's own culture is central to culture sensitivity. Engaging in self-reflection activities (such as journaling, discussion, and exploring resources) reinforces these concepts.

*Behavioral (developing appropriate skills):* Developing skills and abilities to work with clients from a variety of cultures is a dynamic process that involves careful thought, reflection, analysis, and introspection. OT practitioners learn from discussion with persons from the culture (including the client), by examining educational resources, and through sharing experiences with others. Students and practitioners may complete cultural sensitivity assessments (see Learning Activities at the end of the chapter) to develop abilities.

*Organizational (support for cultural competence):* Organizations may provide support to enhance or facilitate cultural competence. For example, an organization may embrace cultural differences. The organization may have workshops, seminars, and resources to support a practitioner's diverse practice.

Munoz (2007)[15] used practitioners' responses and further categorized **culturally responsive care** into the following five constructs:

- Building cultural awareness
- Generating cultural knowledge
- Applying cultural skills
- Engaging in culturally diverse situations
- Exploring multiculturalism[15 (p. 256)]

Building cultural awareness refers to gaining knowledge and understanding of different cultures through reading, discussion, and reflection. Generating cultural knowledge can be achieved by using semistructured interviews and culturally sensitive tools (e.g., Model of Human Occupation and Canadian Occupational Performance Models assessments). Spending time with clients from different cultures allows practitioners to better understand cultural values, beliefs, and customs and apply skills. Engaging in culturally diverse situations promotes learning and encourages the development of skills that can be applied to a variety of situations. Gaining cultural sensitivity and competence is a lifelong journey. Practitioners benefit from exposure to multiple cultures followed by reflection to grow and develop additional skills and abilities.

## CASE STUDY

Thomas, an OT working in a rehabilitation center, enjoyed working with a variety of clients. He prided himself on his ability to provide client-centered intervention and collaborate with clients. At the end of a busy day, he reflected on one particular client, Maria, an older woman, who suffered a traumatic brain injury. She nodded her head with all of Thomas' recommendations, she performed activities upon request, and she was polite throughout the session. However, Thomas did not feel she was engaged in therapy. He had a difficult time getting her to give her opinion on intervention activities. As a result, he was not sure if the intervention sessions were meaningful to Maria and he wondered if there were more he could do.

Maria was new to the United States from the Dominican Republic. After reading about her culture, Thomas found that as a general rule, people in this age bracket from this culture view professionals as the experts and follow their recommendations without question. They do not collaborate regarding their intervention plans as is common in the United States and Canada. Furthermore, the culture reinforces that women listen to men, which explained how Maria responded to him when he questioned her goals. Thomas realized that his attempts to make things "client-centered" may have caused her to be confused. In this circumstance, the client was behaving within her cultural expectations.

After discussing and reflecting on the cultural expectations, Thomas made sure a female therapist was close by during the sessions. He explained to Maria that he wanted to create goals that would most benefit her. Thomas respected her values of listening to the professionals by carefully making suggestions that worked within her culture. For example, Thomas demonstrated techniques to Maria's husband. He asked Maria to describe the cultural activities in which she continued to perform in the states to learn more about her needs. Thomas found out that Maria enjoyed cooking traditional meals, and they incorporated this into the intervention plan. Talking about her traditions allowed her to reminisce and helped her with the transition to the United States.

## Educational Initiatives to Promote a Global Perspective

Faculty and researchers have developed several initiatives to promote collaboration and understanding of different cultures. Global partnerships involve agreements between institutions. These mutually beneficial partnerships enrich student learning and provide resources to

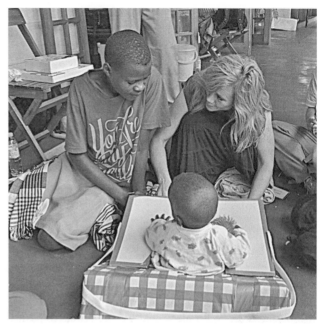

**Fig. 5.3** Developing reciprocal partnerships such as this one, in which the faculty member conducts research and training with staff while also working with children and their families, benefits everyone involved.

communities.[23] Often the goal of these experiences is to promote the health and well-being of individuals in low-resource countries.[20] Yet a partnership works best when it is beneficial to both parties. Fig. 5.3 shows a faculty member providing resources and education to staff in Ethiopia. Thus OT faculty, students, and practitioners work to establish that type of collaboration.[20] For example, the University of Illinois at Chicago partnered with the Ann Sullivan Center of Peru (CASP) to engage in collaborative community-based research.[18] Elliot (2015)[9] examined reflections from students who participated in a short-term international immersion experience. Elliot (2015)[9] found that many students reported a "desire to do good". The desire to do good for others without understanding their culture is a Western culture attitude (i.e., more affluent culture helping out those less fortunate) and may not promote long-standing partnerships.[9] Elliot suggests that partnerships where both parties gain something are both beneficial and sustainable.

Successful partnerships begin with open and honest communication, well-defined goals and objectives, and clear expectations of what each partner offers and requires. Saurez-Balcazar et al. (2013)[18] and Witchger Hansen (2015)[23] outlined the following factors as key to developing and sustaining the partnership:

- Establishing adequate communication
  - Clarifying goals and expectations
  - Establishing open and honest communication
  - Being consistent and client-centered
- Recognizing and celebrating cultural practices
  - Showing respect for the culture and how things are done, valued, and celebrated
  - Building relationships of trust and respect

- Understanding the local and national cultural context of the host country
- Establishing reciprocal learning communities
  - Promoting two-way learning (others refer to this as "doing good")
  - Ensuring equality of resources and learning
  - Doing what the local community requests
  - Sharing power with partners
- Addressing the needs of the community[17,19]
  - Supporting local solutions to local problems
  - Studying local and national government policy on health, education, and disability; local beliefs around health and the stigma of disability; and cultural norms and expectations[25]

**Occupational justice** refers to the belief that all persons (regardless of ability, age, gender, social class, or economic status) are entitled to have access to participation in everyday occupations. Everyone should be able to participate in the full range of meaningful and enriching opportunities for social inclusion. People should have resources to participate in activities that satisfy personal health and quality of life. OT practitioners are often in a position to advocate for access or equal opportunities for all.

## Interprofessional Education and Team Partnerships Reflecting a Global Practice

Today's health-care environment requires that professionals collaborate and work closely together for the best interest of the client. **Interprofessional education** (IPE) is an important part of OT education because it prepares students for practice. Some academic institutions are using global experiences as an opportunity for interprofessional learning[6,7] (Fig. 5.4A and Fig. 5.4B). Whereas some institutions have students travel to other countries to experience global health issues, other academic programs arrange for unique classes, workshops, seminars, and interprofessional experiences emphasizing global topics. Students learn about the culture through IPE.[6,7]

Students who worked in interprofessional teams regarding global health issues reported that "value of sharing similar goals, role blurring, and value of teamwork" were concepts that influenced interprofessional collaboration.[5] Students enjoyed learning about others' professions and teaching others about their own. Because the topic of global health issues is generally new to all students in the groupings, no one profession held the advantage. Students overall felt more confident when they articulated the differences in their own words and listened to one another.[6] By listening to one another, team members learned about the different theories that influence each profession. This required that they understand their own values, philosophy, and theories and use the knowledge as a base in making decisions.[6] The team partnerships strengthened the responses and allowed members to develop important collaboration skills. Such experiences allow students to see the "big picture."

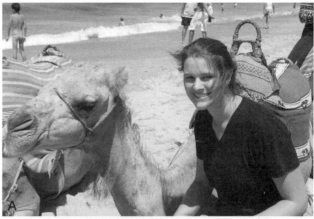
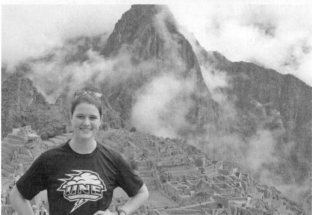

• **Fig. 5.4A, B** A student gains confidence while studying in Morocco.

For example, one IPE event featured a client who recently immigrated to the United States from Sudan. He described his journey and the challenges he faced by coming to the United States. The interprofessional teams discussed the social needs and community resources and then developed a plan, which considered the health-care system and the political, environmental, and personal issues the client faced. They were surprised when they heard that the man was a physician in Sudan, but fled when his village was overtaken and he was left at a refugee camp. He was sent to the United States with other Sudanese boys, none of whom had resources or transportation. He had no family members for support. The interprofessional team learned about global health care by discussing the political nature of this case, which illustrated the complexities influencing human occupation. They learned about the other professions and determined how each could contribute to the intervention plan and provide resources for the man.

## Cultural Immersion

Cultural immersion programs, such as international fieldwork opportunities for OT students, promote personal and professional growth and development[4] (Fig. 5.5). By becoming immersed in another culture, students learn about themselves, reflect upon their own culture, and compare

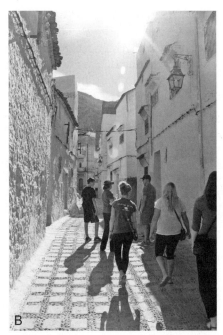

**Fig. 5.5** Living in the country allows students to understand the culture and environment by engaging in daily activities in the same manner as members of the culture. These students walk along the cobblestone streets of Santiago, Chile.

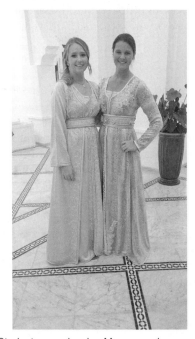

**Fig. 5.6** Students experiencing Moroccan dress.

and contrast political, social, and environmental issues. These immersion programs have been deemed essential in transforming students' thinking (Fig. 5.6). OT students learn firsthand about health-care systems and the culture's view of disability, health, and wellness. Challenging oneself to assimilate to a new culture requires self-reflection, problem solving, and awareness, which build confidence and empower students. Students develop cultural sensitivity

through opportunities to study OT practice in different settings.[23] The awareness, reflection, and maturity of students may increase the quality of care clients receive as students practice in different environments.[23]

### International Fieldwork Experiences

Some students may opt to complete an international fieldwork experience. The Accreditation Council for Occupational Therapy Education (ACOTE) provides standards for international fieldwork placements.[1] Specifically, international placements for OT students "must not exceed 12 weeks" and for OTA students "must not exceed 8 weeks".[1] Students must be supervised by an occupational therapist who graduated from a program approved by WFOT and has 1 year of experience.[1] The fieldwork placement sites must meet the educational program requirements (e.g., immunizations, criminal background checks, professional liability insurance) as well as international requirements. To ensure that students understand and are adequately prepared to complete the requirements (such as NBCOT certification) to practice in their country, an international fieldwork placement is often provided as an additional optional fieldwork.

Specific challenges to an international fieldwork experience include concerns regarding the level and nature of offsite supervision (or remote supervision), costs related to travel and housing, logistics, communication (which may be compromised by time zones), difficulty adjusting to a foreign environment, language issues, and possibly less prior exposure to specific diagnoses or a low caseload.[4] However, critical reflection (through journaling, discussion, and reflection) will facilitate therapeutic reasoning. Box 5.1 provides a list of suggestions to develop successful international fieldwork placements.

---

**• BOX 5.1    Suggestions for International Fieldwork Placements**

- Develop an effective partnership with the site before, during, and after placement.
  - Engage in ongoing dialogue, adjustments, continual feedback, and reexamination of values and beliefs.
  - Identify and document mutual partnership goals.
- Communicate clear and explicit expectations.
  - Communicate requirements regarding living conditions, social supports, levels of maturity, and academic expectations.
- Provide a thorough orientation to setting.
  - Orient regarding food, transportation options, cultural norms, local occupations, and governmental systems.
  - Consider a translator for a period, if needed.
- Communicate effectively between partners.
  - Identify and discuss level of preparation of student and supervisor.

From Cameron, D., Cockburn, L., Nixon, S., Parnes, P., Garcia, L., Leotaud, J., … Williams, T. (2013). Global partnerships for international fieldwork in occupational therapy: Reflection and innovation. *Occupational Therapy International, 20*(2), 85–93. http://dx.doi.org/10.1002/oti.1352

## Practicing Occupational Therapy Around the Globe

OT practitioners enable clients to engage in those things that they find meaningful and culturally relevant. They consider the client's values, beliefs, and cultural expectations when designing occupation-based intervention. Faculty and practitioners often travel to settings to educate or provide resources to practitioners. The intent of expert consultants travelling to places with limited resources is to teach local practitioners skills that they may be able to continue to provide after the consultant returns home. For example, Dr. Patty Coker-Bolt recently taught therapists in Ethiopia the principles of constraint-induced movement therapy and how to make low-cost chairs.[5] Figs. 5.7A and 5.7B show Dr. Coker-Bolt working with the practitioners and family.

Some countries emphasize community practice.[22] Practitioners around the globe contend with the real pressures of health-care funding. This may limit the number of occupational therapists in clinical settings. They must work within the systems that reimburse for services, such as Medicare and Medicaid in the United States. Collaborating on techniques that were effective in one country may help another country justify services. Examining the evidence from around the world strengthens OT practice. Evidence-based OT practice

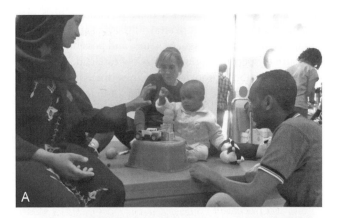

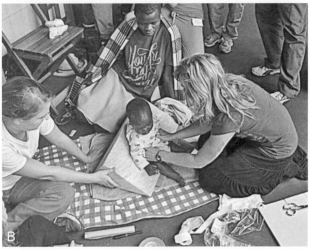

• **Fig. 5.7A, B** Dr. Coker-Bolt working with the practitioners and family to teach them CIMT techniques and low-cost positioning options.

refers to basing practice decisions on an analysis of the current research evidence.[8,13] This requires that OT practitioners carefully examine the research evidence, use therapeutic reasoning to make intervention decisions based upon their analysis, and review the outcomes of the intervention. Practitioners use evidence to support therapeutic reasoning and intervention planning, determine outcomes, and monitor progress. Practitioners use evidence-based research around the world to provide evidence to support intervention.

As people acknowledge the WHO[25] concepts of quality of life and health and wellness, OT practitioners in some countries may shiftservice provision from hospital-based care to community-based. For example, in Denmark, services are provided as social services for home and work environments.[22,25] OT practitioners who work in countries involved in war (such as Iran and Iraq) work with polytrauma and have limited resources.[16,22] **Polytrauma** refers to multiple injuries, which can be life-threatening. Consequently, initial intervention is focused on medical management. These types of injury require intensive, long-term OT services.[16]

Some practice approaches are unique to countries, such as elephant-assisted therapy in Thailand.[22] Via a survey, McGrath and O'Callaghan (2014)[14] gathered data on current practice in dementia care in Ireland. They found that the majority of respondents worked in primary care and provided services for people with early stage or mild dementia. Practitioners ($n = 47$) reported barriers to the delivery of OT services as lack of therapist time ($n = 42$, 89.4%), cost of OT ($n = 12$, 25.5%), role restrictions imposed by the setting ($n = 10$, 21.3%), and lack of knowledge and skills relating to dementia among staff ($n = 7$, 14.9%).

The Canadian Occupational Therapy Association (CAOT) has a comprehensive website that provides current resources for families and highlights current research. The United Kingdom has completed much work on implementing OT into the mental health system, specifically using the Model of Human Occupation.

OT practitioners can find information on the state of the OT practice for a given country through researching the literature. Attending international conferences (such as those of the WFOT) allows practitioners from around the world to network. Learning about practice in other cultures can provide creative solutions that can be useful to other countries. Resources may be shared and benefit clients and their families.

### *World Federation of Occupational Therapists*

WFOT began in 1951 as a way to promote and advance occupational therapy, maintain the ethics and interests of the profession, facilitate the exchange of information, educate and train therapists, and hold international congresses.[24] The mission of WFOT is to "promote occupational therapy as an art and science internationally. The Federation supports the development, use and practice of occupational therapy worldwide, demonstrating its relevance and contribution to society."[24]

OT practitioners and students may become members of WFOT through their national associations, by paying an annual membership fee.[24] WFOT provides an OT international outreach network (OTION) forum for members, publications, and a congress.

## Summary

OT is practiced around the world. Learning about different cultures and developing skills to become culturally responsive to clients creates trusting therapeutic relationships. Understanding the factors that may influence families and clients allows practitioners to advocate for occupational justice and meet the client's needs, while bettering the resources available for other people. In today's global community, it is essential that therapists develop cultural competence and become aware of OT theory and practice around the world.

## Learning Activities

1. Research the cultural practices of a culture outside of your own. Describe how the culture engages in specific occupations. What occupations are unique to this culture?
2. Participate in an interprofessional education experience, either at your school or through and online learning experience. What did you learn about and from the other professionals? How did it enrich the learning experience?
3. Interview someone from another country to explore the individual's perspectives on health and disability.
4. Investigate OT practice in another country. What social, political, or environmental factors influence health care?
5. Complete one of the following cultural sensitivity assessments and reflect on your strengths and weaknesses.

Develop a plan to increase your level of cultural sensitivity.
- Cultural Competence Assessment Instrument (CCAI): http://www.excellenceforchildandyouth.ca/support-tools/measure-profile?id = 362
- Cultural Competence Health Practitioner Assessment: http://www4.georgetown.edu/uis/keybridge/keyform/form.cfm?formID = 277.
- Quality and Culture Quiz: http://erc.msh.org/mainpage.cfm?file = 3.0.htm&modue = provide&language = English
- A Self-Reflection Cultural Sensitivity Scale: http://cirrie.buirfalo.edu/culture/curriculum/activities/scale.php

## Review Questions

1. What is the importance of a global perspective on OT?
2. How does culture influence occupational performance?
3. What activities can a practitioner engage in to develop awareness of skills and attitudes for cultural competence?
4. What is occupational justice? What are some examples of occupational justice in OT practice?
5. How do interprofessional education and practice benefit clients and team members?
6. What are some strategies to develop skills for working in an interprofessional team?

## References

1. Accreditation Council for Occupational Therapy Education. *ACOTE Standards and Interpretive Guide*. 2011. Available online at http://www.aota.org/Educate/Accredit/StandardsReview.aspx.
2. American Occupational Therapy Association. *AOTA's Centennial Vision*. Retrieved from, 2006. http://www.aota.org/News/Centennial/Background/36516.aspx? FT = pdf.
3. American Occupational Therapy Association. Occupational therapy practice framework: domain and process (3rd ed.). *Am J Occup Ther*. 2014;68:S1–S48. Retrieved from, http://dx.doi.org/10.5014/ajot.2014.682006.
4. Cameron D, Cockburn L, Nixon S, et al. Global partnerships for international fieldwork in occupational therapy: reflection and innovation. *Occup Ther Int*. 2013;20(2):85–93. http://dx.doi.org/10.1002/oti.1352.
5. Coker-Bolt P, DeLuca S, Ramey S. A partnership model to adapt and implement pediatric constraint-induced movement therapy (CIMT) in Sub-Saharan Africa. *Occup Ther Int*. 2015;22(3):141–151. http://dx.doi.org/10.1002/oti.1932.
6. Cooper B, MacMillan B, Beck R, Paterson M. Facilitating and evaluating a student-led seminar series on global health issues as an opportunity for interprofessional learning for health science students. *Learning Health Soc Care*. 2009;8(3):210–222.
7. Cooper C. Student perspectives: global health issues fostering interprofessional collaboration at Queen's University. *Occup Ther Now*. 2012;14(2):24–26.
8. Depoy E, Gitlin L. Introduction to research. In: *Understanding and Applying Multiple Strategies*. St. Louis, MO: Elsevier Mosby; 2011:316–318.
9. Elliot ML. Critical ethnographic analysis of "doing good" on short-term international immersion experiences. *Occup Ther Int*. 2015;22(3):121–130. http://dx.doi.org/10.1002/oti.1390.
10. Goode T, Sockalingam S, Bronheim S, Brown M, Jones W. *A Planner's Guide*. Retrieved from, http://nccc.georgetown.edu/documents/Planners_Guide.pdf; 2000.
11. Hilderand K, Lewis L, Pizur-Barnekow K, et al. *How Can Occupational Therapy Strive Towards Culturally Sensitive Practices?* Bethesda, MD: AOTA; 2013.
12. Hume C. Why a global perspective can benefit occupational therapy. *Br J Ther Rehabil*. 2002;9(6):205.
13. Karhula M, Harra T, Kanelisto K, Heiskanen T, Kronlöf GH. An overview of the current status of evidence-based occupational therapy in Finland. *WFOT Bulletin*. 2011;64:24–28.
14. McGrath M, O'Callaghan C. Occupational therapy and dementia care: a survey of practice in the Republic of Ireland. *Aust Occup Ther J*. 2014;61(2):92–101. http://dx.doi.org/10.1111/1440-1630.12081.

15. Munoz JP. Culturally responsive caring in occupational therapy. *Occup Ther Int*. 2007;14:256–280.

16. Quick C, Judkins J, Prudencio T, et al. *Occupational therapy in polytrauma*. Fact Sheet, Bethesda, MD: AOTA; 2014.

17. Suarez-Balcazar Y, Hammel J, Helfrich CA, Thomas J, Wilson T, Head-Ball D. A model of university–community partnerships for occupational therapy scholarship and practice. *Occup Ther Health Care*. 2005;19:47–70.

18. Suarez-Balcazar Y, Hammel J, Mayo L, Inwald S, Sen S. Innovation in global collaborations: from Student placement to mutually beneficial exchanges. *Occup Ther Int*. 2013;20(2):94–101. http://dx.doi.org/10.1002/oti.1341.

19. Suarez-Balcazar Y, Harper G, Lewis R. An interactive and conceptual model of community–university collaborations for research and action. *Health Educ Behav*. 2005;32:84–101.

20. Suarez-Balcazar Y, Witchger Hansen AM, Muñoz JP. Transformative nature of global partnerships. *Occup Ther Int*. 2015;22(3):117–120. http://dx.doi.org/10.1002/oti.1406.

21. National Center for Cultural Competence. (nd). *Curricular enhancement module series: Glossary*. Georgetown University Center for Child and Human Development. Retrieved from). http://www.ncccurricula.info/glossary.html.

22. Waite A. OT around the world: profiles of occupational therapists in South America, Europe, the Middle East, Africa, and Asia. *OT Practice*. 2015;21(1):8–12.

23. Witchger Hansen AM. Crossing borders: a qualitative study of how occupational therapy educators and scholars develop and sustain global partnerships. *Occup Ther Int*. 2015;22(3):152–162. http://dx.doi.org/10.1002/oti.1401.

24. World Federation of Occupational Therapists. *Fundamental Beliefs*. Retrieved from, http://www.wfot.org/AboutUs/FundamentalBeliefs.aspx; 2011.

25. World Health Organization. *World health Report 2004: Changing history*. Retrieved from, http://www.who.int/whr/2004/en/index.html; 2004.

# Occupational Therapy: *The Practitioner*

# 6

# From Student to Practitioner: Educational Preparation and Certification

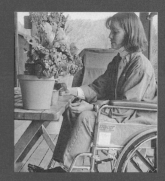

## OBJECTIVES

*After completing this chapter, the reader will be able to do the following:*

- Describe the accreditation process for occupational therapy educational programs.
- Identify the three categories of occupational therapy personnel.
- Define the roles of occupational therapy personnel.
- Delineate the educational and professional requirements for each personnel category.
- Describe the purpose of level I and level II fieldwork experiences.
- Describe the Doctor of Occupational Therapy (OTD) and the Doctor of Philosophy (PhD) degrees.

## KEY TERMS

accreditation
Accreditation Council for Occupational
   Therapy Education
certification
certified occupational therapy
   assistant (COTA)
Doctor of Occupational Therapy

fieldwork
level I fieldwork
level II fieldwork
licensure laws
National Board for Certification in
   Occupational Therapy
occupational therapist

occupational therapy assistant
occupational therapy aide
registered occupational therapist (OTR)
registration
service competency
supervision

(e) Visit *www.evolve.elsevier.com* to access the Evolve student resources that accompany your book.

*The most memorable aspects of my career in occupational therapy (OT) education were the wonderful students I had the privilege of knowing and the opportunity I had to share with them my beliefs and philosophy about the health-giving value of occupation. My students taught me so much about life, teaching, and learning. It was a richly rewarding experience to facilitate and witness the evolution of the OT student to the professional occupational therapist.*

**LORRAINE WILLIAMS PEDRETTI, MS, OTR (RETIRED)**
**Professor Emeritus**
**Department of Occupational Therapy**
**San José State University**
**San José, California**

The personnel who deliver occupational therapy (OT) services to consumers can be divided into three categories that vary in the type and amount of training they receive and the duties they perform. The most highly trained at the professional level is the **occupational therapist**. The **occupational therapy assistant** (OTA) is trained at the technical level and works under the **supervision** of the occupational therapist. A third category of worker, the **occupational therapy aide**, does not receive specialized training before working in the field; rather, OT aides receive on-the-job training.

Consistent with the terminology used by the American Occupational Therapy Association (AOTA), the term *occupational therapy personnel* is used when referring to any personnel (including OT students and aides) who assist in delivering OT services. The term *occupational therapy practitioner* refers to any individual who is "initially certified to practice as either an occupational therapist or an OTA, or licensed or regulated by a state, district, commonwealth, or territory of the United States to practice as an occupational therapist or OTA, and who has not had that certification, license, or regulation revoked due to disciplinary action."[10] When it is necessary to distinguish between the three categories of personnel, the respective titles are used.

This chapter focuses on the educational preparation and certification process for the occupational therapist and the OTA. It describes the roles and responsibilities of the OT personnel.

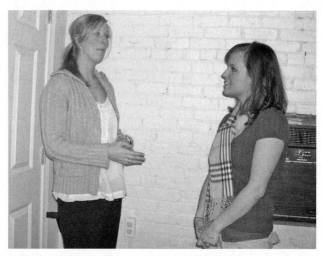

● **Fig. 6.1** The occupational therapist and occupational therapy assistant discuss their findings from a recent observation to develop service competency.

## Role of the Occupational Therapist and Occupational Therapy Assistant

Occupational therapists are autonomous practitioners who deliver OT services.[6] Occupational therapists are responsible for all aspects of OT service delivery, and they are accountable for the safety and effectiveness of OT service. Therapists direct the evaluation process, interpret data, develop intervention plans, and measure outcomes.[6] They supervise OTAs and occupational therapy aides and determine when to delegate responsibilities. Occupational therapists are professionals who seek supervision and mentoring to promote their professional growth. They recognize when they need advanced training and seek out opportunities to advance their abilities to benefit clients and families.[6]

OTAs deliver OT services under the supervision and in partnership with an occupational therapist. They contribute to the evaluation process by conducting parts of the evaluation (once service competency has been established).[6] **Service competency** refers to the occupational therapist and OTA performing a skill in the same way or obtaining the same result when measuring a client's performance[5] (Fig. 6.1). For example, the occupational therapist may ask the OTA to administer parts of an assessment to see if the OTA obtains similar findings. The OTA has achieved service competency when he or she reaches the same findings or performs the task in the same way as the occupational therapist, which allows the occupational therapist and OTA to be confident that they perform consistently. Although the OTA may provide information for the evaluation, he or she is not responsible for the interpretation of the data.[5,6] The occupational therapist is ultimately responsible for developing and implementing the plan. The OTA carries out the intervention plan by determining activities and working directly with the client. The OTA and occupational therapist collaborate throughout the intervention process.[5,6] For example, the OTA may report observations to therapeutically reason through intervention ideas. The OTA may

discuss the client's progress to date to receive feedback or suggestions to increase the effectiveness of the sessions. The occupational therapist may observe the OTA performing new strategies to provide him or her feedback and support. It is the OTA's responsibility to seek and obtain appropriate quality and frequency of supervision so that proper OT services are provided. Both the occupational therapist and OTA follow state practice acts, which provide specific guidelines for supervision, documentation, and intervention.[5,9] If a discrepancy exists between state, professional, or insurance guidelines, practitioners are to follow the most stringent guidelines.[5,9] OT aides provide supportive services to the occupational therapist and OTA. They do not provide skilled OT services but are trained by the occupational therapist or OTA to perform specifically designed tasks or activities.

## Accreditation of Educational Programs

The **Accreditation Council for Occupational Therapy Education** (ACOTE) of AOTA regulates entry-level education for both occupational therapist and OTA programs in the United States. Since 1935, AOTA has set standards for educational programs. The standards are reviewed and revised every 5 years by various constituency groups, educational program directors, and the public at large. The latest revision of the standards for occupational therapist and OTA programs was completed in 2011 and went into effect 2013, (meaning that educational programs must comply with the new standards by 2013). These standards are published in the *Standards for an Accredited Educational Program for the Occupational Therapist*[1] and in the *Standards for an Accredited Educational Program for the Occupational Therapy Assistant.*[1]

ACOTE evaluates each educational program's compliance with the standards as part of the accreditation process.

Each program must meet ACOTE standards to become accredited and to maintain accreditation. Educational programs are reviewed to determine if they meet the minimal compliance with the ACOTE standards. All educational programs must show minimal compliance with the Standards to receive accreditation. The Standards include administration procedures, educational content, and fieldwork processes. For example, institutions must inform ACOTE of their intention to begin a new program, and they must design an educational program with coursework that addresses the standards regarding curriculum. Accreditation requires a review of the program design and an on-site inspection. The on-site evaluation includes interviews with alumni, students, faculty, and administration. After meeting the minimal standards for competency requirements, the program becomes fully accredited and is then reviewed on a regular basis. To maintain accreditation, programs complete a "Report of Self-Study" and undergo a site visit before the end of the period in which accreditation was awarded. The review board has the power to grant or withhold approval.

The Preamble to the ACOTE standards provides an overview of what graduates at the doctorate, masters and associates level must possess. Graduates from doctoral degree programs engage in research and leadership work as well as preparation to provide direct patient care. They are trained to assume positions of consultant, educator, manager, leader, researcher, and advocate for the profession and the consumer.[1] Occupational therapy graduates who earn a masters degree also possess basic skills in patient care, and may act as consultant, educator, manager, researcher, and advocate for the profession and the consumer.[1] The occupational therapy assistant is educated to " possess the basic skills as a direct are provider, educator, and advocate for the profession and the consumer."[1] Each of these professionals offer important services to the profession of occupational therapy.

**Accreditation** of an OT educational program means that the minimal educational standards recommended by the profession have been met and the school has received formal approval by ACOTE. This approval ensures that graduates of an accredited program meet minimal entry-level standards and that they are qualified to take the national certification examination. As of 2016, there were 196 accredited occupational therapist programs, 40 OT doctoral programs and 272 accredited OTA programs in the United States.[7] A current listing of all programs can be found at AOTA's website, www.aota.org.

A number of developing programs are under way (24 for occupational therapist; 47 for OTAs).[7, 2a] In selecting a school, prospective students are advised to seek information about the accreditation status, success of program graduates on the national certification examination, job placement rates, mission statement and philosophy, and the design and focus of the educational program.

## Entry-Level Educational Preparation

Table 6.1 summarizes the characteristics of the different levels of OT educational preparation. In practice, the roles of the occupational therapist and OTA are complementary and collaborative. Therefore the curricula for the entry-level preparation of the occupational therapist and the OTA consist of a similar combination of classroom and clinical learning experiences that reflect current practice. Students in occupational therapist and OTA programs study anatomy, physiology, medical conditions, kinesiology, and general education courses that lead to a degree awarded by the respective college or university. Courses in the professional areas of the curricula are also similar in content. Students at both levels learn OT principles, practices, and processes. Occupational therapist education differs from OTA education in that it provides more detailed theory in the core and professional curricula and a greater emphasis on evaluation, interpretation, and research.

Each level of training requires practical experience, referred to as **fieldwork.** The purpose of fieldwork is to advance students' thinking, reasoning, performance, and professionalism from the role of student to that of practitioner.[4] Participation in fieldwork experiences solidifies and deepens knowledge from academic coursework, allowing students to integrate material so that they may use it in practice. Thus fieldwork is an essential component of the OT curriculum and in developing competent, entry-level practitioners.

Students are expected to increase their technical and therapeutic reasoning skills over time (Fig. 6.2). Therefore both occupational therapist and OTA educational programs require two levels of fieldwork. The initial level is referred to as **level I fieldwork** and is completed concurrently with academic coursework; it involves observation and participation in selected aspects of the OT process[4] (Fig. 6.3). The purpose of level I fieldwork is to introduce the student to the profession and to the various applications of intervention. Level I fieldwork allows students to learn from practitioners, observe client interactions and intervention, engage in practice settings, and complete assignments that reinforce academic learning. For example, students may learn to write notes in the subjective, objective, assessment, plan (SOAP) format in class and complete a SOAP note on a client they observe on level I fieldwork. The amount of time required for level I fieldwork experiences and the type of assignments vary by program.

**Level II fieldwork** experiences are hands-on clinical training opportunities designed to provide students with in-depth experiences in delivering OT services with supervision.[4] Students in occupational therapist programs complete full-time level II fieldwork at a facility for a minimum of 24 weeks, whereas OTA students complete 16 weeks of full-time level II fieldwork. Students engaged in level II fieldwork are immersed in OT practice, and, by the end of the

| TABLE 6.1 | Characteristics of Levels of Preparation in Occupational Therapy |
|---|---|

| Degree | Distinctive Curricular Features | Prerequisites | Average Program Length | Additional Requirements |
|---|---|---|---|---|
| Associate AA/ AS (required to practice as OTA) | Focus is on technical skills related to the methods and procedures used in OT | High school diploma | 2 years | 16 weeks of level II fieldwork |
| Entry-level master's MS/MA/MOT (required to practice as occupational therapist) | In-depth theory; greater emphasis on evaluation, interpretation, and intervention planning; emphasis on critically analyzing research for practice | Baccalaureate degree in preoccupational therapy, health sciences, or another field | 2 years following baccalaureate degree | 24 weeks of level II fieldwork; basic research project or thesis |
| Advanced master's MS or MA | Develop advanced research skills and specialization in practice area | Baccalaureate degree in OT | 1–3 years following baccalaureate degree | Master's thesis or advanced-level research project; may require additional fieldwork |
| Entry-level Doctorate in Occupational Therapy (OTD) | Advanced-practice competencies; clinical leadership; scholarship | Master's degree in any field | 3 years following baccalaureate | Clinical research project or practicum required |
| Postprofessional Doctorate in Occupational Therapy (OTD) | Advanced-practice competencies; clinical leadership; research and scholarship | Master's degree in OT | 2–3 years following master's | Clinical research, leadership, scholarship required |
| Doctoral degree (PhD, EdD, DrPH) | Generate research and knowledge for the profession | Master's degree | 3–5 years | Dissertation |

AA, Associate of Arts; AS, Associate of Science; MA, Master of Arts; MOT, Master of Occupational Therapy; MS, Master of Science; OT, occupational therapy; OTD, Doctor of Occupational Therapy; PhD, Doctor of Philosophy.

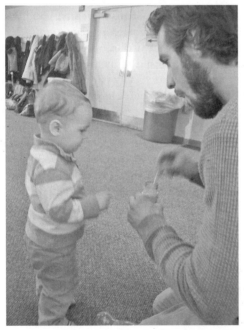

• **Fig. 6.2** Occupational therapy students engage in experiential learning to develop therapeutic reasoning skills for practice.

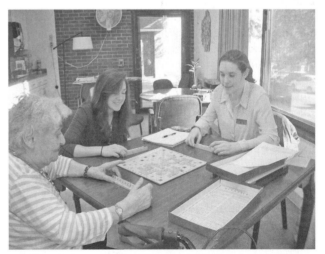

• **Fig. 6.3** As part of level I fieldwork experience, occupational therapy students engage an older adult in a game to facilitate participation in social activities.

experience, students are expected to function as entry-level practitioners. Students complete two separate level II fieldwork experiences. For example, a student may complete one level II fieldwork experience at a large medical facility and another at a community mental health center. The diverse settings provide optimal learning experiences and prepare students to work in a variety of contexts.

## Educational Demographics of Occupational Therapy Practitioners

Workforce data reveal that OT practitioners are primarily women, most OTAs hold associate's degrees (93%), and the majority of occupational therapists have master's degrees (60%).[8] Entry-level doctoral programs are emerging. The passage of the Affordable Care Act has led people to predict that there will be a greater demand for OTAs to fill positions, so that occupational therapists can conduct evaluations. In fact, the projected growth rate of occupational therapist and OTA jobs is "much faster than expected," and this is evidenced in the 70% 5-year growth rate of OTA educational programs.[7,8]

## Educational Preparation for the Occupational Therapist

Since 2007, occupational therapists must complete a master's degree to practice; thus, the percentage of occupational therapists prepared at the master's level has risen in recent years.[8] Practitioners who obtained a baccalaureate degree in OT before 2007 are "grandfathered in" and may continue to practice. Some universities offer programs to help practitioners with baccalaureate degrees in OT progress to earn an advanced master's degree. Often, these courses are offered during evenings and weekends to accommodate the working therapist. Students who earned a baccalaureate degree in a related field (e.g., psychology, child development) may enter an entry-level master's degree OT program (sometimes referred to as the basic master's degree). Students are encouraged to explore the educational options by communicating with local universities and colleges.

### Entry-Level Doctor of Occupational Therapy

Students who have a baccalaureate degree or master's degree in a discipline other than OT may elect to obtain an entry-level **Doctor of Occupational Therapy** (OTD). The OTD degree is expected to educate practitioners so that they can contribute to outcomes research, program evaluation, and evidence-based practice. As such, the OTD may help practitioners participate as interprofessional team members and contribute to the outcomes evidence needed for the profession.[2] This degree is also called the clinical doctorate.

### Postprofessional Doctor of Occupational Therapy

Students who are occupational therapists may decide to enroll in a postprofessional OTD program to advance their clinical expertise, develop research skills, and develop strong leadership and/or educational skills to advance the profession and add to the scholarship of the profession.

### Postprofessional Education

The Doctor of Philosophy (PhD) is the traditional postgraduate degree and is a research-based degree. Doctorates such as the Doctorate of Education (EdD), Doctorate of Science (ScD), and Doctor of Public Health (DrPH) are also research-based degrees. Some academic institutions offer PhDs in OT, occupational science, and other related areas, such as psychology, which are appealing to professionals. An individual with a doctoral degree is trained to be an independent researcher, with importance placed on the discovery of knowledge.

## Entry-Level Degrees in Occupational Therapy

With the increased emphasis on interprofessional team collaboration because of the demands of health care and the profession's need to provide evidence-based research, the AOTA Board of Directors recommended that the entry-level degree for occupational therapists change to a single point of entry at the OTD by 2025.[2] However, after much discussion and input from members and stakeholders, the Board released a statement in August 2015 stating that their position was that the master's and doctoral entry-level degrees should remain entry-level options for occupational therapists.[2] They cited the following reasons for maintaining the two entry levels: limited outcomes exist differentiating the two graduates; academic institutions may not have adequate doctoral-trained OT faculty to meet the needs; issues exist surrounding additional fieldwork expectations; and two levels of entry allow for flexibility of the profession to address changing health-care needs.[2] Only the Representative Assembly can establish official professional policies or standards for occupational therapy.

## Educational Preparation for the Occupational Therapy Assistant

In 1965, AOTA mandated that OTA programs be established in junior or community colleges. Gradually, OTA educational programs were lengthened from 9 to 12 months and then to 2 years. Beginning in 1977, OTA students were required to take the certification examination. Currently, OTA students must complete at least 2 years of postsecondary education in an accredited program, which may be obtained at a community college, junior college, or technical training school. The OTA student must successfully complete level I and level II fieldwork experiences. The type of associate's degree (science or arts) awarded depends on the institution. Students who have completed all of the educational requirements and level II fieldwork are eligible to take the national certification examination for OTAs. Programs for the OTA typically focus less on theory and more on the "doing" aspects of the field, such as methods and procedures used in OT.

OTA students may elect to further their education by seeking a baccalaureate degree in a related field and then obtaining a basic master's degree in OT. Some universities offer special arrangements so that OTAs receive credit for the work they have completed toward advanced degrees. Nontraditional programs, such as weekend and online formats, are available to help OTAs advance their education. Those wishing to advance their education are urged to communicate with faculty and explore options.

The AOTA Board determined that the entry-level degree for OTAs will be offered at both the associate's degree and bachelor's degree levels.[2] The council agreed that the two entry levels may better prepare individuals for further academic achievement and leadership positions, expand opportunities within the scope of practice, and permit additional flexibility to address the changing health-care needs of clients and populations.[2]

## Entry-Level Certification and State Licensure

Certification refers to the acknowledgment that an individual has the qualifications to be an entry-level practitioner, either a registered occupational therapist (OTR) or certified occupational therapy assistant (COTA). After completing the educational and fieldwork requirements, candidates at each educational level are eligible to sit for the national certification examination, administered by the National Board for Certification in Occupational Therapy (NBCOT). The certification examination is a 4-hour multiple-choice examination that covers evaluation and intervention planning for all areas of practice, ethics, delivery systems, and basic OT principles. Those candidates who pass the certification examination are entitled to use the appropriate professional designation after their names—OTR or COTA. Once they pass the examination, candidates may apply for a state license required to practice. Candidates who do not pass the examination may retake the test. However, they must pay for each attempt. Typically, persons working under a temporary license who fail the examination may not continue working as an OT practitioner. They may work as aides until the test is passed.

## State Regulation

The practice of OT is regulated through licensure laws that safeguard the public and protect the public from unethical, incompetent, or unauthorized practitioners. State licensure laws, also called practice acts, provide a legal definition of OT and the domain of OT practice that differentiates it from other professions.[9] These laws provide important guides for consumers, facilities, and providers, especially with regard to the minimum qualifications for practitioners. The state practice acts address supervision, service competency, and scope of practice.[9] State licensure laws may require that professionals show continuing competency by engaging in continuing education.

OT practitioners must remain up-to-date on the status of the licensure laws in their state and any proposed changes to the regulations. Because government leaders and other professional organizations may oppose renewal of licensure laws that protect and support OT practice, OT practitioners must become involved and advocate for these guidelines and practice acts. State licensure is discussed further in Chapter 8.

## History of Certification and Registration

Registration began in 1931 when AOTA listed occupational therapists who completed approved professional training and 1 year of subsequent work experience. Those individuals who qualified were granted the designation registered occupational therapist (OTR).[3] The first National Register, published in 1932, listed 318 occupational therapists. In 1939 the standards for registration included the passage of a written essay examination. In 1947 the essay examination was converted to an objective multiple-choice examination, which is still in use today.

In the late 1950s, registration for OTAs was implemented for those individuals who graduated from an approved educational program. Initially, those individuals who did not graduate from an approved program but worked a minimum of 2 years in one disability area were "grandfathered" into the profession.[3] This plan was eliminated in 1963. The first OTA certification examination was administered in 1977.

In 1980, a category called "certified only" was created for practitioners who wanted to be certified without being a member of AOTA.[3] The certification process underwent a major administrative change in 1986, when an autonomous certification board was created, separating AOTA membership and certification. This board was initially named the American Occupational Therapy Certification Board (AOTCB). In 1988 the AOTCB was incorporated as a separate entity from AOTA.[3] In 1996, AOTCB changed its name to the National Board for Certification in Occupational Therapy (NBCOT). NBCOT consists of a 15-member board of directors composed of eight OT practitioners and seven public members.[3] NBCOT functions independently in all aspects of initial certification. NBCOT has established procedures for and implemented a certification renewal program that includes creating an e-portfolio to determine continued competency. Practitioners are urged to complete the Professional Development Tool provided by NBCOT.

## Summary

Occupational therapist and OTA are the two official levels of professionals in the field of OT, and each receives formal education in OT theory, philosophy, and process.

The formal education of the occupational therapist and OTA is similar in content, but the occupational therapist receives more depth of theoretical knowledge and research. The OTA educational program typically takes 2 years to obtain an associate's degree; the occupational therapist degree requires a master's degree (5–6 years of study). Students who complete the required coursework in an occupational therapist or OTA program are eligible to sit for the national certification examination and apply for state licensure. OT practitioners continue to develop competency for practice by engaging in ongoing education.

## Learning Activities

1. Prepare a report on the logistics of the NBCOT examination.
2. Write a short paper on the history of OT education.
3. Interview an OT practitioner. Determine his or her motivation for entering the field. How did he or she learn about OT? Why did he or she decide to pursue the field? What is his or her educational background? Ask the individual to describe his or her fieldwork experiences.
4. Compare and contrast the OT programs offered at two universities. Describe the levels of education, coursework, and time requirements.
5. Examine the educational requirements for occupational therapist, OTA, OTD, and PhD programs.
6. Complete the AOTA Professional Development Tool (PDT) to create a professional plan.

## Review Questions

1. What are the categories of OT personnel?
2. What are the educational requirements for each personnel category?
3. What are the professional requirements for each personnel category?
4. What is the Accreditation Council for Occupational Therapy Education?
5. What is the certification process for occupational therapist and OTA personnel?
6. What are the fieldwork requirements for occupational therapist and OTA personnel?

## References

1. Accreditation Council for Occupational Therapy Education. *Standards and Interpretive Guide: August 2015 Version.* 2011. Retrieved from, http://www.aota.org/-/media/Corporate/Files/EducationCareers/Accredit/Standards/2011-Standards-and-Interpretive-Guide.pdf.
2. Accreditation Council for Occupational Therapy Education. *ACOTE's Statement on the Entry-Level Degree for the OT and OTA.* 2015, August. Retrieved from, http://www.aota.org/Education-Careers/Accreditation/acote-entry-level-degrees.aspx.
2a. Accreditation Council for Occupational Therapy Education (ACOTE). *ACOTE October 2016 Accreditation Actions.* 2016. Retrieved from, http://www.aota.org/-/media/Corporate/Files/EducationCareers/Accredit/Announcements/Actions/October2016ACOTEActionsforWeb.pdf.
3. American Occupational Therapy Association. Eye on the profession: AOTA: chronology of certification issues dated through January 29. *OT Week.* 1997;11(7):9–12.
4. American Occupational Therapy Association. Occupational therapy fieldwork education: value and purpose. *Am J Occup Ther.* 2009;63(6):821–822.
5. American Occupational Therapy Association. *Advisory Opinion for the Ethics Commission: OT/OTA Partnerships: Achieving High Ethical Standards in a Challenging Health Care Environment*; 2010. Retrieved from, http://www.aota.org/-/media/corporate/files/practice/ethics/advisory/ot-ota-partnership.pdf.
6. American Occupational Therapy Association. Guidelines for the supervision, roles, and responsibilities during the delivery of occupational therapy services. *Am J Occup Ther.* 2014;68(suppl 3):S16–S22.
7. American Occupational Therapy Association. *Academic Programs Annual Data Report: Academic Year 2014–2015.* Bethesda, MD: AOTA; 2015. Retrieved from, http://www.aota.org/-/media/corporate/files/educationcareers/educators/2014-2015-annual-data-report.pdf.
8. American Occupational Therapy Association. *Salary & Workforce Survey: Executive Summary.* 2015. Retrieved from, http://www.aota.org/education-careers/advance-career/salary-workforce-survey.aspx.
9. American Occupational Therapy Association. Standards of practice for occupational therapy. *Am J Occup Ther.* 2015;69(suppl 3):http://dx.doi.org/10.5014/ajot.2015.696506 6913410057p1-6913410057p6.
10. American Occupational Therapy Association. *Reference Manual of the Official Documents of the American Occupational Therapy Association, Inc.* 20th ed. Bethesda, MD: Author; 2015.

# 7

# The Occupational Therapy Practitioner: Roles, Responsibilities, and Relationships

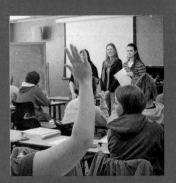

## OBJECTIVES

*After completing this chapter, the reader will be able to do the following:*

- Identify the different roles an occupational therapy practitioner may assume.
- Describe the levels of performance for occupational therapy practitioners.
- Explain the role of activity director.
- Discuss the minimum responsibilities of the occupational therapist and the occupational therapy assistant in service delivery as described in the *Scope of Practice*.
- Understand the levels of supervision and parameters that affect these levels.

- Identify the practices that contribute to successful supervisory relationships.
- Describe service competency.
- Describe the different types of teams in health care and recognize the importance of interprofessional teams.
- Understand the importance of lifelong learning and professional development.
- Describe tools that can be used to maintain and document continuing competency.

## KEY TERMS

activity director
advanced-level practitioner
board certification
career development
client-related tasks
close supervision
continuing competence
direct supervision

entry-level practitioner
general supervision
interdisciplinary team
intermediate-level practitioner
multidisciplinary team
non–client-related tasks
professional development
relationship

roles
routine supervision
service competency
specialty certification
supervision
transdisciplinary team

e Visit *www.evolve.elsevier.com* to access the Evolve student resources that accompany your book.

I like helping people.

Okay, so maybe that sounds a little simplistic, but it is true. I like solving problems, connecting people with resources, working with an individual eye to eye, and setting and meeting goals. I like looking at not only the "forest," but also the "trees," and seeing each "tree" for the individual

that he or she is and recognizing the unique and special characteristics that each person has to offer. I like treating a person with respect and dignity, and through the knowledge and skills that I possess as an occupational therapist, helping that person to achieve a life that is purposeful and meaningful to him or her, not by my definitions, but by *what he or she defines as important. I like looking at the whole person, not just a body part or specific function, but as a precious asset to society, complex and dynamic. I like the look on someone's face when he or she realizes that he or she can accomplish far more than he or she ever thought he or she would be able to do before working with an occupational therapist. I like when "can't" becomes "can" and "doesn't" becomes "done."*

*I like helping people; I love being an occupational therapist.*

**JILL J. PAGE, OTR/L**
**Industrial Rehabilitation Consultant**
**ErgoScience, Inc.**
**Birmingham, Alabama**

Once a student graduates from an accredited educational program and passes the National Board for Certification in Occupational Therapy (NBCOT®) examination, he or she is eligible to apply for state licensure. At this point, the practitioner is considered to be an entry-level practitioner, which signifies a basic level of competence. This is an exciting point in time for occupational therapist and occupational therapy assistant (OTA) students, who have many career opportunities and experiences for learning. This chapter identifies the various roles in which an occupational therapy (OT) practitioner may function. The responsibilities of the entry-level OT practitioner in service delivery are outlined, along with guidelines for supervision. Next, relationships found in service delivery and how the OT practitioner can work effectively within those relationships are discussed. An outline of how an entry-level practitioner may develop knowledge and skills to achieve advanced competency to benefit clients is provided. By understanding the available roles, responsibilities, and requirements, the entry-level OT practitioner may direct his or her career.

## Professional Roles and Career Development

**Professional roles** and relationships refer to positions or sets of stipulated job-related responsibilities.[12] Each **role** holds certain defined expectations for job performance and responsibilities. An individual's ability to function in a role is based on educational preparation, professional responsibilities, and prior experience in the role.[12] OT practitioners working in organizations interact with many professionals and have multiple roles. The connection of different roles to one another is a **relationship.** Working organizations are made up of many relationships. The interactions between health-care members' roles and relationships vary among organizations.[12]

Direct client care is the role most commonly assumed by the OT practitioner who is just entering the field. However, there are an additional 10 roles identified by the profession that can potentially be held by occupational therapists and OTAs: educator, fieldwork educator

in a practice setting, supervisor, administrator in a practice setting, consultant, academic fieldwork coordinator, faculty, academic program director, researcher/scholar, and entrepreneur. Descriptions of the major functions for each of these roles are shown in Table 7.1. OT practitioners may function in more than one role, even within the same job. For example, an occupational therapist may provide direct client services and serve as an administrator; an OTA may hold positions as both a faculty member and clinician.

As the career of an OT practitioner progresses, he or she may wish to advance within the service-delivery path or transition into a role outside of service delivery. This is referred to as **career development.** Career development depends on one's choices regarding job positions, roles, and relationships.[12]

Career development may occur within a setting (vertical movement), across settings (lateral movement), or by developing within a role (maturation).[12] In vertical movement within a setting, the practitioner advances within the organization to progressively higher positions that involve greater responsibilities or skills. For example, a practitioner may move from the role of fieldwork educator to department supervisor, and eventually to manager of a rehabilitation clinic. A lateral movement across settings might involve an expert clinician transitioning to the role of a clinical instructor in a university setting. The third means of career development is the maturation of the individual within a specific role as observed when a practitioner develops from entry level, to intermediate level, to an advanced clinical specialist. Practitioners understand roles and responsibilities so they may develop abilities and make informed choices regarding their individual career paths.

## Levels of Performance

OT practitioners may perform at the entry, intermediate, or advanced level. An individual's level of performance is not based on years of experience but rather on attaining a higher skill level through work experience, education, and professional socialization.[9] The **entry-level practitioner** is expected to be responsible and accountable for professional activities related to the role as defined by state licensure laws. The **intermediate-level practitioner** has increased responsibility and typically pursues specialization in a particular area of practice. The **advanced-level practitioner** is considered an expert or a resource in the respective role. Advanced-level practitioners gain knowledge and expertise through practice and education. They reflect and develop skills through feedback.

Each individual progresses along the continuum at a different pace. Some individuals never progress past the entry level in a particular role. A person may transition to a new role, wherein his or her level of performance is classified as entry level. For example, an individual who has worked as

| TABLE 7.1 | **Occupational Therapy Roles** |
|---|---|
| Role | Major Function |
| Practitioner—occupational therapist | Provides quality OT services, including evaluation, intervention, program planning and implementation, discharge planning–related documentation, and communication. Service provision may include direct, monitored, and consultative approaches. |
| Practitioner—OTA | Provides quality OT services to assigned individuals under the supervision of an occupational therapist. |
| Educator (consumer, peer) | Develops and provides educational offering or training related to OT to consumer, peer, and community individuals or groups. |
| Fieldwork educator (practice setting) | Manages level I or II fieldwork in a practice setting. Provides OT students with opportunities to practice and carry out practitioner competencies. |
| Supervisor | Manages the overall daily operation of OT services in defined practice area(s). |
| Administrator (practice setting) | Manages department, program, or agency providing OT services. |
| Consultant | Provides OT consultation to individuals, groups, or organizations. |
| Academic fieldwork coordinator | Manages student fieldwork program within the academic setting. |
| Faculty | Provides formal academic education for occupational therapist or OTA students. |
| Academic program director | Manages the educational program for occupational therapist or OTA students. |
| Researcher/scholar | Performs scholarly work of the profession, including examining, developing, refining, and evaluating the profession's body of knowledge, theoretical base, and philosophical foundations. |
| Entrepreneur | Entrepreneurs are partially or fully self-employed individuals who provide OT services. |

OT, occupational therapy; OTA, occupational therapy assistant.
Adapted from American Occupational Therapy Association. (1993). Occupational therapy roles. *American Journal of Occupational Therapy, 47*(12), 1087–1099.

an occupational therapist at the advanced level may transfer into an administrative role where he or she functions at the entry level. An OTA at the intermediate level may transition to the role of an entry-level faculty member. Even at the entry level, individuals in new positions may need to acquire additional knowledge and skill to satisfactorily perform the new job functions. It is possible for an individual to function in two roles at different levels. For example, an OTA intermediate-level practitioner may assume new responsibilities as a fieldwork educator. In the new role, this OTA would initially perform the job requirements at the entry level.

For role advancement or transition, the OT practitioner must be aware of the expectations for the new role and prepare accordingly. There are various methods to achieve role advancement, which are discussed further in this chapter in the section on professional development.

## Specialized Roles

There are specialized roles in which OT practitioners can function, including case manager, supervisor of other allied health-care professionals, consultant, and activity director. These roles are advanced-level positions for OT practitioners.

### Case Manager

Case managers work with a variety of practitioners to provide resources and organize the complexity of intervention. They help families and clients receive services and equipment needed. Case managers may help clients arrange for financial reimbursements. They are aware of available resources within the community and skilled at accessing resources. Case managers may facilitate scheduling, appointments, services, and referrals to other professionals. Case managers are vital members of the health-care team. They form relationships with other team members and understand the roles of others so they can best serve clients and their families.

### Supervisor of Other Allied Health Professionals

OT practitioners may assume the role of supervisor of allied health-care professionals. This role involves knowledge of the policy and procedures of the setting. The supervisor provides feedback regarding one's performance. A supervisor must also understand the health-care professional's specific roles and responsibilities. In particular, the supervisor must understand the scope of practice of each team member. Supervisors play a role in negotiating with employees and manage conflicts.

They conduct performance evaluations, advocate for employees, and provide feedback. They may supervise one or more professionals.

### Consultant

A consultant provides specific information regarding a requested topic or issue. For example, an occupational therapist may consult with a school system to design a wellness program for children with and without disabilities. A practitioner may consult with a teacher on handwriting intervention. An occupational therapist may consult with a hospital rehabilitation clinic on new evidence regarding interventions. Occupational therapist and OTA faculty members may consult with practitioners regarding research or program development. The key to providing consultation is to develop expertise in an area. The consultant provides advice, feedback, and education and often follows up to evaluate the outcomes of the consultation.

### Activity Director

The role of **activity director** is one for which the OTA is well qualified and in which the OTA can function independently.[12] Activity directors are typically employed in group homes, institutions for people with intellectual disabilities assisted living facilities, and long-term care facilities for older persons. In these types of facilities, residents may withdraw and become isolated. The activity director is responsible for planning, implementing, and documenting an ongoing program of activities that meet the needs of the residents. The activity director needs to be aware of and adhere to regulations for activity programs and personnel that have been set forth by Medicare, state health departments, and licensing agencies.

The National Association of Activity Professionals classifies activities that are provided to the client as supportive, providing maintenance, or empowering.[14] Supportive activities are commonly provided to individuals who do not have the cognitive or physical ability to participate in a group program. The purpose of these activities is to promote a comfortable environment and to provide stimulation to those individuals. Activity examples include placing meaningful objects in the person's room or providing background music. Maintenance activities are those that provide opportunities for the individual to maintain physical, cognitive, social, emotional, and spiritual health. Examples of maintenance activities are exercise groups, games such as shuffleboard, creative writing, and choir. Empowering activities are geared toward promoting self-respect, and they offer opportunities for self-expression, personal responsibility, and social responsibility. Writing a facility newsletter or forming a council dedicated to resolving residents' issues are examples of empowering activities.[14]

## Roles and Responsibilities During Service Delivery

AOTA has outlined the minimum requirements for OT practitioners working in service delivery according to four areas: (1) professional standing and responsibility; (2) screening, evaluation, and reevaluation; (3) intervention; and (4) outcomes.[6,8] The occupational therapist is responsible for the evaluation process and the OTA may contribute as delegated by the supervising therapist. The occupational therapist is directs all aspects of the evaluation. The therapist develops the OT intervention in collaboration with OTA. The OTA is responsible for selecting, modifying and implementing therapeutic activities and interventions to address client goals. The occupational therapist may provide intervention or supervise the OTA. The therapist reviews the intervention with input from the OTA. The therapist conducts the outcome evaluation. The OTA provides information regarding outcome achievement and discharge resources.[6]

These guidelines are often used by states to form licensure laws. State licensure laws provide a legal definition of practice for that state and specify the responsibilities for the occupational therapist and OTA related to role delineation, supervision, documentation, and advanced practice. The OT practitioner provides services in accordance with the laws or regulations of the state in which he or she practices. Other regulatory agencies, such as the Centers for Medicare and Medicaid Services (CMS), have regulations that may supersede these guidelines.

OT practitioners are responsible for maintaining professional standing and responsibility by: (1) delivering services that reflect the philosophical base of OT; (2) being knowledgeable about and delivering services in accordance with American Occupational Therapy Association (AOTA) standards, policies, and guidelines and state and federal regulations; (3) maintaining current licensure, registration, or certification as required; (4) abiding by the AOTA *Occupational Therapy Code of Ethics*[4] and *Standards for Continuing Competence*;[5] (5) maintaining current knowledge of legislative, political, social, cultural, and reimbursement issues; and (6) being knowledgeable about evidence-based research.[6]

Practitioners are also responsible for screening, evaluation, and reevaluation. An occupational therapist accepts and responds to referrals and initiates the screening, evaluation, and reevaluation process. The occupational therapist is responsible for analyzing and interpreting the evaluation data. The OTA contributes to the process by performing assessments that have been delegated by the occupational therapist. The OTA communicates (verbally or in writing) to the occupational therapist his or her observations of the assessment and the client's abilities. The occupational therapist then completes and documents the evaluation results. The OTA contributes to the documentation of the evaluation results. The occupational therapist recommends additional consultations or refers clients to appropriate sources as needed.[6]

Practitioner responsibilities during the intervention stage of service delivery include documentation and implementation of the intervention, which is based on the evaluation, client goals, best evidence, and therapeutic reasoning. The OTA can select, implement, and modify therapeutic activities (consistent with his or her demonstrated competency, delegated responsibilities, and intervention plan). The occupational therapist, with contributions from the OTA, modifies the intervention plan throughout the process and documents the client's responses and any changes to the intervention.[6]

The occupational therapist selects, measures, documents, and interprets outcomes that are related to the client's ability to engage in occupations. The occupational therapist is responsible for documenting changes in the client's performance and for discontinuing services. A discontinuation plan or transition plan is prepared by the occupational therapist (with contributions from the OTA) regarding the client's needs, goals, performance, and follow-up services. Either practitioner facilitates the transition process in collaboration with the client, family members, and significant others. The occupational therapist evaluates the safety and effectiveness of the OT processes and interventions; the OTA contributes to this evaluation of safety and effectiveness.[6]

## Supervision

AOTA defines **supervision** as a "cooperative process in which two or more people participate in a joint effort to establish, maintain, and/or elevate a level of competence and performance."[7] The supervisor directs, guides, and monitors the supervisee's practice. It is important that the occupational therapist and OTA work collaboratively to develop and implement a plan for supervision that ensures safe and effective service delivery and promotes professional competence and development.[7]

After obtaining certification and state licensure, the entry-level practitioner is able to independently deliver OT services. Entry-level practitioners require supervision and mentoring from a more experienced occupational therapist, to grow professionally and to develop best practice. OTAs require supervision from an occupational therapist to deliver OT services. The occupational therapist is ultimately responsible for all aspects of the services provided by the OTA, the OT aide, or the OT student.

Regarding supervision, OT practitioners adhere to state and federal regulations, the *Occupational Therapy Code of Ethics*[4] (see Chapter 8), and the policies of the workplace. OT practitioners are responsible for familiarizing themselves with state regulations regarding supervision. Outside accreditation bodies and third-party payers also have specific requirements related to supervision. For example, CMS specifies requirements regarding provision of services by students. Any facility that is reimbursed by Medicare needs to abide by specific requirements.

## Levels of Supervision and Parameters That Affect Supervision Levels

Supervision can be quantified by the number of hours and the level or intensity of supervision that is provided. Supervision occurs along a continuum (as shown in Fig. 7.1) ranging from direct face-to-face contact to general.[2,7] At the high end of the continuum is **direct supervision** (or continuous supervision), wherein the supervising occupational therapist is on-site and available to provide immediate assistance to the client or supervisee if needed. **Close supervision** is the need for direct, daily contact. **Routine supervision** involves direct contact at least every 2 weeks, with interim supervision as needed. **General supervision** is described as at least monthly face-to-face contact.[2,9]

Contact between a supervisor and supervisee can be face-to-face or via telecommunication. Some state regulations are specific about the amount of face-to-face contact that is to take place at the different levels. For example, descriptors such as "daily," "once every seventh treatment," "1 hour per 40 occupational therapy work hours," or "every 21 calendar days" may be used by states to define the amount of face-to-face contact. State regulations may specify that when the occupational therapist is not providing direct supervision, he or she must be available via other methods (such as telecommunication) at all times while the OTA is treating clients. Communication may include use of cell phones, voice mail, and laptops with the capability of sharing client data and emailing. See Case Example 7.1.

**Levels of Supervision**

More supervision ⟶ ⟶ ⟶ ⟶ ⟶ Less supervision

| **Direct or continuous supervision:** | **Close supervision:** | **Routine supervision:** | **General supervision:** |
|---|---|---|---|
| Supervising therapist is nearby and observing at all times. Direct supervision is required for students (OT and OTA), and aides. | Direct observation and contact daily at the work site on a regular basis. | Face-to-face contact at least every 2 weeks at the site of work. It may also include regular supervision through telecommunication. | Initial direction and face-to-face contact with the supervising therapist at least once a month, with interim supervision as needed by telecommunication |

**Fig. 7.1** Supervision levels in occupational therapy.

Elaine is an OTA with over 10 years of experience in home health. She works under the supervision of an occupational therapist but only sees her face-to-face once a month. She takes a cell phone and a laptop with her to every home visit. After her first visit of the day is complete, she checks her email using her laptop computer. She has an email message from her supervising occupational therapist that there is a new client whose evaluation has recently been completed, and the client needs to be scheduled for therapy. Elaine then goes into the agency database on her laptop and searches for the new client. In the client's electronic file, Elaine finds and reads the occupational therapist's evaluation report and intervention plan. Elaine locates the client's phone number and schedules an appointment for later that afternoon. Elaine has a question regarding her last intervention session, so she sends an email to her supervisor so that they will be sure to discuss the question before the next scheduled session. This case illustrates direct supervision that is occurring via telecommunication.

State regulations may also specify the number of OTAs whom an occupational therapist can supervise at any one time. In some cases, states also stipulate how many years of experience the supervising occupational therapist needs to have before he or she can supervise an OTA.

Supervision is an ongoing process that changes with the setting and the individuals involved. The frequency, method, and content of supervision depends on several parameters. First, it is important to determine the regulatory requirements and requirements of the practice setting that pertain to supervision. The supervisor and supervisee also need to understand each other's level of competence, experience, education, and credentials. After these parameters have been established, supervision is based on the following factors:

- The complexity of client needs
- The number and diversity of clients
- The skills of the occupational therapist and OTA
- The type of practice setting

A level of supervision that is *more frequent* than the minimum level required by the practice setting and regulatory agencies may be required if (1) the needs of the client and the OT process are complex and fluctuating, (2) a large number of clients with diverse needs are served by OT in the practice setting, and (3) the occupational therapist and OTA determine that additional supervision is necessary for the delivery of safe and effective OT services.[7] Based on these factors, the occupational therapist works with the OTA to determine how much and what type of supervision is appropriate. Collaboratively, they develop and document a plan for supervision.

Supervisory contacts should be documented, including the frequency of supervisory contact, the methods(s) or types(s) of supervision, content areas addressed during the contact, evidence to support areas and levels of competency, and signatures and credentials of the individuals participating in the supervisory process.[7] Keeping such records meets regulatory requirements and allows both the supervisor and supervisee to observe the progress made, to adjust job expectations as needed, and to provide evidence of professional development activities for both individuals.[1,7,10]

The supervising occupational therapist may cosign treatment notes completed by the supervisee as another way of documenting that supervision has occurred. Generally, documentation by either an occupational therapist or OTA student needs to be signed by the supervisor. Individuals (occupational therapists and OTAs) holding a temporary license or limited permit must also have documentation cosigned. OTAs do not necessarily need their documentation cosigned. The supervisory process is an interactive one that requires more than paper review and a cosignature on documentation.

### Service Competency

Because the occupational therapist is responsible for the performance level of the OTA, he or she must have confidence that the OTA will obtain the same results when providing OT services. **Service competency** is a useful mechanism to ensure that services are provided at the same level. Service competency is defined as the determination that two people performing the same or equivalent procedures will obtain the same or equivalent results.[2,7,11] In test development, this is known as interrater reliability.

The methods and standards to establish service competency vary, depending on the task or procedure involved. Methods such as independent scoring of standardized tests, observation, videotaping, and cotreatment can be used. Service competency is more easily established for frequently used procedures (Fig. 7.2). It may take longer to establish competency for uncommon procedures. Service competency is established for a particular procedure when the practitioners meet the acceptable standard

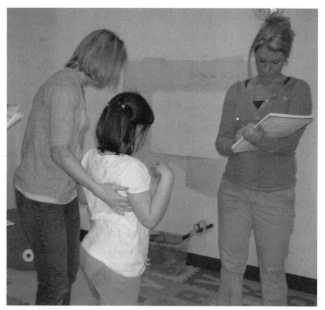

**Fig. 7.2** The occupational therapy assistant and occupational therapist work together to address the client's needs and to establish service competency.

of performance on three successive occasions.[2,7,11] It is important that service competency be established for each procedure.

## Supervision of the Occupational Therapy Aide

An OT aide is an individual who supports the occupational therapist and OTA by performing specifically delegated tasks.[2] OT aides may also be referred to as restorative aides, service extenders, or rehabilitation aides/technicians. Depending on state law, either an occupational therapist or an OTA may supervise the OT aide; however, the occupational therapist is ultimately responsible for the actions of the aide. He or she directs the development, documentation, and implementation of a supervisory plan. The person working as an aide is not required to have any special training; typically, he or she receives on-the-job training from the OT practitioner. Because the level of training is limited, it is important that supervision remain close.

The aide is assigned to perform selected delegated client-related and non–client-related tasks for which the aide has demonstrated competency.[2,7] **Non–client-related tasks** include the preparation of the work area and equipment, clerical tasks, and maintenance activities. Examples of these types of tasks include setting up for a group activity, making the daily schedule, and cleaning equipment. The aide may provide routine **client-related tasks** in which the aide interacts with the client but not as the primary service provider of OT.[2,7] These tasks must have a predictable outcome and occur in a situation in which the client and environment are stable and that does not require the aide to make judgments, interpretations, or adaptations. The client needs to have demonstrated prior ability to perform the task and follow a clearly established task routine and process.[7] The supervisor ensures that the aide is competent in carrying out selected tasks and in using related equipment. The aide must be instructed in how to perform the task with the specific client and be aware of precautions and signs or symptoms the client may demonstrate that indicate that assistance is needed.[7] The practitioner documents the supervision of the aide.

## Strategies for a Successful Occupational Therapist–OTA Supervisory Relationship

Beyond the practical need to determine appropriate duties and supervision, each OT practitioner understands that the roles of the occupational therapist and OTA are intentionally interrelated. The relationship is a partnership. For that partnership to be effective, there needs to be mutual respect and trust.

Many factors contribute to a successful supervisory relationship. The supervisor begins with a solid knowledge base related to the practice of OT and guidelines for supervision.[2] It is important that the supervisor have an understanding of the different ways in which individuals learn as well as an awareness of his or her own learning style and that of the supervisee. Communication is a key element in successful supervisory relationships. Both parties must listen actively, give and receive constructive feedback, be assertive

and tactful, and resolve conflicts.[2,5–7] Instead of providing quick and easy answers to concerns brought up by the supervisee, the supervisor provides resources and direction that facilitate problem solving and therapeutic reasoning.

Several practices can promote the success of supervision. Setting a designated time for meetings and having a written agenda to identify the issues and priorities promotes the effective communication needed for supervisory relationships. It is helpful to create a list of topics that occur during the week. Successful supervision requires active participation by both the supervisor and supervisee. Both parties should be involved in actively evaluating and discussing levels of competency, seeking feedback on performance, setting goals for the future, and maintaining records of professional development.[7,8,10,12,13] Establishing clear and open communication promotes effective supervision and helps each practitioner develop professionally.

## Health-Care Teams and Teamwork

Practitioners also navigate many relationships within the health-care team. Box 7.1 lists some common professionals who may be on a team with the OT practitioner. In health-care environments today, working as a member of an **interprofessional team** is the norm. Entry-level practitioners first establish a solid identity in their own profession and its uniqueness.[13] The OT practitioner learns the roles

---

> **• BOX 7.1   Professionals Who Team with Occupational Therapy Practitioners**
>
> Activity director
> Adapted physical educator
> Audiologist
> Biomedical/rehabilitation engineer
> Case manager
> Dentist
> Dietician
> Durable medical equipment provider
> Mobility specialist
> Nurse
> Orthotist and prosthetist
> Pharmacist
> Physical therapist
> Physicians (primary care provider, physiatrist, neurologist, psychiatrist, ophthalmologist, orthopedist, cardiologist)
> Physician assistant
> Psychologist
> Rehabilitation counselor
> Respiratory therapist
> Recreation therapist
> Social worker
> Special educator
> Speech–language pathologist
> Vocational counselor
> Vision specialist
>
> Adapted from Cohn, E.S. (2009). Interdisciplinary communication and supervision of personnel. In E. B. Crepeau, E. S. Cohn, & B. A. B. Schell (Eds.), *Willard and Spackman's occupational therapy* (11th ed.), Philadelphia, PA: Lippincott Williams & Wilkins.

and responsibilities of other health professionals and develops good interpersonal, communication, and team-building skills.[5-8] The practitioner builds productive relationships with members of other disciplines.[13] An experienced OT practitioner may be responsible for coordinating the interprofessional treatment team and supervising team members. This role includes organizing and leading team meetings, managing client data, and communicating results to doctors and administrators.

Teams may function as multidisciplinary, interdisciplinary (also known as interprofessional), and transdisciplinary teams. In a **multidisciplinary team,** a variety of disciplines or professions work together in a common setting. However, the relationship between the team members is not interactive. The **transdisciplinary team** involves members who cross over professional boundaries and share roles and functions.[12] In this approach, there is a blurring of traditional practitioner roles. Members of an **interdisciplinary team** maintain their own professional roles while using a cooperative approach that is interactive and centered on a common problem to solve.

In the **interprofessional team** approach, various disciplines meet and plan the overall care of the client and maintain an awareness of the client's needs, responses, and goals. Team members are mutual sources of information and support in treatment. It is not uncommon for team members using this approach to cotreat a client (treatment provided by each team member at the same time). For example, the team occupational therapist and speech–language pathologist may both treat a client with a swallowing disorder at mealtime. The occupational therapist focuses intervention on the client's skill of bringing the food to his mouth and chewing it, whereas the speech–language pathologist may focus on producing an effective swallow. In this case professionals all work to remediate the client's swallowing disorder for feeding. Each member focuses on what he or she does best and supports the other during the intervention.

Team members function well when each member demonstrates effective communication skills and understands the roles of others, professional boundaries, and group processes (Fig. 7.3).

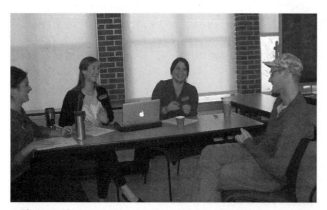

• **Fig. 7.3** Team meetings involve a variety of professionals working together to develop a plan for a specific client.

Teams whose members are open-minded, willing to hear and try new things, and tolerant of change are the most effective.[13]

## Lifelong Learning and Professional Development

The focus of this chapter has been on the roles and responsibilities of the entry-level practitioner who has a minimum skill base. Health-care environments are constantly changing. Changes in technology, new research, and current evidence influence clinical reasoning and practice. Practitioners must remain current with the changes to provide best practice to clients. Employers, third-party payers, and consumers seek out practitioners who use current research evidence to conduct practice. Each practitioner is responsible for remaining up-to-date on current best-practice methods to provide optimum care.

OT practitioners continually acquire new knowledge and skills. This influences intervention strategies. OT practitioners are responsible for achieving and maintaining continuing competency to practice them ethically. **Continuing competence** is a dynamic process that involves many factors in which the professional develops and maintains the knowledge, performance skills, interpersonal abilities, therapeutic reasoning skills, and ethical reasoning skills necessary to perform his or her professional responsibilities. Thus OT practitioners commit to lifelong learning to ensure that they are competent to practice. Organizing and personally managing a cumulative series of work and educational experiences to add to one's knowledge, motivation, perspectives, skills, and job performance is referred to as career development or **professional development**[1,5,9,10] (Fig. 7.4).

AOTA has developed standards for continuing competence in the areas of knowledge, critical reasoning, interpersonal abilities, performance skills, and ethical reasoning; Table 7.2 provides an outline of these standards. Practitioners examine the standards and reflect on their performance in relationship to their position. This reflection serves as the basis for professional development.

### Strategies for Professional Development and Continuing Competence

The mission of AOTA, NBCOT®, and state regulatory boards is to protect the public and ensure quality services. The OT practitioner demonstrates continuing competence through participation in continuing education activities, state association activities, or other professional activities. The practitioner earns a certain number of contact hours or continuing education units. The number of contact hours required is specified in each state's licensure regulations. There are many avenues and resources available to practitioners for professional development. It is the practitioner's responsibility to determine what to do and which resources to use.

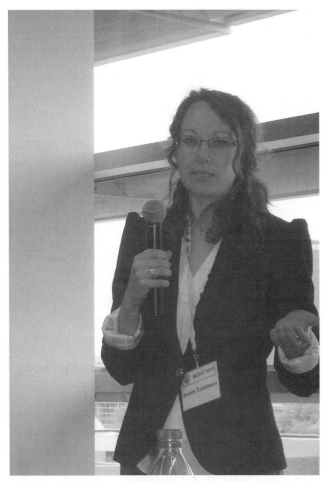

• **Fig. 7.4** Occupational therapy students and practitioners may enjoy educating the next generation of practitioners. This student takes on an educator's role as she provides an informative talk to conference attendees.

Each OT practitioner is responsible for managing his or her professional development and continuing competency activities. The OT practitioner develops goals for his or her career path and designs activities to address the goals. Various activities are available that meet professional development and continuing competency requirements. For example, the practitioner can participate in professional development activities through his or her place of employment, conferences, universities, or online. Practitioners also maintain competency by reading literature, engaging in research projects, reviewing abstracts, and providing feedback on scholarship. They receive professional development units for attending state, regional, and national conferences.[1] Attending conferences allows one to network with other practitioners and learn about the latest practice and research influencing the profession. Examples of professional development activities are listed in Box 7.2.

AOTA developed the Professional Development Tool (PDT) to facilitate the process.[1] The PDT provides a way for the practitioner to organize his or her professional activities and can help the OT practitioner to do the following:

- Assess learning needs and professional growth activities that address self-identified professional or career outcomes
- Identify and pursue professional development opportunities that will improve practice and career opportunities
- Promote quality in the profession and contribute to the growth of the profession
- Fulfill one's responsibility for continuing competence

Practitioners use the PDT to identify personal and professional development interests and needs, create a professional plan, and document completion of activities in

| TABLE 7.2 | Standards of Continuing Competence for Occupational Therapists and OTAs |
|---|---|
| **Standard** | **Description** |
| Knowledge | Understand information required to fulfill responsibilities such as OT theory and principles, OT process, evidence for practice, conditions and populations served, legislative, legal and regulatory issues. |
| Critical Reasoning | Develop sound reasoning to make decisions related to roles and responsibilities, including analyzing occupational performance, reflecting on one's performance, synthesizing information for practice, problem-solving, and applying evidence, research findings and outcomes. |
| Interpersonal abilities | Develop professional relationships with colleagues and clients, including using effective communication, interacting with people from diverse backgrounds, responding to feedback, collaborating with others and sustaining team relationships. |
| Performance skills | Demonstrate expertise, aptitude, proficiency and ability to fulfill roles and responsibilities. Develop skills required to practice occupational therapy, including therapeutic use of self, occupations and activities, consultation, and education to bring about change. Integrate current practice techniques and technologies and update performance based on up current evidence. |
| Ethical Reasoning | Identify, analyze and clarify ethical issues or dilemmas to make reasonable decisions. Understand and adhere to the AOTA Code of Ethics and use ethical principles in practice. Make and defend decisions based on ethical reasoning. |

Adapted from American Occupational Therapy Association. (2015). Standards for continuing competence. American Journal of Occupational Therapy, 69, (Suppl. 3). 6913410030. doi: http://dx.doi.org/10.5014/ajot.2015.696303

---

### • BOX 7.2   Examples of Professional Development Unit Activities

Examples of professional development activities that qualify for PDUs from the NBCOT® are as follows:

- Attend outside workshops, seminars, lectures, and professional conferences
- Complete self-assessment and professional development plan
- Develop instructional materials, such as a training manual
- Complete external self-study series or telecommunication course
- Find fellowship training in specific area
- Teach academic courses in occupational therapy or occupational therapy assistant program as a guest lecturer
- Complete independent learning/study with or without assessment component (e.g., continuing education article, video, audio, and/or online courses)
- Present at state, national, or international workshops, seminars, and conferences
- Make presentations for local organizations/associations
- Make peer presentations on specific treatment approaches or case studies
- Become a primary investigator in scholarly research
- Review a professional manuscript for journals or textbooks
- Join a professional study group/online study group
- Provide professional in-service training
- Publish an occupational therapy article in a non–peer-reviewed publication (e.g., *OT Practice*, *SIS Quarterly*, *Advance*, *Community Newsletters*)
- Publish chapter(s) in occupational therapy or related professional textbooks
- Do reflective occupational therapy practice in collaboration with an advanced-certified occupational therapy colleague
- Volunteer services to organizations, populations, or individuals

Refer to the NBCOT® website for complete and updated information: http://www.nbcot.org.
NBCOT®, National Board for Certification in Occupational Therapy; PDU, professional development unit.

---

a professional development portfolio. Many practitioners start the development of a portfolio while they are students.

## NBCOT® Certification Renewal

NBCOT® certification renewal is another mechanism that facilitates professional development and continuing competency. Practitioners must renew NBCOT® certification every 3 years to continue to use the registered occupational therapist (OTR) or certified occupational therapy assistant (COTA) credential. Although NBCOT® certification renewal is voluntary, it may be required by employers or for state licensure. To renew, practitioners submit proof of having completed a minimum of 36 professional development units (PDUs) within each 3-year certification renewal cycle. At least 50% of those units must be directly related to the delivery of OT services.[1] Box 7.2 lists professional development activities that may apply to NBCOT® renewal.

## Specialty Certification

Obtaining an advanced-practice credential or specialty certification is another avenue for pursuing and documenting competency. Many OT practitioners gain advanced knowledge, skills, and experience in a specialized area of practice. The OT practitioner who completes the requirements for an advanced-practice credential or specialized certification can represent himself or herself to employers, payers, and consumers as having a certain level of expertise and the qualifications to practice in the specialized area. Table 7.3 provides a listing of credentials for advanced practice or specialty certification that OT practitioners may obtain.

AOTA currently provides **specialty certification** for both occupational therapists and OTAs in driving and community mobility; environmental modification; feeding, eating, and swallowing; and low vision.[3] Competencies unique to each of these areas of practice have been defined. Generally, practitioners must document number of hours of experience in the certification area to clients over the last 3 calendar years. The applicant submits an application, verification of employment, and a reflective portfolio demonstrating achievement of defined competencies.

AOTA also offers **board certification** for occupational therapists in the areas of gerontology, mental health, pediatrics, and physical rehabilitation.[3] Certification is based on the completion and peer review of a portfolio, a professional development plan, and a rigorous self-assessment. To apply for board certification, the practitioner must have completed a minimum of 5000 hours of experience as an occupational therapist in the certification area in the last 7 calendar years and a minimum of 500 hours of experience delivering OT services (paid or voluntary) in the certification area to clients in the last 5 calendar years.

Several other organizations offer certification based on the passage of an examination, evidence of experience, or both (see Table 7.3). Sensory Integration International offers a specialty certification in sensory integration (SI). The American Society of Hand Therapists certifies individuals in hand therapy, and those who pass the examination are

| TABLE 7.3 | Specialty Certification/Advanced-Practice Credentials | | |
|---|---|---|---|
| **Examples of Advanced-Practice and Specialty Certification Credentials** | | **Credential Awarded** | **Granting Organization*** |
| Advanced practitioner (for OTAs) | | AP | AOTA |
| Board certified in pediatrics (for occupational therapists) | | BCP | AOTA |
| Board certified in mental health (for occupational therapists) | | BCMH | AOTA |
| Board certified in gerontology (for occupational therapists) | | BCG | AOTA |
| Board certified in rehabilitation (for occupational therapists) | | BCPR | AOTA |
| Assistive technology practitioner | | ATP | RESNA |
| Certified case manager | | CCM | CCMC |
| Certified driving rehabilitation practitioner | | CDRS | ADED |
| Certified hand therapist | | CHT | ASHT |
| Certified professional ergonomist | | CPE | BCPE |
| Certified vocational evaluation specialist | | CVE | CCWAVES |
| Trained in neuro-developmental therapy | | NDT | NDTA |
| Certified to administer the Sensory Integration and Praxis Tests | | SIPT | WSP/USC; SII |
| **Specialty Certification (OT and OTA):** | | | |
| Driving and Community Mobility | | SCDCM or SCDCM-A | AOTA |
| Environmental Modification | | SCEM or SCEM-A | AOTA |
| Feeding, Eating, and Swallowing | | SCFES or SCFES-A | AOTA |
| Low Vision | | SCLV or SCLV-A | AOTA |
| School Systems | | SCSS or SCSS-A | AOTA |

*ADED, Association for Driver Rehabilitation Specialists; AOTA, American Occupational Therapy Association; ASHT, American Society of Hand Therapists; BCPE, Board of Certification in Professional Ergonomics; CCMC, Commission for Case Manager Certification; CCWAVES, Commission on Certification of Work Adjustment and Vocational Evaluation Specialist; NDTA, Neuro-developmental Training Association; OTA, occupational therapy assistant; RESNA, Rehabilitation Engineering and Assistive Technology Society of North America; SII, Sensory Integration International; WSP/USC, Western Psychological Service/University of Southern California.

Adapted from Schell, B. A. B., Crepeau, E. B., & Cohn, E. S. (2003). Professional development. In E. B. Crepeau, E. S. Cohn, & B. A. B. Schell (Eds.). (2003). *Willard and Spackman's occupational therapy* (10th ed., p. 143). Philadelphia, PA: Lippincott Williams & Wilkins.

allowed to use the designation of certified hand therapist (CHT) after their names. The Rehabilitation Engineering and Assistive Technology Society of North America (RESNA) offers a specialty certification in assistive technology. Those who submit verification of a certain amount of work experience and pass the examination are allowed to use the designation of assistive technology provider (ATP) after their name. These are just a few examples of the many specialty certifications currently available.

## Summary

The primary role for the entry-level OT practitioner is service delivery. Once a practitioner increases his or her level of expertise and knowledge, he or she can assume or transition to other roles within and outside of OT. For health-care professionals, involvement in lifelong learning and professional development is important to maintain competency for practice.

## Learning Activities

1. Develop a career plan based on your education. In what role(s) and at what level of performance do you want to be functioning in 5 years? 10 years? 15 years?
2. AOTA has published papers that describe the specialized knowledge and skills needed to practice in specific areas.

Find these documents and identify the areas of practice that have developed a special knowledge base and skills. Define the knowledge and skills required.
3. Some state licensure laws delineate advanced areas of practice in which the OT practitioner is required to have

specialized knowledge and skills. Research the regulations for the state in which you live, and identify any areas requiring advanced knowledge and skills.

4. Box 7.1 lists a number of professionals with whom OT practitioners may team. Describe each professional's role and define the primary functions of each within the health-care team.

5. Interview an OT practitioner. Describe his or her job requirements, supervision, and role within the team. Provide examples of the level of performance in which the practitioner functions.

6. Observe an occupational therapist and OTA working together. Describe the relationship and the type of supervision the OTA receives from the occupational therapist. Interview each practitioner to gain insight on how this relationship works or could be improved. Write a summary of your findings, and present it to the class.

7. Compare and contrast in a short paper the role of the OT practitioner when working in a multidisciplinary, transdisciplinary, or interdisciplinary team.

8. Develop a presentation on professional development opportunities in your state. Complete the AOTA Professional Development Tool.[1] Provide a summary of your findings.

## Review Questions

1. Describe the three levels of performance that OT practitioners progress through as they obtain experience.

2. What are the minimum requirements (hint: standards) for occupational therapists and OTAs working in service delivery?

3. What is meant by service competency, and how may it be achieved?

4. Describe the occupational therapist/OTA relationship.

5. Describe the OT practitioner's role in multidisciplinary, transdisciplinary, and interdisciplinary teams.

## References

1. American Occupational Therapy Association. *Professional Development Tool*. Bethesda, MD: AOTA; 2015. Retrieved from, http://www.aota.org/education-careers/advance-career/pdt.aspx.

2. American Occupational Therapy Association. *Occupational Therapy Assistant Supervision Requirements*. Retrieved from, 2014. http://www.aota.org/-/media/corporate/files/secure/advocacy/licensure/stateregs/supervision/occupational%20therapy%20assistant%20supervision%20requirements%202014.pdf.

3. American Occupational Therapy Association. *AOTA Board and Specialty Certification Programs*. 2016. Retrieved from, http://www.aota.org/education-careers/advance-career/board-speciality-certifications.aspx.

4. American Occupational Therapy Association. Occupational therapy code of ethics. *Am J Occup Ther*. 2015;69(suppl 3): 6913410030. http://dx.doi.org/10.5014/ajot.2015.696303.

5. American Occupational Therapy Association. Standards for continuing competence. *Am J Occup Ther*. 2015;69(suppl 3): 6913141055. http://dx.doi.org/10.5014/ajot.2015.696516.

6. American Occupational Therapy Association. Standards of practice for occupational therapy. *Am J Occup Ther*. 2015;69(suppl 3):691341007. http://dx.doi.org/10.5014/ajot.2015.696506.

7. American Occupational Therapy Association. Guidelines for supervision, roles, and responsibilities during the delivery of occupational therapy services. *Am J Occup Ther*. 2014;68(suppl 3):S16–S22. http://dx.doi.org/10.5014/ajot.2014.686S03.

8. American Occupational Therapy Association. Scope of practice. *Am J Occup Ther*. 2014;68(Suppl. 3):http://dx.doi.org/10.5014/ajot.2014.686S04.

9. American Occupational Therapy Association. Occupational therapy roles. *Am J Occup Ther*. 1993;47(12):1087–1099. http://dx.doi.org/10.5014/ajot.47.12.1087.

10. American Occupational Therapy Association. Career exploration and development: a companion guide to the occupational therapy roles document. *Am J Occup Ther*. 1994;48:844–851.

11. American Occupational Therapy Association. Entry-level role delineation for registered occupational therapists (OTRs) and certified occupational therapists (COTAs). *Am J Occup Ther*. 1990;44(12):1091–1102.

12. Crist P. Roles, relationships, and career development. In: Johnson M, ed. *The Occupational Therapy Manager*. Bethesda, MD: American Occupational Therapy Association; 1996:327–348.

13. Gilkeson GE. *Occupational Therapy Leadership: Marketing Yourself, Your Profession, and Your Organization*. Philadelphia: F.A. Davis; 1997.

14. National Association of Activity Professionals. *Standards of Practice: Section A—Standards of Care*. Washington, DC: Author; 1991.

# 8

# Practicing Legally and Ethically

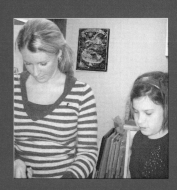

## OBJECTIVES

*After reading this chapter, the reader will be able to do the following:*

- Understand the purpose of a code of ethics.
- Identify the six principles in the Occupational Therapy Code of Ethics.
- Describe the function of the Ethics Commission.
- Outline the steps to ethical decision making.
- Distinguish between ethical and legal behavior.

- Explain the purpose and implementation of state laws regulating occupational therapy.
- Describe the disciplinary processes developed by state regulatory boards and the professional association.
- Discuss the similarities and differences of morals, ethics, and laws and their connection to the practice of occupational therapy.

## KEY TERMS

autonomy
beneficence
clinical reasoning
code of ethics
confidentiality
ethical dilemma
ethical distress

ethics
fidelity
informed consent
justice
law
licensure
locus of authority

mandatory reporting
morals
nonmaleficence
regulations
statutes
veracity

ⓔ Visit *www.evolve.elsevier.com* to access the Evolve student resources that accompany your book.

*I chose the field of occupational therapy because the profession seemed limited only by the individual professional. As an occupational therapist, I have had numerous choices of work settings and ages of clients with whom I have interacted. I have worked in acute care hospitals, comprehensive outpatient and adult day-care settings, public school settings, regular day-care settings, preschool settings for children with special needs, and home environments. I have had the pleasure of working with clients of all ages from diverse cultural backgrounds. I taught for many years at a community college. Our typical occupational therapy assistant student was nontraditional in age and historical background. Now I am providing services to children throughout the school district.*

*I am rewarded on a regular basis as my clients progress, gaining more active interaction with others and control of themselves and their environment. I believe I have been able to significantly influence the quality of life of my clients. In essence, it is not how long we live (quantity), but rather how we live (quality). Occupational therapists are in a unique position to assist in improving the quality of life of the persons whom we serve.*

**JEAN W. SOLOMON, MHS, OTR/L, FAOTA**
**Berkeley County School District**
**Charleston, South Carolina**

Health care today is very complicated, and practitioners often face ethical dilemmas. The need for increased productivity, managed care policies, and an increase in consumer activism require practitioners be skillful at making ethical decisions. Occupational therapy (OT) practitioners are confronted daily with situations that require decisions. Morals, ethics, and laws have the potential to affect the clinician's decision making in practice.

**Morals** are related to character and behavior from the point of view of right and wrong. Morals develop as a result of background, values, religious beliefs, and the society in which a person lives. Thus OT practitioners bring their individual morals to situations, and those morals may or may not be in agreement with the client's morals. Professional decisions may or may not agree with the practitioner's morals; rather, practitioners are required to comply with professional ethics and legal mandates.[13]

**Ethics** is the study and philosophy of human conduct. Ethics is "a systematic reflection on and an analysis of morals."[12] Ethics guide how a person behaves and makes decisions so that the best or "right" conduct is carried out. **Law** is defined as "a binding custom or practice of a community: a rule of conduct or action prescribed or formally recognized as binding or enforced by a controlling authority."[12] Laws are established by an act of the federal or state legislature. Laws are intended to protect citizens from unsafe practice, whereas ethics compel the professional to provide the highest level of care.

Ethics and laws are closely intertwined. However, ethics differ from laws and rules in that ethical standards are more general, and their intent is to give positive guidance rather than impose binding and negative limits to specific situations. However, because ethics are blended with laws to form professional standards, ethical misconduct may also constitute a violation of the law.[13]

In this chapter, the Occupational Therapy Code of Ethics of the American Occupational Therapy Association (AOTA) and an approach to ethical decision making are described. State licensure laws and regulations of the profession are also discussed, including potential sanctions when a practitioner violates the regulations.

## Practicing Ethically

Frequently, OT practitioners encounter situations in which they must weigh alternatives and make decisions about a course of action. Some situations are easy to resolve, whereas others may challenge one's decision-making abilities. Clinicians frequently rely on their own values and morals when deciding on a course of action. However, professional decision making relies on a systematic ethical problem-solving process.

**Clinical reasoning** involves understanding the client's diagnoses, strengths, weaknesses, prognosis, and goals. Practitioners use clinical reasoning to develop and provide interventions to address goals and make necessary adaptations. Clinical reasoning requires problem solving and professional judgment; therefore, it improves with experience, reflection, and critical analysis. Practitioners use

clinical reasoning along with morals and ethics when making professional decisions.

A professional **code of ethics** provides direction to members of a profession for mandatory behavior and protects the rights of clients, subjects, their significant others, and the general public.[4,13] For example, the code of ethics dictates that OT practitioners treat each client equitably which is a basic principle of the OT profession. Ethical codes provide guidelines for making correct or proper choices and decisions of health-care practice in the field.[4,12] These guidelines are usually stated in the form of principles.

## American Occupational Therapy Association Code of Ethics

AOTA's Occupational Therapy Code of Ethics[4] was recently updated in 2015 (see Appendix A). This code provides practitioners with guidelines to help them recognize and resolve ethical dilemmas, to practice at the expected standard using guiding principles, and to educate the public. The Code of Ethics is meant to inspire professional conduct for quality and empathetic OT while respecting the diversity of clients. The Code of Ethics is based on the core values of the profession.[9]

The Occupational Therapy Code of Ethics consists of six principles, each addressing a different aspect of professional behavior.[4] Following is a brief description of each principle and an example to illustrate professional application.

## Principle 1: Beneficence

In general terms, the principle of **beneficence** means that the OT practitioner will contribute to the good health and welfare of the client. This principle highlights the need for OT practitioners to (1) treat each client fairly and equitably, (2) advocate for recipients to obtain needed services, (3) promote public health and safety and well-being, and (4) charge fees that are reasonable and commensurate with the services provided.[4] Beneficence requires that practitioners maintain competency, refer to other providers when needed, and take steps to ensure proficiency.

Mr. Parker can no longer pay for OT services. His occupational therapist, Karen, started a daily self-feeding program for Mr. Parker before his funds ran out. Karen visits Mr. Parker at mealtime and explains the proper use of the adaptive equipment to the aide. She discusses how to work on independence and what assistance may still be needed upon discharge. The therapist advocates for this additional meeting at a discounted rate, knowing that Mr. Parker will receive better care after she has personally addressed the issues.

This example illustrates the principle of beneficence in that the OT practitioner shows concern for the client by ensuring that the aide is properly trained in feeding techniques. The OT practitioner advocates for the client to receive the services he needs.

When serving as a consultant to a residence facility for individuals who have severe intellectual disability, Judy, the occupational therapist, becomes aware that another therapist, Sam, is billing for 1/2-hour individual intervention sessions. In reality, Sam only passes through the unit and briefly talks with the clients and does not provide intervention. After observing the pattern for several weeks, Judy speaks with Sam, who brushes off the inquiry, saying, "Look, we all have plans on file, but these clients are not going to progress no matter what we do." Judy documents the situation and brings the matter to the attention of the administrator.

In this case Judy must address the breech of ethical conduct by Sam. Sam is financially exploiting the client by charging for intervention services that do not take place. This is both a legal and ethical breech of conduct.

## Principle 2: Nonmaleficence

The principle of **nonmaleficence** means that the practitioner should not inflict harm on the client. This principle ensures that OT practitioners maintain therapeutic relationships that do not exploit clients physically, emotionally, psychologically, socially, sexually, or financially. Furthermore, the OT practitioner is obligated to identify and address problems that may affect professional duties and bring concerns regarding professional skills of colleagues to the appropriate authority.[4] In that OT practitioners work with a variety of clients, it is the practitioner's responsibility to address concerns and foresee possible harmful situations so that harm can be avoided. The principle of nonmaleficence requires practitioners avoid any relationships, activities, or undue influences that may interfere with services.[4]

Tonya, a 15-year-old teen attending an outpatient group for eating disorders, becomes exceptionally attached to the OT practitioner, Mark. The teen calls Mark at home to discuss her intervention plan, telling Mark she got his phone number from her cousin, whom Mark knows from school. Mark limits the call and speaks to Tonya the next day at group, explaining to Tonya that it is inappropriate to call him at home and reiterating the professional nature of their relationship. Tonya is upset, but agrees that she will not call him. Mark asks a colleague to work with Tonya. He does not completely stop working with Tonya because he does not want her to feel rejected, but rather reinforces professional boundaries.

This example illustrates nonmaleficence (i.e., do no harm). Mark believes the relationship between himself and the teen may be harmful to the teen's intervention plan. Tonya has become too attached and is unsure of the boundaries. Mark is truthful with the teen and brings the situation up with the team so that no emotional harm will come to Tonya. The team supports him in continuing to serve on the

team so that he does not completely reject Tonya. The team fears that complete rejection may harm Tonya emotionally and result in slower progress or regression in her treatment.

## Principle 3: Autonomy

Principle 3 protects the client's right of **autonomy** and **confidentiality**. Autonomy is the freedom to decide and the freedom to act.[4] This principle includes self-determination and one's duty to treat the client according to the client's desires. Confidentiality refers to the expectation that information shared by the client with the OT practitioner, either directly or through written or electronic forms, will be kept private and shared only with those directly involved with the intervention (under conditions expected by the client).[2,11] Confidentiality also stipulates that the client will determine how and with whom information may be shared. This principle requires OT practitioners to respect a client's right to refuse treatment, and it protects all privileged communication.[11]

According to Principle 3, the OT practitioner (1) collaborates with clients and caregivers to determine goals; (2) informs clients of the nature, possible risks, and outcomes of services; (3) receives informed consent for services; (4) respects a client's decision to refuse treatment; and (5) maintains confidentiality concerning information.[4]

**Informed consent** refers to the "knowledgeable and voluntary agreement by which a client undergoes intervention that is in accord with the patient's values and preferences."[12] Thus, clients have the right to refuse intervention and the right to be made aware of the risks, benefits, and cost of OT intervention.

Mrs. Jones, who lives in a skilled nursing facility, resists going to OT but rather constantly asks to return to her room. The therapist, Andrea, learns that Mrs. Jones is afraid someone will steal her things. Andrea deals with the issue by making an intervention plan to address Mrs. Jones's fear that she will lose her hairbrush, an old mirrored compact, a change purse, a bottle of water, and a pair of underpants. Mrs. Jones does not want to tell anyone, but with her consent Andrea obtains a wheelchair carrier. Part of Mrs. Jones's intervention plan is the use of a checklist to pack her carrier with these treasured belongings each morning and to unpack it at the end of each day. The staff is informed that using a daily checklist is part of her OT program. Now Mrs. Jones goes to activities and therapy without protest.

This example illustrates a respect for the rights of autonomy. The therapist allowed Mrs. Jones the freedom to choose to keep her treasures with her. This autonomy gave Mrs. Jones the assurance and comfort to participate in OT activities. The therapist respected her confidences by being careful to only discuss the contents of the carrier with Mrs. Jones, but informing the team of the intervention plan. The therapist respected Mrs. Jones's right to decide if and how she would participate in therapy and allowed her to contribute to the intervention planning process. The practitioner respected Mrs. Jones's right to confidentiality by not discussing with others the reasons she refused to go to therapy.

## Principle 4: Justice

Principle 4 stipulates that OT practitioners provide services in a fair and equitable manner to all. Accordingly, individuals and groups should receive fair treatment and be afforded the same opportunities. Therefore OT practitioners advocate for their clients and provide opportunities for their clients to participate equally in occupations. This principle suggests that practitioners advocate for clients, promote activities for all patients, provide services to all (regardless of race, socioeconomic status, religion, or culture), and take responsibility to educate the public and society about the value of OT services.

Brie is an occupational therapist working in private practice. The recent economic crisis has made it difficult for Brie's clients to continue coming to OT weekly. She is concerned for her clients, and at the same time, she has to keep her business afloat. She meets with her employees, and they decide to offer rates on a sliding scale so that the clients continue to receive therapy. She also contacts a local university to inquire if the OT students could conduct home visits as a classroom project (while being supervised by a therapist). She is aware that some of her clients need home adaptations. The students will make the adaptations under the supervision of the therapist to assure safety and fit.

In this example, the therapist is seeking services for her clients in a fair and equitable manner. She is making adjustments to provide fair and equitable services for all clients. By using the university resources, Brie is able to provide additional services to her clients while maintaining her practice.

**Justice** also refers to the obligation to comply with the laws and regulations that guide the profession. The OT practitioner must be aware of and follow federal, state, and local laws, in addition to institutional policies. The practitioner may also need to inform employers, employees, and colleagues about these laws and policies. OT practitioners must accurately report and document information related to professional activities.[4]

Before Kaitlin, an OTA, moves to a new state, she requests a copy of the licensure law and notes that the new state limits some treatment modalities. Once employed, she reads the employer's policies and procedures manual regarding facility records and acquaints herself with the department's style of recordkeeping. The facility uses a specific style for documenting intervention. Although not familiar with the style of charting, Kaitlin refreshes her understanding with the format and implements it in her documentation.

The OT practitioner in this example is in compliance with state laws related to intervention procedures and with the documentation policies delineated by the facility where she works.

## Principle 5: Veracity

**Veracity** refers to the duty of the health-care professional to tell the truth. OT practitioners must accurately represent their qualifications, education, training, and competence.[2,4] Practitioners may not use any form of false advertising or exaggerated claims. The OT practitioner must disclose instances that pose actual or potential conflicts of interest. Furthermore, the OT practitioner must accept responsibility for actions that reduce the public's trust in OT services. Veracity refers to the principle of honesty in all interactions. Students in occupational therapist and OTA programs must follow the principle of veracity by giving credit and recognition when using the ideas and work of others in written, oral, or electronic media (i.e., avoiding plagiarism).[4]

Kevin, a therapist who is opening a private practice, makes certain that the advertising circulars promoting his private practice center do not the make any exaggerated claims about the center's ability to "cure" or make unrealistic promises of creating a "new life."

This example illustrates the principle of veracity because the clinician ensures that advertisements for his private practice are truthful while promoting its services.

## Principle 6: Fidelity

**Fidelity,** or faithfulness, in professional relationships describes the interactions between OT practitioners and their colleagues. They must treat clients, colleagues, and other professionals with respect, fairness, and integrity.[4] Such aspects as the importance of maintaining confidentiality in matters related to colleagues and staff; accurately representing qualifications, views, and findings of colleagues; and reporting any misconduct to the appropriate entity are considered part of fidelity.[4] This principle includes statements concerning taking measures to discourage, prevent, expose, or correct any breeches of the code.[4]

Lindsay, an occupational therapist student, just completed her thesis for her master's degree, and her faculty advisor wants to present the results at a national conference. The faculty advisor asks Lindsay for permission to submit a conference proposal describing the results of her thesis with the understanding that Lindsay will be listed as the principal author. Lindsay is also encouraged to present the paper with the faculty advisor, if the proposal is accepted.

In this example, the professor demonstrates the principle of fidelity to her student colleague. By ensuring that both the faculty advisor's name and the student's name are on the paper, she is accurately reporting who has been involved in both gathering the data and reporting the findings.

## Solving Ethical Problems

Ethical problems may be divided into three categories: ethical distress, ethical dilemma, or locus-of-authority problems.

**Ethical distress** situations challenge how a practitioner maintains his or her integrity or the integrity of the profession.[12] Ethical distress involves feelings that something is amiss and often signifies the need to work through the ethical decision-making process. An **ethical dilemma** is a situation in which two or more ethical principles collide with one another, making it difficult to determine the best action. Ethical dilemmas involve two courses of actions. The OT practitioner must make a decision about which course of action to take. Problems with **locus of authority** require decisions about who should be the primary decision maker.[12] The OT practitioner considers who is entitled to make the decision by systematically working through the case. These situations rely on the ethical decision-making process.

Generally, six steps are used to resolve an ethical problem:[12]

1. Gather all of the relevant facts about the situation. Describe the clinical, contextual, individual, and personal preferences concerning the situation.
2. Identify the type of ethical problem (e.g., distress, dilemma, locus of authority). Determine the ethical principles involved (e.g., beneficence, nonmaleficence, justice, veracity, autonomy, fidelity).
3. Clarify professional duties in this situation that may be outlined in the Code of Ethics (e.g., do no harm, tell the truth, keep promises, and be faithful to colleagues). What is the conduct required of each professional (including yourself)?
4. Explore alternatives, including the desired outcome and consequences of actions.
   a. Describe features that are pertinent to this situation, including facts, laws, wishes of others, resources, risks, Code of Ethics, degree of certainty of the facts on which a decision is based, and predominant values of the others involved.[3,12]
   b. Who are the other people involved? What are the consequences of the actions for the interested parties?
5. Complete the action.
6. Evaluate the process and the outcome.

The ability to decide which action to take may be developed by understanding the steps and discussing situations in which there are conflicting elements. Examining ethical distress, dilemmas, and locus-of-authority problems provides the opportunity to base professional decisions on ethical reasoning. Examining situations systematically benefits clients, professionals, and the employer.

The case application in Box 8.1 provides an example of the ethical decision-making process.

## Practicing Legally

Laws at the state and federal levels govern certain aspects of OT practice. The US Constitution and state constitutions are the primary sources of legal authority. After the

---

**• BOX 8.1    Dave: A Case Application of the Ethical Decision-Making Process**

Dave, a 13-year-old boy, has reached his OT* goals. He was injured in an automobile accident wherein the driver had excellent insurance coverage, so coverage for OT services is still available. Reportedly, his home situation is not good; both parents are alcoholics and have difficulty staying employed, and there is concern for his welfare. Dave enjoys the attention he receives in therapy and works hard on his goals. In the time the OT practitioner has worked with him, his whole attitude has improved. He wants to keep coming to occupational therapy, but he has achieved the OT goals. The OT practitioner is meeting with the team and must make a recommendation as to whether or not to continue intervention. The practitioner enjoys working with Dave and has established a meaningful and positive therapeutic relationship.

Following is a description of how to work through this case using the ethical decision-making process.

| Steps in the Ethical Decision-Making Process | Consideration and Analysis of the Steps |
| --- | --- |
| 1. Gather all of the relevant facts about the situation. Describe the clinical, contextual, individual, and personal preferences concerning the situation. | • Dave will be returning home to a less-than-optimal situation.<br>• Dave's parents are both alcoholics who have difficulty keeping employment.<br>• Dave has moved frequently.<br>• Dave's parents are inconsistent in visiting him.<br>• Dave loves the attention he gets during OT intervention.<br>• Dave is well liked by his older peers in the rehabilitation setting.<br>• If Dave continues to come to OT services, he may become dependent on a support structure that is not readily available to him upon eventual discharge. The team is concerned for the welfare of the child; social workers are involved in the case.<br>• Dave has a tutor who will make home visits upon discharge. The teacher, school psychologist, and family physician are all important members of the team. |

*Continued*

| • BOX 8.1 | Dave: A Case Application of the Ethical Decision-Making Process—Cont'd |
| --- | --- |

| Steps in the Ethical Decision-Making Process | Consideration and Analysis of the Steps |
| --- | --- |
| 2. Identify the type of ethical problem (e.g., distress, dilemma, locus of authority). Determine the ethical principles involved (e.g., beneficence, nonmaleficence, justice, veracity, autonomy, fidelity). | • Ethical distress is illustrated as the OT practitioner examines whether Dave should continue to receive OT services after meeting his goals. The OT practitioner, experiencing ethical distress, wonders if her integrity would be compromised by providing services to a child who may not require them.<br><br>• The ethical dilemma can be defined as discharging Dave now that he has reached his goals or continuing OT services, which may require new goals.<br><br>• A locus-of-authority problem is depicted in that the child (a minor) wants to continue with therapy, yet his parents (who have substance abuse issues) may not serve his best interest. The OT practitioner must decide if she will rely on the wishes of the parents, the child, or the institution (which supports continued treatment due to insurance funding) to determine intervention. |
| 3. Clarify professional duties in this situation that may be outlined in the Code of Ethics (e.g., do no harm, tell the truth, keep promises, and be faithful to colleagues). | • The OT practitioner may hypothesize that OT services could still help the child and that returning home to an unsupportive environment may do more harm. Thus the principle of beneficence (do well) is being challenged. Furthermore, the professional issue of providing services to a child who has reached his goals may challenge the principle of veracity (truthfulness). The OT practitioner may view it as less than truthful in saying the child requires OT services. Fidelity is challenged by not trusting other colleagues to serve the child. |
| 4. Explore alternatives, including the desired outcome and consequences of actions. | • The OT practitioner is responsible for helping Dave return to the occupations that he desires, including school, community activities, and activities of daily living. Although the child has reached the physical and social goals, as per his intervention plan, the practitioner believes Dave may require some modifications to be successful in school. The OT practitioner also remains concerned that Dave's support system (e.g., his parents) may not adequately assist him. After careful consideration, the practitioner acknowledges that other professionals, such as the social worker and school psychologist, may be able to address these issues.<br><br>• The OT practitioner could develop new goals for OT intervention. This way Dave would stay in the current system. He may become attached to the center and have difficulty transitioning to home, school, or the community.<br><br>• Dave could be discharged from OT services and attend a new program for children with learning issues (resulting from head injuries), which takes place close to his community. The social worker may be able to secure transportation. However, the child may still be in a chaotic home environment and benefit from outside support. The school psychologist recommends a Big Brother/Big Sister program and a parent support group for the parents (who may be willing, with encouragement from the team). |
| 5. Complete the action. | • The team meets to discuss the courses of action and the consequences for each. After a thorough analysis, the OT practitioner feels informed and prepared to discuss the options that are in Dave's best interest. Although the initial reaction of the practitioner was to continue Dave's occupational therapy by reworking several goals, the practitioner realizes that the other alternatives might benefit him. In this case the team members work together to address the issues and discharge the client to a successful situation. Dave will attend a support program in his local area for teens. This program will address his emotional needs and help him transition to school. The OT practitioner will consult with the director and staff members concerning Dave's physical and social needs. The OT practitioner agrees to attend a session with Dave so that he feels some continuity of care. |
| 6. Evaluate the action. | • The OT practitioner felt supported by the team. The careful analysis of the alternative plans provided a solution that maintained the integrity of the profession and supported the child. Dave benefited from the work of all members and saw the team members as advocates. The school and community support provided the child with the independence to engage in activities with his peers. |

*OT, occupational therapy.

federal and state constitutions, statutory law is the next source of legal authority.[3,13] **Statutes** are laws that are enacted by the legislative branch of a government. There are federal and state statutes. The federal Congress or state legislature votes to pass a law, which then is assigned to an agency. The agency itself, or a designated board, follows up with the development of regulations to implement and enforce the law. The **regulations** describe in specific terms how the intent of the law will be carried out. In this section, we discuss both statutes and regulations that affect the practice of OT.

## Federal Statutes

Federal statutes, which are passed by Congress, pertain to all 50 states. Federal statutes can be enforced through the federal court systems. Violating a federal statute may result in fines, injunctions, or prison time. Examples of some of the important federal statutes that affect the practice of OT include the following:

- The Health Insurance Portability and Accountability Act (HIPAA) established national standards for electronic health-care transactions and addressed the security and privacy of health-care data.[10]
- The Individuals with Disabilities Education Act (IDEA) requires public schools to make available to all eligible children with disabilities a free, appropriate public education in the least restrictive environment appropriate to their individual needs. OT practitioners working in school systems practice under this act. Thus the role of the OT practitioner is to provide intervention that will allow the child to engage in education.
- The Americans with Disabilities Act (ADA) provides protection from discrimination on the basis of disability. The ADA upholds and extends the standards for compliance set forth in Section 504 of the Rehabilitation Act of 1973 to employment practices, communication, and all policies, procedures, and practices that affect the treatment of students with disabilities.[16]
- The Social Security Amendments of 1965 established, among other provisions, the foundation for the Medicare and Medicaid programs. Medicare is a federally subsidized health insurance program for individuals aged 65 and older. Medicaid is a joint federally and state-funded program that provides health-care services to the poor. OT services are covered under both of these programs.

## State Statutes

State statutes are passed by state legislatures. Accordingly, regulations vary from state to state. Most state statutes are organized by subject matter and published in books referred to as codes. Typically, a state has a family or civil code, a criminal code, a welfare code, and a probate code, in addition to many other codes dealing with a wide variety of topics.

States are permitted by the federal constitution to regulate areas such as education, insurance (private and public), and licensing. Consequently, state statutes may affect the practice of OT through regulation of the insurance industry, including health maintenance organizations, workers' compensation insurance programs, and health-care services for the indigent. Child abuse and elder abuse laws are also within the state purview. All states have passed some form of law requiring **mandatory reporting** of suspected child abuse and neglect. Mandatory reporting requires that certain professionals, including health-care providers, report suspected child abuse. A health-care provider who fails to report suspected abuse may be criminally liable.[14]

One of the most significant statutes affecting OT practice is the state occupational therapy practice act. With the recognition that laws and regulations vary from state to state, the next section focuses on general principles of state regulation of OT.

## State Regulation of Occupational Therapy

State regulation of OT practice has been in place since the 1970s and includes licensure, statutory certification laws, registration, and trademark laws. OT is regulated in all 50 states, the District of Columbia, Puerto Rico, and Guam.[1] The primary purpose of regulation is to protect the consumer from practitioners who are unqualified or unscrupulous.

Under statutory certification and registration, a person may not use the title of or proclaim to be *certified* or *registered* unless he or she has met specific entry-level requirements. State trademark laws (also called *title control*) are similar to statutory certification in that they prevent non–OT practitioners from representing and charging for OT services. Neither statutory certification nor trademark laws define the scope of practice of the profession.

**Licensure,** the most stringent form of regulation, is "the process by which a government agency grants permission to an individual to engage in a given occupation upon finding that the applicant has attained the minimal degree of competence required to ensure that the public health, safety, and welfare will be reasonably protected."[15] State licensure is one way to assure the public that the person delivering services has obtained a degree of competency required by the profession and has permission to engage in that service.

In addition to listing the qualifications needed for a person to practice, licensure laws also define the scope of practice of a profession and therefore are often referred to as practice acts. The scope of practice defined in the licensure law is a legal definition of OT's domain of practice. This is another step toward ensuring consumer protection. The scope of practice also defends OT from challenges of other professions that may question the qualifications of practitioners to provide particular services or that may infringe upon OT's scope of practice.[8] Most states use the *Definition of Occupational Therapy Practice for the AOTA Model Practice Act*[6] and the *Scope of Practice*[8] as model language for state licensure laws and regulations. These documents are not statutes and do not have the force of the law, but they are intended to support state laws and regulations that govern the practice of OT.

Occupational therapists are legally responsible for services provided by OTAs or aides under their supervision. The roles and supervision of OTAs and aides are also delineated in state regulations. AOTA provides guidelines that describe the minimum standards of practice and the parameters for the supervision of OT personnel.[5,7]

An appointed state regulatory board carries out the tasks involved in implementing the licensure law and regulations. Licensure boards are responsible for writing the regulations that govern the license, collecting fees and issuing licenses, investigating complaints, and delineating requirements for continuing competency. Licensure boards cannot change the scope of practice enacted through state legislation. They may advise the legislature or make suggested amendments. In some states, OT practitioners are appointed to serve on the board. OT practitioners can provide input into the regulatory process through their state association or by attending hearings, which are typically announced ahead of time and open to the public.

To be licensed in a state generally requires that the practitioner provide proof that he or she has completed the academic and fieldwork requirements of an occupational therapist or OTA program accredited by the Accreditation Council for Occupational Therapy Education (ACOTE) and has passed the National Board of Certification for Occupational Therapy (NBCOT) certification examination. An application is completed, fingerprints are submitted for a background check, and a fee is paid. Upon satisfying all requirements, the practitioner is issued a license to practice in that state. Each state requires its own licensing, and it is not permissible to practice OT without a state license. A practitioner may become licensed in as many states as he or she wishes.

States require practitioners to renew their license at regular intervals, usually every 1 to 2 years. Many state regulations require that practitioners complete a number of continuing education hours or continuing competence requirements to renew licensure. It is the responsibility of the practitioner to keep his or her knowledge up to date with current practice. Practitioners need to be aware of the continuing competency requirements in their states of practice.

## Disciplinary Processes

Law and professional ethics are often intertwined. Consequently, the potential to process violations in a number of different ways exists. Box 8.2 presents a case study that illustrates the blending of ethics and law.

The Occupational Therapy Code of Ethics applies to individuals who are or were members of AOTA.[4] Therefore,

---

| • BOX 8.2 | Case Study: Ethics and Law |
|---|---|

An occupational therapy student is completing her level II fieldwork in a mental health setting. Her clinical supervisor repeatedly asks her if she would like to join him in activities outside of work hours. She makes up excuses or manages to avoid the questions. During a group session, he jokes with a client about how attractive he finds the student. They give her a flirtatious look and both smile. The student is afraid to say anything to her supervisor or the department manager for fear that it will affect how she will be evaluated on her fieldwork. She had some difficulty on her previous fieldwork and is very anxious regarding her performance. The student keeps quiet about the situation until the end of her fieldwork, when she reports the situation to the academic fieldwork coordinator. Preceding her statement to the coordinator, she asks that the information she is about to divulge remain confidential.

- Use the steps of ethical decision-making process to review and understand all the aspects of this case.
- Identify the legal aspects of this case and the steps the student could consider.
- Describe the ethical issues illustrated in this case.
- Identify actions the academic fieldwork coordinator may take at this time.
- Discuss options that the student may consider and describe possible outcomes.

---

AOTA has jurisdiction over complaints against members who are suspected of unethical conduct. The Ethics Commission (EC) of AOTA ensures compliance with the Code of Ethics, and it establishes and maintains enforcement procedures. Any individual, group, or entity within or outside of AOTA may file a formal, written complaint against a member of AOTA for unethical conduct.[3] The EC conducts a preliminary assessment and determines whether there is sufficient ground to carry the complaint forward to a full investigation. If the member is found to have committed an ethical violation, one of the following disciplinary sanctions is imposed: reprimand, censure, probation of membership subject to terms, membership suspension, or revocation of membership in AOTA.[3] It is the policy of AOTA to communicate with NBCOT and state regulatory boards when disciplinary actions have been taken against an OT practitioner.

It is the responsibility of the licensure board to protect the public from direct or potential harm that may be caused by unqualified or incompetent practitioners. The regulatory board follows established disciplinary processes and guidelines that are clearly outlined in each state's regulations. In cases in which there is not direct or potential harm to the public, the licensure board may assess a fine, which would vary depending on the gravity of the situation. An abatement, or order of correction, may be given to the practitioner and completed in a designated amount of time. In situations in which there is clear evidence of direct or potential harm to the public, the consequences for the practitioner are more severe. Disciplinary actions that could be taken against the practitioner include public censure, suspension, or revocation of licensure or practice privileges. Each state has jurisdiction only over practitioners licensed in the state.

## Summary

AOTA's Occupational Therapy Code of Ethics provides standards of conduct for OT practitioners. The Ethics Commission enforces the principles of the Code of Ethics. The six principles are beneficence, nonmaleficence, autonomy, justice, veracity, and fidelity. Using ethical decision-making guidelines helps practitioners make professionally sound decisions.

Standards of practice provide guidelines for the delivery of quality OT services to the consumer. State licensure is the legal means of regulating OT practice. Both the Code of Ethics and state licensure laws have procedures for processing disciplinary actions. OT practitioners are responsible for understanding and following the ethical and legal standards of practice.

Ethics, laws, and regulations serve primarily to protect the public from unqualified or unscrupulous practitioners. Laws and regulations establish a legal scope of practice for the profession and differentiate it from other professions. OT practitioners obtain rights and protection as a result of these laws and regulations, but they must also assume the responsibilities and limits imposed by regulation.

## Learning Activities

1. Obtain a series of ethical situations, including suggested solutions, from faculty members or practicing therapists. In small groups, discuss the scenarios, then, using the ethical decision-making guidelines, develop a solution. Discuss each scenario, and use the suggested solutions to provide alternatives.
2. Compare and contrast AOTA's Occupational Therapy Code of Ethics to the ethical codes of two other allied health professions.
3. View a film such as *The Kevorkian Files, The Tuskegee Study,* or the *Life of David Gale* to promote discussion

on ethical decision making. Identify one or two ethical issues from the film, define them, and discuss the stakeholders and alternatives.
4. Find an ethical issue in the current news media. Using the ethical decision-making process, discuss this issue and possible solutions.
5. Research the licensure laws from three states. Compare and contrast the OT practice guidelines for each of these states.

## Review Questions

1. What is a code of ethics?
2. What are examples of ethical distress, ethical dilemmas, and locus-of-authority problems?
3. What are the six principles in AOTA's Occupational Therapy Code of Ethics? Describe each principle.
4. What are the six steps to ethical decision making?

## References

1. American Occupational Therapy Association. *Issues in licensure.* Retrieved from, http://www.aota.org/advocacy-policy/state-policy/licensure.aspx; 2016.
2. American Occupational Therapy Association. Guidelines to the occupational therapy code of ethics. *Am J Occup Ther.* 2006;60:652–658.
3. American Occupational Therapy Association. Enforcement procedures for occupational therapy code of ethics. *Am J Occup Ther.* 2014;68:(suppl 3): S3–S15.
4. American Occupational Therapy Association (2015). Occupational therapy code of ethics. *Am J Occup Ther.* 2015;69(suppl 3), 1–8.
5. American Occupational Therapy Association. Standards of practice for occupational therapy. *Am J Occup Ther.* 2015;69(Suppl. 3):691341007. http://dx.doi.org/10.5014/ajot.2015.696506.
6. American Occupational Therapy Association. *Definition of Occupational Therapy Practice for the AOTA Model Practice Act.* Bethesda, MD: Author; 2015.
7. American Occupational Therapy Association. Guidelines for supervision, roles, and responsibilities during the delivery of occupational therapy services. *Am J Occup Ther.* 2014;68(suppl 3):S16–S22. http://dx.doi.org/10.5014/ajot.2014.686S03.
8. American Occupational Therapy Association. Scope of practice. *Am J Occup Ther.* 2014;68(suppl 3):http://dx.doi.org/10.5014/ajot.2014.686S04.
9. American Occupational Therapy Association. Core values and attitudes of occupational therapy practice. *Am J Occup Ther.* 1993;47:1085–1086.
10. Centers for Medicare and Medicaid Services. *HIPAA—General Information.* 2013. Retrieved from, https://www.cms.gov/Regulations-and-Guidance/HIPAA-Administrative-Simplification/HIPAAGenInfo/index.html.
11. Davis CM. *Patient Practitioner Interaction: An Experiential Manual for Developing the Art of Health Care.* In: 4th ed.Thorofare, NJ: Slack; 2006.

12. Purtilo R, Doherty R. *Ethical Dimensions in the Health Professions.* 5th ed. Philadelphia, PA: WB Saunders/Elsevier; 2011.

13. Scott R. *Professional Ethics: A Guide for Rehabilitation Professionals.* St. Louis, MO: Mosby; 1998.

14. US Department of Health and Human Services. *Mandatory Reporters.* 2016. Retrieved from, http://www.childwelfare.gov/topics/systemwide/laws-policies/statutes/manda/.

15. US Department of Health, Education, and Welfare, Public Health Service. *Credentialing Health Manpower.* [Publication No. [OS] 77-50057]. Bethesda, MD: Author; 1977.

16. US Department of Justice, Civil Rights Division. *Disability Rights Section: A Guide to Disability Rights Laws.* 2005, September. Retrieved from, http://www.ada.gov/cguide.pdf.

# 9

# Professional Organizations

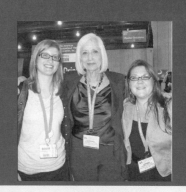

## OBJECTIVES

*After reading this chapter, the reader will be able to do the following:*

- Describe the mission and major activities of occupational therapy professional associations.
- Describe the activities of the American Occupational Therapy Association, World Federation of Occupational Therapists, and state associations.
- Describe how professional associations assure the delivery of quality occupational therapy services.

- Identify ways professional organizations contribute to the professional development of their members.
- Outline the importance of being involved in professional organizations.

## KEY TERMS

American Occupational Therapy
 Association (AOTA)
American Occupational Therapy
 Foundation (AOTF)

American Occupational Therapy
 Political Action Committee (AOTPAC)
American Student Committee of the
 Occupational Therapy Association
 (ASCOTA)

professional association
World Federation of Occupational
 Therapists (WFOT)

I stumbled upon the profession of occupational therapy (OT) quite serendipitously. I had originally intended to pursue a law degree in college but found myself drawn to courses in the sciences and arts. A university counselor recommended that I take a series of career tests, and the profession of OT appeared. Because I had never heard of this profession, the counselor provided me with information and names of individuals to contact regarding OT. I was amazed at the range of the profession and the creativity of the occupational therapists I encountered. This profession offered such variety!

As I reflect on over 25 years as an occupational therapist (I stopped counting after the quarter-century mark!), I am so grateful to that counselor who opened my eyes to a profession that has provided me with such a tremendous opportunity for growth. This profession has allowed me to be a clinician, supervisor, educator, and researcher. Throughout the years, I have been so fortunate to learn from my clients, students, and colleagues in OT and other professions. They have taught me the true importance of occupation, whether

playing a card game with friends, jumping rope on a playground, studying for an examination, or discussing the efficacy of various intervention methods. I have never ceased to be thankful that I found a profession as rewarding and fulfilling as OT.

WINIFRED SCHULTZ-KROHN, PHD, OTR/L, SWC, BCP, FAOTA
Professor of Occupational Therapy
Department of Occupational Therapy
San José State University
San José, California

When Mary was a first-year occupational therapy (OT) graduate student, she joined American Occupational Therapy Association (AOTA) upon the recommendation of, Joe, an occupational therapist she met while completing her level I fieldwork experience. Joe had just returned from an AOTA national conference and showed her many new materials and information he found at the conference that he could now use with his clients.

Mary found that the evidence-based critically appraised papers and resources helped her read research more easily for her academic work. She also joined a student group so she could network for housing for level II fieldwork. Mary made connections with students across the country, and they decided to meet at the next AOTA conference. These early networks provided Mary with the idea to practice in another state. Mary found other materials that she used for her classes, and she even compiled some of the AOTA Tip and Fact sheets into a notebook to use during fieldwork.

Mary attended the Student Conclave at AOTA, where she met leaders in the profession and heard about pressing issues. Mary pursued student scholarships and presented her research work with a faculty member at the next AOTA conference. Mary received funding through her university to present nationally. She made connections at the poster session with other OT students and faculty interested in her topic area. Mary also decided to present her research at the state conference. She was recognized by the state for presenting and enjoyed networking with practitioners. This helped her focus her job search and feel comfortable interviewing. She also used her AOTA membership to look for job opportunities and find facts about the areas in which she would practice. Mary decided she would become active in her state association early so she could meet practitioners throughout the state, remain current regarding upcoming issues, and develop an understanding of the resources available to her clients.

This example shows the importance of joining one's professional organization early and exploring the membership benefits.

Professional associations create, promote, and support the vision of the profession and its members. Stronger associations provide greater benefits for their members. A **professional association** is organized and operated by its members for its members. It exists to protect and promote the profession it represents by (1) providing a communication network and channel for information, (2) regulating itself through the development and enforcement of standards of conduct and performance, and (3) guarding the interests of those within the profession.[1]

The professional organization for occupational therapy (OT) practitioners in the United States is the **American Occupational Therapy Association (AOTA).** Originally incorporated in 1917 as the National Society for the Promotion of Occupational Therapy, the association's name was changed to its present version in 1923. The **World Federation of Occupational Therapists (WFOT)** was established in 1952 to help OT practitioners access international information, engage in international exchange, and promote organizations of OT in schools in countries where none exists.[3,5] Each state also has a professional organization for OT practitioners living in the state. Although there is frequent collaboration between AOTA and individual state associations, state associations are funded and operated independently from the national association. Furthermore, state associations may divide into smaller regions to meet the needs of local members. It is beneficial for OT practitioners

to have a good understanding of the professional organizations and the services they provide. Because it would be impossible to discuss each state association in this text, this chapter describes the international and national associations. Readers are encouraged to join and support their professional associations at the international, national, state, and local levels.

## American Occupational Therapy Association Mission

The mission of AOTA is "to advance the quality, availability, use and support of OT through standard-setting, advocacy, education, and research on behalf of its members and the public."[1] In keeping with this mission statement, AOTA directs its efforts to (1) assure the quality of OT services, (2) improve consumer access to health-care services, and (3) promote the professional development of its members.[1]

## Membership

Three professional membership categories exist in AOTA: occupational therapist, occupational therapy assistant (OTA), and occupational therapy student (OTS). Persons interested in the profession who are not OT professionals may join the organization as organizational or associate members. Membership categories determine the fees paid for membership and conferences and who can attend special meetings, hold office, and vote. For example, organizational and associate members do not have voting privileges. Membership fees are higher for occupational therapists. Student membership fees are lowest to encourage them to become involved in the organization and familiarize themselves with membership benefits.

Members at all levels are encouraged to become actively involved in AOTA by serving on committees, attending the annual conference, reviewing journal articles, presenting at conferences, and holding elected and volunteer positions.

The Coordinated Online Opportunities for Leadership (COOL) database was developed to encourage membership participation at a variety of levels. Members complete a profile and indicate areas of expertise and interest. AOTA staff and committee chairpersons use the database to find volunteers for a variety of organization and membership activities. Active membership helps OT practitioners become informed, which benefits them professionally while also benefitting clients and their families.[1] Members are able to access professional information to advocate for their clients and the profession. Materials that support intervention planning are readily available. For example, AOTA Tip and Fact sheets regarding best practice related to a variety of situations are available (e.g., driving, cognition, vision). OT members benefit from becoming aware and using the resources available through AOTA. They learn about new opportunities that may benefit them professionally and enhance their practice, thereby benefitting clients and their families.

## Organizational Structure

AOTA is made up of a volunteer sector and paid national office staff. The paid office staff is employed at the headquarters in Bethesda, Maryland, and performs the day-to-day operations under the management of the executive director. The national office staff is organized into five divisions:

- Membership (marketing, communication, AOTA press and periodicals, sales, instructional technology)
- Human resources (finance, administration, general counsel)
- Conferences (continuing professional development, practice)
- Accreditation (research, academic education)
- Federal affairs (reimbursement and regulatory policy, state affairs, affiliate relations, special policy activities)

The volunteer sector consists of all of the members of the association and is represented by the executive board and the Representative Assembly. The executive board is charged with the administration and management of the association and includes elected officers. There are several standing committees of the executive board, including the Representative Assembly (RA), which is the legislative and policymaking body of AOTA. The RA is composed of elected representatives from each state, elected officers of the assembly and the association, a representative from the student committee, an OTA representative, the first delegate of the World Federation of Occupational Therapists (WFOT), and the chairpersons of the commissions. The standing commissions of the RA include the Commission on Education, Commission on Practice, Ethics Commission, and Commission on Continuing Competence and Professional Development.[1]

Many OT educational programs have a club or organization for students. Student groups may participate in the **American Student Committee of the Occupational Therapy Association (ASCOTA),** a standing committee of the executive board of AOTA (Figs. 9.1A and 9.1B). This standing committee provides feedback to AOTA regarding student issues. It meets at the AOTA conference annually and through online committee work.

AOTA also provides opportunities for its members through multicultural networking groups. These national groups meet to discuss current issues, develop resources, advocate for services, and educate consumers and other professionals regarding current topics as related to the specific culture and occupational therapy. The groups may offer scholarships, support, and ideas for promoting multiculturalism within the profession. (See AOTA website for more information regarding these groups). The networking groups include:

- Asian/Pacific Heritage Occupational Therapy Association (APHOTA)
- National Black Occupational Therapy Caucus (NBOTC)

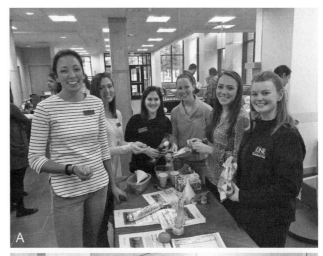

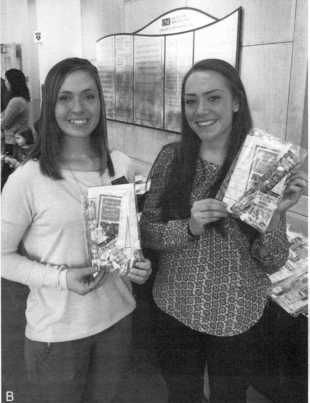

• **Fig. 9.1  A,** Members of the student association support a community service project during Occupational Therapy Month. **B,** Members of the student association give out dental kits to help children enjoy the experience.

- Network for Lesbian, Gay, Bisexual and Transgender Concerns in Occupational Therapy (The Network)
- Network of Occupational Therapy Practitioners with Disabilities and Their Supporters (NOTPD)
- Occupational Therapy Network for Native Americans (OTNA)
- Orthodox Jewish Occupational Therapy Chavrusa (OJOTC)
- Terapia Ocupacional para Diversidad, Oportunidad y Solidaridad (TODOS) Network of Hispanic Practitioners

## Assuring Quality of Occupational Therapy Services

AOTA is responsible for ensuring the delivery of quality OT services. To this end, the association develops standards, produces official documents that identify the standards, and reviews the standards on a regular basis. Standards ensure that educational programs prepare students properly, that guidelines are in place articulating OT practice, and that a code of conduct is provided to clarify ethical issues. AOTA has developed standards of education, standards of practice, and ethical standards.

Standards for occupational therapist and OTA educational programs are developed and reviewed on a regular basis by the association's Accreditation Council for Occupational Therapy Education (ACOTE). Educational programs are accredited based on their compliance with these standards (see Chapter 6). These standards help ensure the delivery of quality educational programs in OT.

AOTA lends its support to states for the regulation of practice through licensure and other state laws. The *Occupational Therapy Scope of Practice,* developed by AOTA, is used by states as a model for their licensure laws.[6] State regulatory laws help ensure that practitioners meet specific competencies. AOTA addresses issues as they arise, such as insurance issues, and raises funds to advocate for the profession. The association monitors actions of members by investigating complaints and developing plans. Advocating for the profession may involve creating publicity, case studies, and news announcements.

## Professional Development of Members

AOTA also promotes the professional development of its members through a number of activities, including publications, continuing education, and practice information. The Commission on Continuing Competence and Professional Development (CCCPD) of the Representative Assembly is responsible for developing standards for continuing competency and for communicating these standards to the various stakeholders.

## Publications

The association contributes to the professional development of OT practitioners through a variety of publications. The organization's official publication, *American Journal of Occupational Therapy (AJOT),* serves as a source of research information for the profession. *AJOT* is distributed monthly to all AOTA members, and it is also available through subscription to nonmembers and libraries. Subjects may include approaches to practice, programs and techniques, research, educational and professional trends, and areas of controversy in the OT field. Articles are written by professionals in OT or related fields and must meet the rigid standards set by its editors.

As a part of AOTA membership, each member receives online access to 11 Special Interest Sections (SISs), voting privileges in three SISs, and one printed SIS quarterly sent by mail.

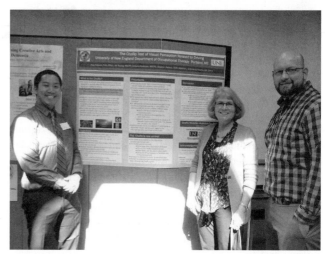

**Fig. 9.2** OT students present a poster with faculty at the national AOTA conference.

The SISs are as follows: Administration and Management, Developmental Disabilities, Education, Gerontology, Home and Community Health, Mental Health, Physical Disabilities, School System, Sensory Integration, Technology, and Work Programs. Members are eligible to participate in activities (such as meetings) held by three SISs.[1]

*OT Practice* is a biweekly publication designed to keep members informed about the profession in general. *OT Practice* (available as an e-journal) publishes useful clinical information to members. AOTA also publishes Critically Appraised Papers (CAPs), which are concise evidence-based reviews of current research that may be applied to OT practice. AOTA publishes books, videotapes, audiotapes, brochures, official documents, and materials on a broad range of topics related to OT.

## Continuing Education

AOTA sponsors continuing education activities, including workshops, continuing education articles (in *OT Practice*), self-paced clinical courses, and online courses. The annual meeting, held in a different city each year and hosted by the area's local or state association, provides a variety of continuing education opportunities. All members are encouraged to attend. The conference hosts presentations ranging from poster sessions, panel discussions, and workshops to formal presentations (Fig. 9.2). The national conference conducts business meetings and also includes an awards ceremony to recognize contributions to the field. The latest materials, equipment, and books are displayed. The national conference provides members with current information and a chance to network with OT practitioners around the country. The association also sponsors an Educational Summit and a Student Conclave as well as other conferences and online learning experiences.

## Practice Information

AOTA has developed resources for information on all of the practice areas, including published practice materials, staff experts, and volunteers who provide consultation. These resources include standards for practice, handouts for families and consumers, and fact sheets concerning OT. Information regarding research, opportunities (clinical and academic), intervention planning, student resources, scholarships, and tip sheets are available. Although some information is available to the general public, much of the information is restricted to use by AOTA members.

## Improving Consumer Access to Health-Care Services

The national association ensures that services are accessible to consumers through an ongoing process of communication with state and federal lawmakers, regulatory bodies, third-party payers, health-care professionals, the media, and the public. For example, AOTA keeps abreast of proposed legislation within the government, ensuring that new laws affecting practice are not passed without the voice of the profession having been heard. The association is in communication with its political action committee (PAC), the legally sanctioned vehicle through which organizations can engage in political action. The **American Occupational Therapy Political Action Committee (AOTPAC)** furthers the legislative aims of the profession by attempting to influence the selection, nomination, election, or appointment of persons to public office.[2]

For example, when the federal government developed legislation outlining what services the Patient Protection and Affordable Care Act (PPACA) must provide, AOTA provided information on OT services and successfully lobbied for the inclusion of OT. This professional vigilance applies not only to the government but also to the private sector. When major insurance companies write or rewrite policies regarding the health services they will cover, AOTA works to ensure that OT is included. AOTA also has a toll-free hotline for consumers to access information regarding OT.

## American Occupational Therapy Foundation

The **American Occupational Therapy Foundation (AOTF)** is a national organization designed to advance the science of OT and increase public understanding of the value of OT. AOTF was incorporated as a separate not-for-profit organization in 1965.[4] It is a vehicle for providing resources to programs and individuals for the purpose of carrying out OT education and research. AOTF also operates a library that contains books and journals related to OT. The foundation provides grant opportunities, scholarships, and research support.[4] AOTF supports its program through donations and bequests from AOTA members, corporations, and private foundations. The foundation supports projects such as the doctoral support group, scholarships, emerging leaders program, and future scientists.

Since 1980, AOTF has published the *Occupational Therapy Journal of Research (OTJR)*, now named *OTJR:*

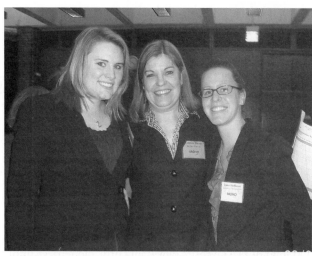

**Fig. 9.3** Practitioners from the United States network with faculty from Chile at an international conference.

*Occupation, Participation and Health,* to address the need for more publication opportunities. This journal is published quarterly and is available for a subscription fee.

## World Federation of Occupational Therapists

The World Federation of Occupation Therapists (WFOT) was developed in 1952 with the objectives to promote and advocate for OT and establish minimum educational standards for member countries.[5] WFOT also serves as a vehicle for international information exchange among OT associations, practitioners, and other allied health personnel. The organization is responsible for publishing the WFOT journal. WFOT is organized into five program areas: standards and quality, education and research, promotion and development, international cooperation, and executive programs.[5] An international conference is sponsored by WFOT every 4 years (Fig. 9.3). As the worldwide practice of OT continues to grow and develop, WFOT is a valuable mechanism for exchange of information with OT practitioners in other countries.

## State Organizations

State OT associations meet the needs of the practitioners within the state. These organizations hold conferences, stay alert to legislative issues that may affect OT services in the state, and provide networking and support for practitioners throughout the state. For example, some states have developed Community of Practice networking groups in which practitioners meet on a regular basis to discuss topics of interest to practice (e.g., pediatrics, rehabilitation, mental health). State associations have elected officers, and the state presidents and representative assembly members meet at the national association to discuss state issues. State OT associations provide information on the state of practice within the state and help advocate for services. They serve as a networking and support system for practitioners, educators, and students.

## Summary

AOTA is the national organization representing OT practitioners. Its major activities include assuring the delivery of quality OT services, improving consumer access to health care, and promoting the professional development of its members.

AOTA ensures the delivery of quality services through the development and enforcement of standards, accreditation of educational programs, research, and support for regulation. To encourage the professional development of its members, AOTA conducts continuing education programs, publishes materials, and provides practice information. AOTA distributes information to federal and state lawmakers, insurance providers, the media, the public, and other health-care providers.

At the international level, WFOT provides an information exchange and advances the practice and standards of OT around the world. OT practitioners are encouraged to participate in professional organizations at the international, national, state, and local levels.

## Learning Activities

1. Go to AOTA's website (www.aota.org) and retrieve information on an aspect of AOTA that is of special interest to you; write a brief paper on your findings.
2. Gather information on the next AOTA conference (e.g., when, where, cost, theme), then prepare a bulletin board display or poster.
3. Hold a class brainstorming session to compile a list of topics appropriate for a 15-minute conference short paper.
4. Gather information on your state OT association; prepare an informational handout for your class.
5. Prepare an overview of a topic from the most recent WFOT conference. Discuss the current issues and topics with classmates.
6. The following is a recommended series of exploratory *American Journal of Occupational Therapy* investigations. Each stage is a bit more demanding and thus builds an increasing familiarity with both the publication and research techniques. Each class member is to do the following:

- Read an article of interest from *American Journal of Occupational Therapy;* give a 5-minute oral report on the topic, the source information, and the point of interest.
- Research an article on an assigned topic; give a 5-minute oral report. (Further research may be required to gain information on the topic before the article search.)
- Read an article from any OT reference source; write a half-page summary of the topic.
- Gather information on an intervention technique by summarizing and critiquing at least three research articles.
- Using Critically Appraised Paper (CAP) guidelines from AOTA, and complete a CAP of a research article of interest. Discuss this in class.
7. Find the contacts and board members for your state association. Determine the next conference and try to attend.

## Review Questions

1. What are the purposes of a professional organization?
2. List five benefits of membership in AOTA, WFOT, and state organizations.
3. How can members participate in professional organizations?
4. What resources are available to OT practitioners through professional organizations?
5. What is your local OT association? Describe the activities of this association.

## References

1. American Occupational Therapy Association. *About AOTA.* (2016). Retrieved from, http://www.aota.org/Aboutaota.aspx.
2. American Occupational Therapy Association. *AOTPAC.* (2016). Retrieved from, http://www.aota.org/Advocacy-Policy/AOTPAC/Fact.aspx.
3. World Federation of Occupational Therapists. *Fundamental Beliefs of the World Federation of Occupational Therapists (WFOT).* (2016). Retrieved from, http://www.wfot.org/About Us/FundamentalBeliefs.aspx.
4. American Occupational Therapy Foundation. *Did You Know? Facts about the American Occupational Therapy Foundation.* 2016. Retrieved from, http://www.aotf.org/aboutaotf/visionmissiongoals.
5. World Federation of Occupational Therapy. *WFOT.* (2016). Retrieved from, http://www.wfot.org/AboutUs/History.aspx.
6. American Occupational Therapy Association. Scope of practice. *Am J Occup Ther.* 2014;68(3):S34–S40.

# SECTION III

# The Practice of Occupational Therapy

# 10

# Occupational Therapy Practice Framework: Domain and Process

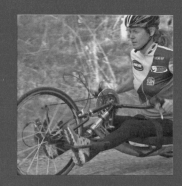

## OBJECTIVES

*After reading this chapter, the reader will be able to do the following:*

- Define the domains of occupational therapy practice.
- Outline the occupational therapy process.
- Analyze activities in terms of occupation, performance skills, performance patterns, and client factors.

- Provide examples of how contexts influence occupations.
- Describe intervention approaches.
- Describe activity demands.

## KEY TERMS

activities of daily living
activity demands
body functions
body structures
client-centered approach
client factors
client satisfaction
consultation
context
education

evaluation
health
instrumental activities of daily living
intervention plan
occupation-based activity
occupational justice
occupational performance
participation
performance patterns
performance skills

preparatory methods
prevention
purposeful activity
quality of life
role competence
therapeutic use of occupations and activities
values, beliefs and spirituality
well-being
wellness

(e) Visit *www.evolve.elsevier.com* to access the Evolve student resources that accompany your book.

My entrance into the profession was influenced and sustained by the efforts and examples of some very remarkable mentors. My mother, a registered nurse, regaled my sisters and me with tales of her nursing experiences in the Army Nurse Corps during World War II. I read every Cherry Ames book (nurse/detective à la Nancy Drew), and I loved my stint as a candy striper at the local hospital, but somehow I knew that nursing wasn't quite what I was looking for in my career future. I remember first hearing about occupational therapy (OT) from Dr. Marian Diamond, the esteemed professor of anatomy and physiology at the University of California at Berkeley and my instructor. Based upon my high regard for her and her suggestion that I would be a perfect occupational therapist (whatever that was), I followed suit and met with

Doris Cutting, the chair of the OT department at San José State University, who made me want to be a part of whatever it was she was. Armed with my bachelor's in humanities from Berkeley, I smiled as I picked up my OT class schedule and saw neuroanatomy, psychology, and weaving on my list—now this was a program that was meant for me!

OT school was a dream—each of the assignments a step closer to my newly chosen profession. Professors Amy Killingsworth, Lorraine Pedretti, and many others further nourished my enthusiasm for OT through their obvious passion for the profession, conveyed through stories of their caring and creative interactions with clients. I was privileged to begin my career at Rancho Los Amigos Medical Center with incomparable role models of superb OT practice, including

*Dottie Wilson, Lois Barber, Doris Heredia, Sarah Kelly, and numerous others who mentored their colleagues, facilitating and celebrating each other's successes. I remember driving to work with a smile on my face and eagerly looking forward to each day and the new stories I would be developing with my clients—a wish I have for every budding occupational therapist.*

*All of these mentors, through their example, inspired pursuit of further learning and scholarship as a commitment to furthering excellence in client care as well as advancing the knowledge base of the profession. In response, I chose to study at the graduate level and subsequently seek an academic position—both environments where I was again treated to the supportive mentoring climate I have come to know throughout my OT experience. Elizabeth Yerxa, Florence Clark, Lela Llorens, and Ruth Zemke—among many others in academia—exemplified for me the importance of nurturing and celebrating the accomplishments of others to strengthen and enrich the profession we love so well. In tribute to these generous and amazing mentors, I encourage my OT colleagues and strive myself to reach out, encourage, and support developing occupational therapists.*

**HEIDI MCHUGH PENDLETON PHD, OTR/L, FAOTA**
**Professor**
**Department of Occupational Therapy**
**San José State University**
**San José, California**

The American Occupational Therapy Association (AOTA) developed the *Occupational Therapy Practice Framework (OTPF)* to help practitioners use the language and constructs of occupation to serve clients and educate consumers.[1] The *OTPF* describes the occupational therapy (OT) profession and process, for students, clinicians, and consumers. The emphasis is on occupation, client-centered care, and the dynamic nature of the therapy process. This chapter provides readers with an overview of the *OTPF* (3rd edition), along with clinical examples to clarify content.

## Occupation

The goal of OT is to help clients engage in occupation.[1,5,6] Occupations are the everyday things that people do and that are essential to one's identity.[1,4,6] Occupation includes activities of daily living, instrumental activities of daily living, rest and sleep, education, work, play, leisure, and social participation.[1] The following paragraphs provide descriptions of the areas of occupation along with clinical examples to help readers understand the breadth of occupations that OT interventions address.

## Activities of Daily Living

**Activities of daily living** (ADLs) refer to activities involved in taking care of one's own body and include such things as dressing, bathing/showering, personal hygiene and grooming, toileting and toilet hygiene, functional mobility, eating, feeding, personal device care, and sexual activity.[1]

Craig is a 2-year-old boy, small for his age, whose mother is concerned that he does not like many foods. Upon evaluation, the occupational therapist determines that Craig exhibits oral-motor control issues (e.g., tongue thrusting) and oral hypersensitivity that interfere with his eating. The occupational therapist develops an intervention plan to address this ADL.

## Instrumental Activities of Daily Living

**Instrumental activities of daily living** (IADLs) refer to activities that involve multiple tasks in the environment. IADLs include care of others, care of pets, childrearing, communication management, driving and community mobility, health management and maintenance, financial management, home establishment and management, meal preparation and cleanup, safety and emergency maintenance, religious and spiritual activities and expression, and shopping.[1]

Raiser is a 19-year-old man with mild intellectual deficits. He recently graduated from a group home and will be living alone in the next few months. The OT practitioner works with Raiser on living independently by practicing how to purchase, use, and maintain household equipment (e.g., toaster, microwave). In another session, the practitioner works with Raiser on using the telephone to call the landlord for assistance with the household. These IADL skills are considered part of home management.

## Rest and Sleep

Rest and sleep are restorative activities that support healthy participation in occupations.[1] These activities include all of those tasks and routines to get ready for sleep, such as grooming, undressing, and establishing sleep patterns. This includes sleeping through the night and taking care of one's sleep needs and routines.

Tom is a 5-year-old boy who is having difficulty sleeping through the night. His parents report that he sleeps only 2 to 3 hours a night. During the day, Tom takes frequent naps. The OT practitioner works with Tom and his family on establishing healthy routines for sleep and rest.

## Education

Education is an occupation that includes formal (e.g., school, university, coursework) and informal (e.g., obtaining topic-related information or skills, instruction/training in areas of interest) learning. OT practitioners examine all the skills and tasks required to engage in education, such as reading, writing, and sitting in class.

David is a 7-year-old second grader who is experiencing difficulty with handwriting. His teacher is concerned that David is falling behind others in his class and makes a referral to OT. The OT practitioner evaluates David's handwriting skills and begins intervention to improve strength and coordination for handwriting. Because children spend approximately 30% of the school day writing,[8] this is a necessary ability for his education.

## Work

Work refers to paid or volunteer activities and includes the entire range of employment activities, such as interests, pursuits, job seeking, and job performance, to retirement preparation and adjustment, to volunteer exploration and participation.[1]

Kylie is experiencing difficulty returning to her job as a legal secretary after being involved in a motor vehicle accident, which resulted in a traumatic brain injury. The OT practitioner emphasizes work habits such as getting to work on time, organizing her workspace, limiting conversation with others, and completing her work. The OT practitioner arranges a meeting with Kylie and her supervisor to review the firm's standards and the necessary job skills. The supervisor agrees to provide the OT practitioner with a description of Kylie's "typical day" so the OT practitioner may adequately prepare her for the job requirements.

## Play

Play refers to "any spontaneous or organized activity that provides enjoyment, entertainment, amusement, or diversion."[1,9] OT practitioners work with clients to facilitate engagement and exploration of play activities.

Karl is a 12-year-old boy who does not engage in play activities with his peers at school or at home. His teachers and parents are concerned that Karl does not find any enjoyment in his childhood. The OT practitioner works with Karl to identify play activities and invites two friends to a session in which they engage in a variety of outdoor games as a means of exploring the types of play that Karl may enjoy.

## Leisure

Leisure refers to nonobligatory activity in which people engage. Leisure may provide diversion, amusement, and interest. This occupation includes planning as well as participating in the activity. Exploring areas of interest is considered part of leisure occupations. As people engage in leisure, they develop skills and abilities. Leisure becomes part of a person's identity and adds to one's quality of life. It has been found to have restorative functions and helps people regain energy.

Jana is a 66-year-old woman who is dealing with the loss of her husband. She and her husband retired to a new state just before his death. Jana has not established new leisure interests and does not find pleasure in her old leisure interests. Upon evaluation, the occupational therapist discovers that Jana participates in few enjoyable activities. In fact, Jana cannot articulate any leisure interests. The occupational therapist invites Jana to several community outings that she thinks Jana may enjoy. The practitioner watches for nonverbal or verbal indication of enjoyment so that she may elaborate or expand on areas of interest. Exploring one's options is often the first step in developing leisure occupations.

## Social Participation

Social participation refers to activities involving interactions with others, including family, community, and peers/friends.[1] OT practitioners examining social participation analyze the behaviors and standards for given social situations. Social participation involves interactions, codes of conduct, reading and responding to cues, and consideration of the context in which the participation occurs. Social participation standards vary among cultures.

Gloria is a 52-year-old woman with a diagnosis of schizophrenia. She has difficulty in many social settings. The OT practitioner begins intervention to help Gloria succeed in community settings by reviewing basic social manners, including dress, language, and how close she stands to others. As part of the intervention, Gloria attends several outings in the community, including the art museum, library, and a coffee shop. Standards of behavior vary with the type of social participation activity.

The previous examples illustrate the variety of occupations in which people engage. OT practitioners consider the client's age, motivation, interests, culture, and abilities when analyzing occupational performance. Further analysis of occupations is necessary to fully understand how to provide meaningful intervention.

## Analysis of Occupational Performance

The *OTPF* supports a top-down approach in that the OT practitioner evaluates the occupations in which the client hopes to engage first, followed by an analysis of the performance skills and client factors interfering with performance. This approach differs from reductionistic approaches that analyze components first and subsequently design intervention based upon deficits. The *OTPF* encourages practitioners to keep occupation central to practice. See Table 10.1 for an overview of the domain of OT.

Once the practitioner has identified the occupations in which the client would like to engage, the practitioner analyzes **performance skills,** which include the motor, process, and social interaction skills required to complete the

## TABLE 10.1    Domain of Occupational Therapy

| Occupations | Client Factors | Performance Skills | Performance Patterns | Contexts and Environments |
|---|---|---|---|---|
| Activities of daily living (ADLs)* | Values, beliefs, and spirituality | Motor skills | Habits | Cultural |
| Instrumental activities of daily living (IADLs) | Body functions | Process skills | Routines | Personal |
| Rest and sleep | Body structures | Social interaction skills | Rituals | Physical |
| Education | | | Roles | Social |
| Work | | | | Temporal |
| Play | | | | Virtual |
| Leisure | | | | |
| Social participation | | | | |

*Also referred to as basic activities of daily living (BADLs) or personal activities of daily living (PADLs).
From American Occupational Therapy Association. (2014). Occupational therapy practice framework: Domain and process (3rd ed.). *American Journal of Occupational Therapy, 68*(Suppl. 1), S4.

occupation. Performance skills are small units of performance. When an OT practitioner examines performance, he or she identifies performance skills that are effective or ineffective.[1] For example, the practitioner may decide that the client's deficits in fine motor skills are interfering with the ability to get dressed in the morning. The client may have difficulty using problem-solving skills to determine how to make breakfast or be unable to make eye contact with peers. Performance skills may need to be addressed before the client can engage in desired occupations. Performance skills are dependent on client factors, activity demands, and context.[1]

**Client factors** are even more specific components of performance that may need to be addressed for clients to be successful. Figs. 10.1A–C illustrate some examples of how an OT practitioner examines client factors required to complete activities. Client factors include **values, beliefs, spirituality**, body functions, and body structures. Values, beliefs, and spirituality refer to those things that motivate clients to engage. **Body functions** refer to the body's physiological functioning (such as vision).[1] Body functions include mental functions (such as affective, cognitive, and perceptual) as well as higher-level cognition, attention, memory, thought, sequencing, emotion, and experience of time.[1] Practitioners also examine global mental functions, such as awareness, consciousness, orientation, personality and temperament, energy and drive, and sleep. They also evaluate client factors such as sensory functions (e.g., visual, hearing, vestibular, taste, smell, proprioception, touch and pain, temperature, and pressure). Body functions include such things as reflexes, range of motion, muscle tone, strength, endurance, posture, visual acuity, and tactile functions. OT practitioners analyze occupational performance at the basic level

so that they can help clients fine-tune their skills and obtain the standards they wish. Furthermore, client factors include an analysis of the cardiovascular, hematological, immunological, and respiratory systems.

**Body structures** refer to the anatomical structures themselves, such as organs and limbs.[1] This includes an evaluation of the client's musculoskeletal system, proportions, and anatomical makeup. For example, the practitioner considers how missing fingers will influence occupational performance.

OT practitioners examine client factors as they evaluate what may be interfering with a client's ability to perform a desired occupation. Understanding the influence of the client factor on the performance allows the practitioner to design effective intervention. OT practitioners may target multiple client factors during intervention. The goal of the intervention is the occupational performance, which may be accomplished by changing the client factor. The goal may also be reached by compensating for the weak client factor or providing assistive technology. A thorough analysis of client factors allows the practitioner to understand how to intervene most effectively. The practitioner does not just consider client factors, but rather evaluates the client's patterns, motivations, activity demands, and the context in which the occupation occurs.

Patterns of performance are another component of occupational performance analyzed by the OT practitioner. **Performance patterns** refer to the client's habits, routines, roles, and rituals.[1] Three types of habits are described in the *OTPF*: useful habits that support occupations, impoverished habits that do not support occupations, and dominating habits that interfere with occupations.[1] Habits that support occupations may include walking to meet with

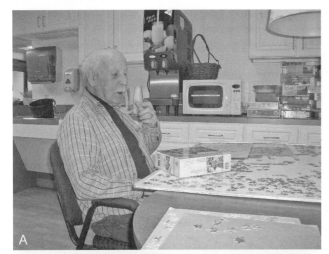

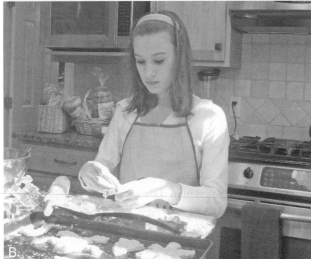

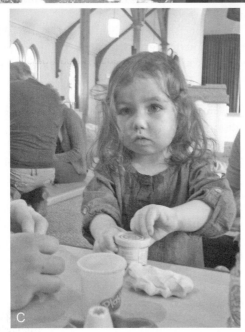

• **Fig. 10.1 A,** Visual perception, attention to details, concentration, memory, problem solving, and fine motor skills are all required for completing a puzzle. **B,** Baking cookies requires concentration, memory, problem solving, measuring (cognition), and fine motor skills. **C,** Playing with Playdoh requires concentration, attention, planning, problem solving, and fine motor skills.

friends each morning, as illustrated in Fig. 10.2. Examining performance patterns helps the OT practitioner understand how the occupation is actually accomplished for the individual client. An example of a client with an impoverished habit is one who has difficulty consistently getting up on time and performing morning self-care in a timely manner. As a result of this, the client will have a poorly established or ineffective routine and experience difficulty carrying out his or her desired roles.

When choosing an activity to help a client reach his or her goals, OT practitioners carefully examine the **activity demands,** which include the relevance and importance to the client, objects used and their properties, space demands, social demands, sequencing and timing, required actions, required body functions, and required body structures.[1] For example, Mrs. Salazar is a client in OT who finds the occupation of baking for her family very meaningful. Because of her recent stroke, she has difficulty sequencing the steps for baking a cake. The OT practitioner modifies the demands of the activity by writing each step out very clearly on a sign that is placed in front of Mrs. Salazar while she bakes a cake. Evaluating activity demands allows the OT practitioner to match appropriate activities to the client's needs and to determine how to modify, adapt, or delete aspects of the activity so the client can be successful.

The activity demands change as a result of the **context** or setting in which the occupation occurs. Fig. 10.3 shows how context changes the requirements and demands of the activity of writing. It also shows how adaptations can make

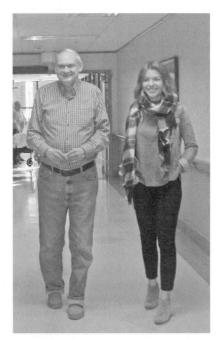

• **Fig. 10.2** As part of this man's daily morning routine (performance pattern), he walks to the coffee station, reads the paper, and socializes with friends. The OT practitioner accompanies him on this morning to evaluate his occupational performance.

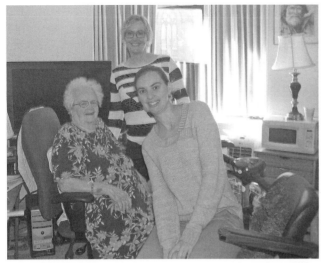

● **Fig. 10.3** The OT practitioner examines the space, computer setup (and adaptations), and tasks required for this author to type her story on the computer. Although the physical space is small, the large-screen monitor and adapted mouse make it possible for the woman to write her stories despite low vision and limited mobility.

## Case Application

The following case provides an overview of how the *OTPF* is used in clinical practice.

An occupational therapist working at a home health agency evaluates 2-year-old David, who has developmental delays, and finds out the following:
- The parents are concerned because David does not "play like other children."
- David does not sleep through the night, does not eat a variety of foods, and is small for his age.
- David drools and is difficult to understand. He talks using one-word sentences. He still sucks his thumb.
- David reaches with and uses a palmar grasp to hold objects. He walks with a wide-based gait.
- David smiles on approach and makes brief eye contact.
- David lives at home with three siblings (ages 7, 5, and newborn).

occupations possible. Context changes the requirements, patterns, and demands of the activity and the performance skills needed. For example, cooking a meal at home for one is much different than having five friends over for a holiday dinner. According to the *OTPF*, contexts include aspects related to the cultural, personal, physical, social, temporal, and virtual areas.[1] Table 10.2 provides definitions of each context.

Using the *OTPF* as a guide, the occupational therapist decides to focus intervention on play and feeding issues. Play and ADLs are occupations within the domain of OT. The practitioner determines that David plays every day for several hours at home with his older sisters. He eats three meals a day, but his parents report that David enjoys snacking while playing. After considering the patterns of performance, the OT practitioner examines David's motor, processing, and social interaction skills (performance skills). The practitioner explores the contexts in which the activities will occur. Specifically, the practitioner finds out that David will play with his

| TABLE 10.2 | Types of Contexts | |
|---|---|---|
| **Context** | **Definition** | **Example** |
| Cultural | Customs, beliefs, activity patterns, behavior standards, and expectations accepted by the society of which the individual is a member. Includes political realm, such as laws that affect access to resources and affirm personal rights. Also includes opportunities for education, employment, and economic support. | Ethnicity, family, attitude, beliefs, values |
| Physical | Nonhuman aspects of contexts. Includes the accessibility to and performance within environments having natural terrain, plants, animals, buildings, furniture, objects, tools, or devices. | Objects, built environment, natural environment, geographical terrain, sensory qualities of environment |
| Social | Availability and expectations of significant individuals, such as spouse, friends, and caregivers. Also includes larger social groups that are influential in establishing norms, role expectations, and social routines. | Relationships with individuals, groups, or organizations; relationships with systems (political, economic, institutional) |
| Personal | "[F]eatures of the individual that are not part of a health condition or health status." Personal context includes age, gender, socioeconomic status, and educational status. | 25-year-old unemployed man with a high school diploma |
| Temporal | "Location of occupational performance in time." | Stages of life, time of day, time of year, duration |
| Virtual | Environment in which communication occurs by means of airwaves or computers and an absence of physical contact. | Realistic simulation of an environment, chatrooms, radio transmissions |

From American Occupational Therapy Association. (2014). Occupational therapy practice framework: Domain and process (3rd ed.). *American Journal of Occupational Therapy, 68*(Suppl. 1), S1–S48.

7- and 5-year-old sisters, who enjoy playing musical games and pretend. The family has a safe and well-stocked playroom. David will get plenty of practice if the sisters participate in the sessions.

Contextually, the practitioner identifies that mealtimes may be very stressful because Dad has an inconsistent work schedule, leaving mealtimes to Mom (with four small children). Thus the practitioner decides to focus on feeding intervention strategies for snack times and subsequently provides adaptations (e.g., finger foods) to compensate for poor skills to ensure successful independent mealtimes. The activity demands of the feeding intervention are changed by modifying the types of food served to David, for example, by having him eat finger foods instead of foods that require a utensil. Furthermore, David is gaining weight and not experiencing any malnutrition. The OT practitioner examined body functions and structures to determine how they may be influencing David's performance.

This example provides an overall look at how to use the *OTPF* to guide intervention. Much more detail can be uncovered by examining each aspect of the framework. Furthermore, many OT models of practice also provide comprehensive guidelines that are congruent with the framework (see Chapter 15).

## Occupational Therapy Process

The *OTPF* provides a description of the process involved in OT. Specifically, OT practitioners are involved in evaluation, intervention, and outcome of services.[1] The occupational therapist is primarily responsible for the evaluation and interpretation of assessments. However, the occupational therapy assistant (OTA) may assist the occupational therapist, and he or she contributes to the evaluation by providing data, after service competency has been determined. Service competency refers to verifying that the OTA is able to produce results that are similar to and consistent with those of the occupational therapist. The OTA is not responsible for the interpretation of the results. The occupational therapist is responsible for developing the intervention plan.[2,3] The *OTPF* emphasizes an OT process that is client-centered and focused on enabling the client to engage in desired occupations. The process is dynamic and involves using occupation to meet goals and as outcome of therapy.

The **evaluation** includes an occupational profile and analysis of occupational performance. An occupational profile provides background information on the client's goals, habits, occupations, and history.[1] Generally, the occupational profile is obtained through an interview. However, the OT practitioner may also administer assessments to obtain the information. Box 10.1 presents the information collected for an occupational profile.

The evaluation process involves a **client-centered approach** whereby the OT practitioner determines the client's viewpoint, narrative, and desires. Because the aim of therapy is to help the client reengage in occupations, the client, if possible, identifies the occupations of interest. A client-centered

---

**• BOX 10.1  Occupational Profile**

- Background information: Client's name, age, diagnosis, medical history and pertinent information
- *Reason for referral:* Client's concerns, daily life activities. What does the client want to accomplish? What are the client's priorities?
- Goals: What are the client's goals and measurements of success?
- *Client's occupational history:* What is the client's background of occupational performance? In what type of activities did the client engage?
- What is supporting or interfering with the client's ability to complete desired occupations? (Does the environment support or interfere with performance?)
- How does the client view his/her current occupational performance? How does client define his/her quality of life?
- Is client able to fulfill his/her roles? Is client satisfied with current performance?
- Does client require modifications or adaptations to engage in occupations?

---

approach involves working collaboratively with clients and is considered a foundational component of OT practice.[1,6]

During the evaluation, the occupational therapist analyzes the client's performance skills and client factors to determine strengths and limitations for the client. The occupational therapist may choose to use formal assessments, including standardized tests or protocols, when evaluating clients. The OTA may assist in the process, once he or she has demonstrated competency in administering the assessment or protocol. However, the occupational therapist is responsible for the interpretation of the data.

## Intervention Plan

An intervention plan is developed once the occupational therapist has completed the evaluation, determined the client's strengths and weaknesses, and analyzed the areas of performance and contexts in which the occupations are performed. The intervention plan is developed with the client to address those areas important to him or her.[1,6]

The **intervention plan** includes a description of the goals and objectives of intervention. Although the occupational therapist develops the plan, the OTA may also contribute to its development (upon establishment of service competency). Goals are designed to be meaningful, relevant to the client, measurable, and occupation-based.

Once the goals and objectives have been established, the intervention approach is developed. The *OTPF* identifies five general approaches to intervention: create, establish, maintain, modify, and prevent. The following paragraphs describe each approach and provide a clinical example.

### Create/Promote (Health Promotion)

Intervention focused on creating and promoting provides opportunities for people with and without disabilities. The OT practitioner sets up a program or activity so that all those who participate will benefit by engaging in the activity. For example, activity programs that organize community outings for older persons benefit all participants.

> Mary, the occupational therapist at a local school, developed an after-school handwriting program to help third through fifth graders. The program provided fun strengthening and coordination activities, along with games to do at home. Mary created this program as a service to the children. OT students from the local university helped run the groups.

## Establish/Restore (Remediate)

The OT practitioner uses strategies and techniques to change client factors to establish skills that have not yet developed or to restore those that have been lost.[1] OT practitioners learn a variety of techniques designed to improve a client's skills, abilities, and function.

> Brian, the OT practitioner in a local rehabilitation hospital, worked with Jasmine, a 54-year-old woman who lost use of her right side after a cerebral vascular accident. The goal of the therapy sessions included increasing the use of her right hand and arm so she could prepare meals for her children again. Brian helped Jasmine improve right arm range of motion, strength, motor control, and eye–hand coordination. Remediation of these client factors ensures that Jasmine is able to meet her goals and cook for her family.

## Maintain

Using maintaining as an intervention approach supports the client to continue to perform in the manner in which he or she is accustomed. OT practitioners using this approach help clients keep the same level of performance and not decline in functioning. This type of approach may be chosen when the client has a prognosis that worsens over time. In this case the OT practitioner provides supports so the client can continue to perform at his or her current functioning level as long as possible.

> Harry is an 89-year-old man who still lives on his own in a small first-floor apartment. Harry experienced a mild heart condition that resulted in a brief hospitalization. The physician requested an OT evaluation to determine how to help Harry. Harry informed the OT practitioner that he wants to remain living alone; his family is close by for support. The OT practitioner conducted a home evaluation and made some changes in the environment to ensure safety (e.g., removed some scatter rugs, installed grab bars, added a call button for safety). These changes allowed Harry to maintain his current living situation, despite his decreased endurance and other natural effects of the aging process.

## Modify (Compensation, Adaptation)

Intervention aimed at compensation or adaptation involves modifying activities so that clients may continue to perform them despite poor skill level. Compensation refers to changing the demands of the activity or the way the client performs the activity.[1] Intervention focusing on compensatory or adaptation strategies is useful when client factors are not changeable in a practical amount of time and the client wishes to engage in the activity before remediation is possible.

> Gerard, a 60-year-old man, recently suffered a severe burn, which interferes with his ability to use his dominant right arm and hand. The OT practitioner provides Gerard with a one-handed knife for cutting, a Dycem mat to hold his bowl steady, and a cup with an adapted handle. These adaptations make it possible for Gerard to feed himself with his nondominant hand. These adaptations allow him to compensate for his inability to use his right upper extremity.

## Prevent

OT practitioners make it possible for clients to engage in those things that they find meaningful. Practitioners may help clients engage in activities to prevent or slow down disease, trauma, or poor health. The practitioner may design activity to prevent clients from losing function and allow them to continue to participate in daily activities as desired.

> Conrad is the OT practitioner in a rural community with a high percentage of families with obesity. Conrad and his colleagues develop a program for adults to engage in physical activity and to educate them in nonintimidating and interesting ways about nutrition. The OT practitioner adapts the physical activity as necessary and provides group activities to enhance self-esteem, self-concept, and healthy choices. This program is designed to prevent the complications that arise from obesity.

These intervention approaches show the range of possibilities for servicing clients. OT practitioners use clinical judgment, experience, and research to determine which type of approach works for the specific client within the particular setting. The OT practitioner considers the context(s), client factors, performance skills, performance patterns, and activity demands when determining the intervention approach. Once the approach is identified, the practitioner develops the intervention plan, which involves therapeutic use of occupations. The following section describes the types of OT interventions.

## Types of Occupational Therapy Interventions

The *OTPF* lists therapeutic use of self (see Chapter 17), therapeutic use of occupations and activities, consultation, and education as the types of OT interventions.[1] The evaluation process helps the OT practitioner determine what type of intervention strategy he or she will use. The OT practitioner also bases these decisions on models of practice (ways to organize one's thoughts[7,10]) and frames of reference (ways to implement therapy) (see Chapter 15). Upon determining the client's goal for therapy, the OT practitioner decides the best strategy for meeting the goals.

## Therapeutic Use of Self

Therapeutic use of self refers to the practitioner's interactions with clients and, in particular, how the therapist uses his or her own self to motivate and facilitate therapeutic goals. Therapeutic use of self involves paying attention to the client's needs and responding in a manner that promotes the client's goals. (See Chapter 17 for more detail.) Practitioners consider eye contact, humor, body position, and timing of interactions when interacting with clients. They facilitate through touching and gentle cuing, encouraging, and using their own self during the intervention. By understanding the client's needs, practitioners are able to adjust responses to promote client communication. Taylor found that practitioners used six modes when interacting with clients: *advocating, collaborating, empathizing, encouraging, instructing, and problem solving*.[11]

## Therapeutic Use of Occupations and Activities

**Therapeutic use of occupations and activities** refers to selecting activities and occupations that will meet the therapeutic goals.[1] OT practitioners may use **preparatory methods** or activities designed to get the client ready to engage in occupations.[1,5] Preparatory activities may include such methods as stretching, range of motion, exercise, and applying heat or ice; they are designed to get the client ready for purposeful or occupation-based activity. Preparatory activities should be conducted as one part of the intervention session rather than making up the entire session.[5]

Purposeful activities involve choice, are goal-oriented, and do not assume meaning for the person. **Purposeful activity** leads to occupation and may be a part of the occupation. For example, practicing folding towels is considered purposeful activity for the occupation of household maintenance.

The goal of OT is for clients to engage in occupations that they find meaningful. Therefore **occupation-based activity** refers to participation in the actual occupation, which has been found to be motivating and results in better motor responses and improved generalization. Occupation-based activity requires that the activity be completed in the actual context in which it occurs.

## Consultation

**Consultation** involves "a type of intervention in which practitioners use their knowledge and expertise to collaborate with the client. The collaborative process involves identifying the problem, creating possible solutions, and altering them as necessary for greater effectiveness. When providing consultation, the practitioner is not responsible for the outcome of the intervention."[1]

## Education

**Education** involves imparting knowledge to the client.[1] This intervention type involves providing clients with information about the occupation, but it may not result in actual performance of the occupation. For example, an OT practitioner who is treating a young child for a feeding problem may be at the house on one visit when it would be inappropriate to have the child eat. The practitioner can educate the mother by using pictures of the proper way to position the child during feeding.

## Outcomes

OT intervention is designed to help clients engage in occupations. It is important for OT practitioners to measure the outcomes of their interventions and to determine whether the overarching goal of engagement in occupations has been met. OT practitioners create specific measureable and meaningful goals with clients. They use these goals to determine the outcomes of the OT intervention.

The client's ability to engage in occupations is called **occupational performance.** The OT practitioner measures improvement or enhancement of the client's ability to engage in occupation. For example, a client at admission to a skilled nursing facility following hip replacement may not have been able to dress himself as a result of decreased endurance and prescribed precautions because of the surgery. The client receives OT intervention to improve his ADLs, and upon discharge he is independent in dressing with the use of assistive devices. The outcome in this case is his ability to independently function in the activity of dressing. Occupational performance outcomes are the most commonly used outcomes in OT. **Participation** in one's desired occupations is the ultimate outcome for OT intervention.

As clients improve skills and perform occupations, they show improved **role competence,** that is, the ability to meet the demand of roles.[1] Furthermore, clients become more able to adapt or change in response to varying situations. Another outcome that can be measured following OT intervention is **client satisfaction.** This is a measure of the client's perception of the process and the benefits received from OT services. Because OT is a client-centered approach, one hopes that the clients are pleased with the outcomes and the process. Furthermore, the outcomes of OT intervention may lead to a feeling of overall **well-being.** As clients reengage in meaningful occupations, they develop a sense of self, self-esteem, and a sense of belonging.

Engagement in occupations and activities influences a client's **health** and **wellness.** Health refers to the state of physical, mental, and social well-being, whereas wellness refers to the condition of being in good health.[1] OT practitioners may develop goals related to health and wellness. Clients may participate in programs to improve their health and wellness after discharge from

OT or as part of the OT intervention. For example, a client may benefit from a support group to encourage walking each day.

Because clients often become active in their lives again after OT intervention, **quality of life** may improve, and this is a desired outcome of intervention. Quality-of-life measures determine the client's appraisal of his or her satisfaction with life at that given time. Finally, another goal of OT intervention is **prevention** of further disability and the promotion of a healthy lifestyle. OT practitioners educate clients on ways to prevent further disability or decline. They may provide resources and adaptive equipment to support clients so that they can continue to participate in desired occupations. For example, the OT practitioner may create a support group to promote healthy choices and activities upon discharge from the hospital.

**Occupational justice** refers to allowing all persons (with and without disability) access to meaningful occupations.[1] OT practitioners may provide intervention to increase opportunities for people to engage in meaningful activities. For example, the OT practitioner may lead a community effort to create a playground that is accessible to children with disabilities. A practitioner may support adults in the community who have mobility issues by advocating for new sidewalks. Ensuring that there are additional seats at the ice rink may allow older persons to engage in a community ice-skating event by watching their grandchildren and socializing.

Outcomes are identified from the very beginning of the OT process, during the evaluation. Practitioners select the types of outcomes and measures they will use to determine success. They focus intervention on meeting the desired outcomes and reevaluate the client's progress toward the desired goal(s) throughout. Modifications to interventions and decisions about further intervention (i.e., continue intervention, discontinue intervention) are based on the client's needs and performance.

## Summary

The *OTPF* provides a description of the OT domain and process for OT practitioners, students, and consumers. The framework emphasizes occupation-based intervention. This framework may be used with a variety of models of practice and frames of reference. Together, the occupational therapist and OTA (upon reaching service competency) develop intervention goals by collaborating with the client. Once an intervention plan has been developed, the occupational therapist and OTA provide intervention that may include therapeutic use of self, therapeutic use of occupation or activity, preparatory methods, consultation, or education. The outcomes of OT include improving occupational performance, role competence, and quality of life. OT intervention may promote client satisfaction, health and wellness, adaptation, and prevention.

## Learning Activities

1. Match a list of activities with the occupations under which they fall.
2. Select an occupation that is important to you. Analyze the performance skills, client factors, and performance patterns required to engage in the occupation. Describe the context(s) in which you most frequently engage in this occupation.
3. Provide a clinical example for each of the five general approaches to intervention. Present these to your classmates.
4. Review research articles exploring OT intervention. Present a review of how the current literature describes therapeutic use of occupation and activities. Write a three-page paper describing therapeutic use of occupations.

## Review Questions

1. What are the differences between occupations, performance skills, and client factors?
2. How is the OT process described according to the *OTPF*?
3. Describe an occupation in terms of the activity demands.
4. What are the types of OT interventions?
5. What are the five general approaches to intervention?

## References

1. American Occupational Therapy Association. Occupational therapy practice framework: domain and process (3rd ed.). *Am J Occup Ther*. 2014;68(suppl 1):S1–S48.
2. American Occupational Therapy Association. Guide for supervision of occupational therapy personnel. *Am J Occup Ther*. 1994;48:1045.
3. American Occupational Therapy Association. Entry-level role delineation for registered occupational therapists (OTRs) and certified occupational therapy assistants (COTAs). *Am J Occup Ther*. 1990;44:1091.
4. Christiansen CH, Baum CM, eds. *Occupational Therapy: Enabling Function and Well-Being*. Thorofare, NJ: Slack; 1996.
5. Fisher AG. Uniting practice and theory in an occupational framework. *Am J Occup Ther*. 1998;52(7):509–519.

6. Law M, Cooper B, Stewart D, et al. The person-environment-occupation model: a transactive approach to occupational performance. *Can J Occup Ther*. 1996;63(1):9–23.

7. MacRae N. *OT 301 Foundations of Occupational Therapy*. Unpublished lecture notes, University of New England; 2001.

8. McHale K, Cermak S. Fine motor activities in elementary school: preliminary findings and provisional implications for children with fine motor problems. *Am J Occup Ther*. 1992;46:898–903.

9. Parham LD, Fazio LS, eds. *Play in Occupational Therapy for Children*. St. Louis: Mosby; 1997.

10. Solomon J, O'Brien J. Scope of practice. In: Solomon J, O'Brien J, eds. *Pediatric Skills for Occupational Therapy Assistants*. 4th ed.St. Louis: Mosby; 2016:1–10.

11. Taylor RR. *The Intentional Relationship Model: Use of Self and Occupational Therapy*. Philadelphia, PA: F.A. Davis; 2008.

# 11

# Occupational Therapy Across the Life Span

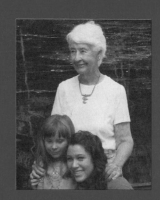

## OBJECTIVES

*After reading this chapter, the reader will be able to do the following:*

- Understand the changes that occur in occupation across the life span.
- Outline the developmental tasks throughout the life span.
- Understand how client factors progress throughout the life span.
- Describe the types of clients with whom occupational therapy practitioners work.
- Understand the unique services provided by occupational therapy at each developmental stage.

## KEY TERMS

| | | |
|---|---|---|
| adolescence | developmental frame of reference | learned helplessness |
| adulthood | family-centered care | least restrictive environment |
| aging | hospice | play |
| cerebral palsy | infancy | reflexes |
| childhood | Interprofessional team | |
| developmental delays | later adulthood | |

e Visit *www.evolve.elsevier.com* to access the Evolve student resources that accompany your book.

*As a boy scout, the moments that I loved most were those where you knew you made a difference in the lives of others. I have always wanted a career where I could re-create those moments, and I found that with occupational therapy. I love promoting independence and self-efficacy, being creative, and helping individuals fix the problems most important to them. I am still a student in graduate school, and I can't wait to get out into the field and make a difference in someone's life. Whether it's helping someone relearn how to eat independently or advocating for a client to productively age at home; I am so excited to positively influence people's lives and help them rediscover or engage in their meaningful occupations.*

PETER DASILVA
Class of 2017
Master of Science in Occupational Therapy
University of New England
Portland, Maine

**Case 1:** Evan is a premature infant weighing 4 pounds, 5 ounces, at birth. The occupational therapy (OT) practitioner works with him in the neonatal intensive care unit (NICU) to facilitate feeding, sleep–wake cycles, and regulation. The practitioner considers the medical context of Evan's intervention sessions along with parent and family needs. Evan's family travels far to see him each day, and the toll of the long drive to the hospital begins to show on his parents' faces. The OT practitioner carefully negotiates suggestions so as to support the family and client.

**Case 2:** Meanwhile, an OT practitioner works with Grace, a 98-year-old woman who hopes to remain at home despite a recent fall. Grace has lived alone since her husband died 25 years ago. She maintains a small house and entertains family on occasion. Grace walks to the post office for her mail daily. She has lived in the small rural town all her life. The occupational therapist evaluates the safety of her home and makes suggestions to Grace and the family so that Grace may remain at home.

Case examples 1 and 2 illustrate the varied approaches an OT practitioner may take with clients who range in age and ability. Because OT practitioners work with clients of all ages, practitioners need to understand the progression of developmental tasks throughout the life span. The following section provides descriptions of the developmental tasks expected of typical age groupings. Not all persons fit exactly into these groupings. Individuals may not complete all tasks in a given age range before moving to the next stage. There is variability in how and when individiduals complete the tasks. Thus practitioners view each person individually. The author provides an overview of diagnoses that may be associated with certain stages and a review of the settings in which OT practitioners may practice given a specific stage of development. These are just examples; OT practitioners provide intervention for clients of all ages and abilities in a variety of settings.

## Infancy

How big was your child at birth? At what age did your child roll, sit, crawl, walk, talk, or feed himself or herself? When did your baby sleep through the night? What are your child's favorite playthings? With whom does your child like to play? Is your child a picky eater? How would you describe your child's temperament?

OT practitioners ask these questions to learn about infants. Frequently, parents of infants wonder if their child is developing "typically." Because a wide range of "typical" behavior exists, OT practitioners must understand the typical range of development to provide parents with answers for promoting infant development and to provide effective intervention.

### Developmental Tasks of Infancy

**Infancy** represents the period of birth through 1 year (Fig. 11.1A and B). During this period, infants grow rapidly and achieve motor, social, and cognitive skills (Box 11.1). Gross and fine motor skills develop as infants begin to voluntarily reach, grasp objects, roll, sit, crawl, and eventually walk. Notably, infants grow in size, height, and weight. Frequently, pediatricians chart the infant's growth pattern as a sign of early development. Pediatricians also test an infant's reflexes. Primitive reflexes are present at birth or soon after, which is an indication of the infant's neurological development.[1] **Reflexes** are motor responses to sensory stimuli, such as moving one's foot when the sole of the foot is stroked or quickly putting one's hands in front to avoid falling. Infants possess a variety of reflexes. For example, the sucking reflex, which promotes nutrition, is present at birth.[1] Over the course of the first year, some primitive reflexes disappear while others (such as protective extension, righting, and equilibrium) remain. Thus the practitioner evaluates for the presence or absence of reflexes as an indicator of development. An infant who continues to have reflexes past the "typical" age may have sustained neurological trauma.[1]

Typically developing infants establish a sleep–wake cycle, and they experience periods of playfulness and express discom-

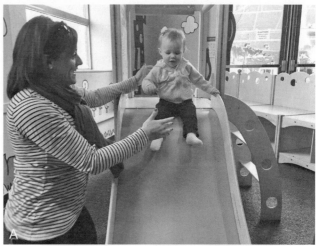

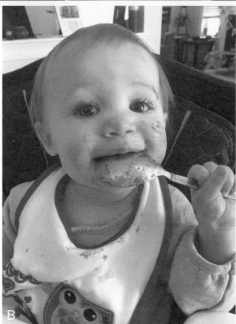

• **Fig. 11.1 A,** Infant sliding down a child slide, with mom close by. **B,** Infants begin to feed themselves, but are very messy.

---

| • BOX 11.1 | Developmental Tasks of Infancy (0–1 Year of Age) |
| --- | --- |

Exploration phase: Child explores self and environment
- Sensory solitary play
- Exploration phase: child explores self and environment
- Regulates sleep-wake cycle
- Rapid physical growth and development
- Motor: Integration of primitive reflexes, rolling, prone-on-elbows, sitting, pull to stand, crawling, walking
- Oral motor: manages different textures and types of food (liquid, pureed, chopped, some whole foods); suck-swallow-breathe, drink from straw, cup drinking
- Language: cooing, babbling, first words
- Fine motor: gross grasp, radial digital, inferior pincer, neat pincer; holding and releasing objects
- Social: smiles, interacts with others, peek-a-boo
- Cognitive: cause and effect, object permanence

fort through crying.[2] They can be consoled and stop crying once their needs are met. Infants who are not consolable may benefit from OT to help them learn to regulate their behaviors.

Socially, infants interact by smiling and expressing emotions to family members. Infants play pat-a-cake, make eye contact, and smile. Between 8 and 10 months, infants develop stranger anxiety and may cry when approached or held by strangers. Social language begins in infancy with sounds, vocalizations such as cooing, listening, speaking words, and learning to respond to simple verbal directions.[3] Infants begin to reciprocate by taking turns vocalizing or smiling, which is observed when they play peek-a-boo.

Activities of daily living develop as infants learn to recognize food sources and begin to hold utensils. They may allow caregivers to dress them, and they may enjoy bath time. Infants may begin to pick up food and put it in their mouths. However, infants are dependent on adults to maintain their self-care tasks.

Cognitively, infants develop awareness of objects, and they recognize familiar people. They begin to use toys and bring their hands to their mouths. The infant responds to his or her parent or caregiver. As infants begin to reach for and grasp objects, they learn cause and effect, an important concept for future learning. Infants learn by observing their surroundings. As they engage in their surroundings, they acquire the cognitive skills of object permanence (e.g., the object may be there even if it is out of sight). At this stage, infants begin to look for hidden objects.

## Diagnoses and Settings

OT practitioners working with this age group work in the Neonatal Intensive Care Unit (NICUS) hospitals, early intervention programs, community-based programs, outpatient clinics, and home health agencies. The NICU is a specialized environment with the main concern being the medical condition of the client. OT practitioners working in the NICU must receive advanced, specialized training. Refer to AOTA document Specialized Knowledge and Skill for Occupational Therapy Practice in the Neonatal Intensive Care Unit for more information.[1a] Pediatric hospitals serve children with numerous medical conditions for brief or extended times. Many pediatric hospitals offer outpatient care for children. This care is intended to maximize the child's development or monitor his or her progress. Some infants discharged from the hospital may receive periodic check-ups at outpatient clinics to monitor their development and growth. Early intervention programs provide services for children from 0 to 3 years of age and may provide services in the home or in specialized day-care settings. Children may receive early intervention services from a team of professionals. The focus of early intervention is on family-centered care; therefore, empowering parents to advocate for their children is an emphasis of these programs. Infants may be also treated in the home by OT practitioners who work for home health agencies.

Because infants are developing, many OT practitioners work in diagnostic clinics to evaluate and provide input into the diagnoses of children. Diagnosing children early may help with payment, care, course of intervention, and support for parents. Diagnosing is meant to help parents and caregivers understand and consequently intervene on behalf of children. However, children will function at different levels despite being given particular diagnoses.

OT practitioners work with infants who may have experienced birth trauma, disease, or genetic conditions that affect their development. Infants with **cerebral palsy** continue to be the largest referral to OT practitioners working in pediatrics. These children experience motor abnormalities caused by an insult to the brain before, during, or soon after birth. Infants with cerebral palsy do not reach milestones as expected for their age. Their motor deficits may result in slow, awkward, or asymmetrical movements. Although the progression of the disorder does not worsen, the child may appear to get worse as he or she ages because more is expected as children age. Other diagnoses requiring OT services include autism spectrum disorder, Down syndrome, spina bifida, Erb's palsy, and a host of genetic disorders.

Infants may experience **developmental delays,** which refers to a slower acquisition of skills over the first several years of life. Children with syndromes may be treated by OT practitioners and frequently exhibit developmental delays, cardiac difficulties, and intellectual delays (previously referred to as *mental retardation*). OT practitioners also work with infants who have failure to thrive, traumatic brain injury, HIV, or congenital anomalies, such as cleft palate.

The OT practitioner does not treat the diagnosis but rather intervenes with infants and families to help the child function at the highest possible level and actively participate in infant occupations.

The OT practitioner works with a variety of team members, such as physicians (neonatologist, developmental pediatrician, neurologist, etc.), nurses, social worker, case managers, speech language pathologists, physical therapists, physician assistants, dietitians, nutritionists, day care workers and family. Working as part of an **inter-professional team** is an essential part of occupational practice. This requires clear and respectful communication, teamwork, interpersonal skills, and knowledge of one's profession and that of the other professions.

## Intervention

The OT practitioner works with the infant and the family to facilitate development or, as Llorens suggests, "close the gap."[5] OT practitioners frequently use the developmental frame of reference to evaluate infants.[4,5] The **developmental frame of reference** postulates that practice in a skill set will enhance brain development and help the child progress through the stages. The OT practitioner using a developmental frame of reference begins by evaluating the current level of skill development. Once the practitioner has determined the skill level, the underlying client factors that may influence development are examined.[5] Factors such as muscle tone, coordination, symmetrical movements, and posture may influence motor development. Intervention is aimed at improving the underlying factors so the infant may perform the desired skill.[3] However, the goal of OT intervention is to improve the infant's participation in occupations. OT intervention with children is generally playful in nature, but it can include medically based intervention such as splinting, positioning, or cardiac rehabilitation.

OT practitioners working with infants provide **family-centered care,** requiring that they collaborate closely with the family. Family-centered care involves working with family members on goals that are considered important to them. This collaboration works best when members of the team respect and listen to one another. This philosophy of care supports parents as being "experts" on their child and urges practitioners to listen and respond to family requests.

OT intervention with infants frequently targets play, behavior regulation, feeding, motor skill development, and sensory regulation. Intervention involves playing with the child and providing activities to stimulate development in a variety of areas. OT practitioners also intervene through consulting and educating parents. Consulting with parents to address questions and concerns regarding the infant's development requires the expertise of an experienced OT practitioner. Consulting involves providing suggestions that the OT practitioner is not directly responsible for, such as suggesting an infant and parent attend an infant massage program. The OT practitioner discusses strategies to enhance the infant's success in activity. The OT practitioner may consult with other programs to collaborate on strategies that will benefit the infant.

Parents may need education about caring for their infant and addressing the special needs of the infant. OT practitioners frequently teach parents how to hold, handle, and calm their infant. Education on feeding techniques and developmentally appropriate activities is common practice. Education may include providing parents with information on the infant's diagnosis, prognosis, and intervention strategies. OT practitioners are skillful at providing this information in a language and format that is understandable to the parents and sensitive to their emotional needs. OT practitioners may also have to educate parents on the data supporting a given intervention. This may involve teaching parents what to look for in terms of outcomes or service from providers. Not only do OT practitioners consult and educate others, but they also provide parents with resources. For example, OT practitioners may provide specialized equipment to help infants with positioning, feeding, bathing, and mobility. Infants may require adapted toys that make it possible for them to grasp or manipulate. Practitioners may help support parents by recommending support groups, respite care, and assistance in making things easy at home. OT practitioners must consider the demands of parents when providing home programs. Box 11.2 provides a list of suggestions for home programs.

## Childhood

**Childhood** includes early childhood (1–6 years) and later childhood or school-aged children (6–12 years). Childhood represents a time of growth and refining of skills.[5] Children

---

| • BOX 11.2 | Suggestions When Providing Home Programs |

- Keep it simple; parents are busy and may be overwhelmed with demands.
- Provide playful, fun, and easy suggestions that can easily be incorporated into the day.
- Provide suggestions that will make things easier for the parent.
- Provide suggestions when asked.
- Limit suggestions.
- Write down home program suggestions.
- Be sure the parent will be successful when implementing the suggestion (adjust the activity so that it is easy to accomplish).
- Ask the parent to demonstrate the activity to you before suggesting it as a home program.
- Request that the parent demonstrate it to you when the family returns for the next session, and make sure you ask how it went. Let the parent show you how well the infant is doing. Praise the parent for being successful, and thank him or her for following through.
- If the parent did not follow through with the program, be sure to empathize and ask what interfered with the ability to do this. See if you can adapt the activity or provide a suggestion that will be more easily implemented.
- Try to provide the parent with activities for carry-through, not activities that are therapy. If the child does not like doing something with you, do not give that as a home suggestion. However, you may give a portion of the activity (in which the child is successful) so that the child is more prepared for the next session.

---

develop more coordination and strength and are therefore able to perform such skills as running, jumping, and more coordinated games. **Play** is the occupation of childhood; it is characterized as a spontaneous, enjoyable, rules-free, internally motivated activity in which there is no goal or purpose.[2] For example, children may spontaneously engage in playing and singing joyfully in the rain or at the beach (Fig. 11.2A). They will play pretend by dressing up in costumes and developing stories that become more complex with age (Fig. 11.2B). Furthermore, children progress from playing independently (solitary play) to playing alongside peers (parallel play) in early childhood. After parallel play, children gain more abilities and engage in cooperative play (play toward an end goal), and in later childhood, games with rules become important. The stages of childhood development are continuous and influenced by culture, family, and environmental variables (Box 11.3).

## Developmental Tasks of Childhood

Motor skills develop during early childhood as children learn to sit, walk, run, climb, and jump. School-aged children refine motor coordination and develop strength and endurance for activities.

Play is the occupation of childhood and the manner in which children learn and practice social, cognitive, and motor abilities.[4,5] Early childhood is a time of intense play.

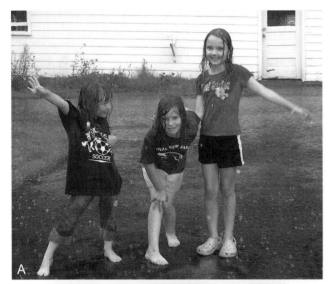

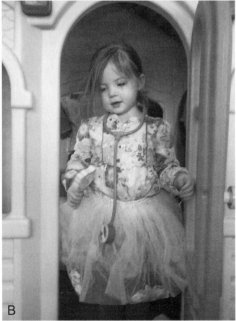

• **Fig. 11.2 A,** Children enjoy playing and singing in the rain. **B,** Preschool children enjoy playing dress-up.

• **BOX 11.3   Developmental Tasks of Childhood**

### Early Childhood (1–6 Years of Age)

- Competency phase:  Children begin to regulate behaviors and refine skills from earlier
- Fluctuations in behavior ("terrible twos") may be observed as child tries to assert self
- Begin to regulate behavior
- Refine motor, cognitive, and social skills
- Play: dramatic, construction, pre-games
- Fantasy play
- Develops conscience
- Learns to relate emotionally to parents, siblings, and others
- Distinguish between right and wrong

### Late Childhood (6–12 Years of Age)

Achievement stage:  Children refine skills and become proficient. There is concern for standard of performance.

- Student role is emphasized
- Develops skills in reading, writing, calculating)
- Physical skills for games and sports
- Increase speed, accuracy and coordination
- Social: Develops friendships with peers (outside of home)
- Develops attitude towards self
- Achieves personal independence
- Separates from family environment
- Develops consciences, morality, and values
- Independent in self care skills
- Develops IADL skills
- Identifies social roles of self and others (male and female roles)
- Begins to develop self-awareness and identity

role-play concerns and consequently deal with stressful situations through play. Imaginative play may help the child work through daily issues. Thus OT practitioners promote creativity and the problem-solving skills that come with imaginative play.

As children go to school, they engage in the occupation of education, which involves interacting with others, following rules, reading, writing, playground activities, and socialization. Children must follow school routines and communicate their needs to a new authority figure (i.e., teacher). They must pay attention to verbal directions, take turns, and transition to new activities. Remembering the rules, routines, and tasks associated with learning may challenge children. Such tasks as remembering sneakers for gym, the note from the teacher, or the homework assignment may appear straightforward to an adult, but may be stressful to a child and difficult to remember. However, these tasks are part of childhood, and therefore all children must have the opportunity to show they can complete them. In school, children must remember academic facts to participate in the cognitive processes entailed in learning.

Cognitive skills for learning require memory, attention, problem solving, sequencing, calculation, categorizing, language, and communication. Children must be able to show their cognitive skills through verbal and written communication. In addition, sensory perception is necessary for making sense of one's environment. For example, children

Children move from parallel play to cooperative play activities. The nature of play changes as the child develops expertise. This is easily observed when comparing the difference between 2-year-olds trying to share toys (something that may not be easily accomplished) and the behavior of 4-year-olds (who are able to skillfully negotiate sharing). As children enter school, they begin to participate in cooperative play. For example, school-aged children spend large amounts of time working out the "rules" to games and developing elaborate themes and scenarios for their play.[2] Sports and competitive games become important as children begin to test their new skills.

Imaginative play develops around 3 to 5 years of age. This type of play involves "pretending" or make-believe scenarios, which requires cognitive problem solving and sequencing. As children develop storylines, they may actually must not only identify the letters but also be able to use visual perception to ascribe meaning to them so that they can read.

Asserting one's needs is necessary to be successful in the classroom. Children need to ask questions when they are confused or curious. Furthermore, they need to hear answers and make sense of what they hear. Children with special needs may need help indicating their wants. Advocating for oneself is an important educational and life skill.

Along with the cognitive skills required for education, children engage in motor skills such as writing, tying their shoes, and carrying a book bag. Children move around the classroom. Motor requirements of gym or singing may pose difficulties for children. Children must be able to independently use the bathroom and eat in the lunchroom. Frequently, adaptations are needed to allow all children to participate in these activities. OT practitioners help children in schools who may have difficulty with these tasks. Childhood can be an exciting time for children. Yet children may require support and assistance in learning how to work with their strengths and weaknesses. Empowering children through play and successful experiences lay the foundation for a strong sense of self and lead to positive self-esteem and self-concept.

Social participation is an important occupation of childhood. Children learn to get along with others through play as they express emotions, communicate, negotiate, and work out play issues. Children learn to take turns, listen to others, and express their needs. Through play, they begin to realize that everyone is different, with their own strengths and weaknesses. In addition, children begin to figure out how social systems work; consequently, children may be "best friends" on one day and not speaking to each other the next day. These issues are important and emotional, and children may require support from the OT practitioner, parent, or teacher.

## Diagnoses and Settings

OT practitioners working with children provide intervention to children with such diagnoses as cerebral palsy, autism spectrum disorder, Down syndrome, intellectual disabilities, developmental coordination disorder, developmental delay, and others. Some children experience childhood illnesses, such as cancer, asthma, or sickle cell anemia, or have rare medical conditions such as William's, Angelman's, or Tourette's syndrome. Still others may experience physical disabilities such as spinal cord injuries, head injuries, amputations, burns, or orthopedic deformities. Finally, children may experience a host of behavioral and psychological disorders that may affect their ability to function in a school, such as attention deficit hyperactivity disorder, conduct disorder, learning disorder, or posttraumatic stress disorder.

Children receive OT in school systems, clinics, community settings, and hospitals. OT practitioners working with children and youth interact with a variety of other professionals, including teachers, teacher aides, resistants, school administrators (such as principals) and coaches. They may work with mobility specialists, speech-language therapists, psychologists, physical therapists, and adapted physical education teachers. OT practitioners must understand the roles of other professionals within the specific setting. As such, practitioners must understand the policies and procedures within the setting.

## Intervention

Intervention is designed to facilitate a child's participation in occupations. Interventions may require the OT to target foundational skills. While OT practitioners target foundational skills, they remain focused on occupations, such as the child's ability to feed, dress, bathe, toilet, play, engage in school, and socialize. OT practitioners working with children focus intervention on play development.[2] Through play, children learn motor, cognitive, social, psychological, and language skills. Children who exhibit play deficits may have difficulty interacting with others, sharing toys, maneuvering around objects, and exhibiting signs of joy.

OT practitioners may use play as the end goal of therapy or as a means to improve motor, social, or cognitive skills.[2,6] When play is the goal of the therapy session, the practitioner focuses on improving the child's play skills. When play is the means used in the session, the practitioner targets another goal through play.[2,4,6]

Donovan is a 3-year-old boy whose parents are concerned that he does not play well with other children, does not share his toys, and frequently throws toys at others instead of manipulating them. The OT practitioner using play *as a means* may design a play session aimed at improving Donovan's ability to pick up objects and use them as they are intended. The practitioner begins by playing a game of catch with large balls, showing Donovan that this is fun. Next, the practitioner introduces a variety of large-sized Lego pieces and playfully tries to get Donovan to build. Play is the means used to improve Donovan's reaching and grasping skills.

The OT practitioner may use play as the *goal* of the therapy session by focusing the session on improving Donovan's ability to engage in play. The goal of the session may be for Donovan to share his toys with the practitioner. In this scenario, the practitioner plays ball and a variety of games involving sharing of toys. Play is the goal of this session (specifically, sharing).

School-aged children spend a majority of their day in school. Therefore OT practitioners help children obtain the necessary foundational skills for sitting at a desk, reading, writing, eating in the cafeteria, playing on the playground, and participating in music, gym, and other academic learning. OT services provided in the schools are considered related services, and the role of the OT practitioner is to help the child function within the classroom in the **least restrictive environment.** The least restrictive environment is the classroom closest to a regular classroom in which the student can be successful. Inclusive environments, in which children are in regular classrooms as much as possible, are considered ideal for children with special needs, although some children require specialized classrooms for at least part of the academic day.

Practitioners working with children are creative, playful, and able to promote structure while setting firm limits. They are sensitive to the child's and parents' needs and attentive to the family. Intervention is aimed at play; school-aged tasks; and independence in playground behavior, handwriting, skills for learning (e.g., perception), and self-care skills.

OT practitioners working in schools are skillful at consulting with teachers and providing overall suggestions that may benefit students. For example, the OT practitioner may suggest that the teacher promote handwriting warm-up exercises in the middle of the day before writing. The OT practitioner provides the warm-up exercises and reviews them with the teacher but does not directly implement the intervention. An OT practitioner may work with children in the classroom or provide direct service to prepare children to be more successful.

## Adolescence

**Adolescence** may be considered a time of turmoil as the person tries to develop a sense of self that is independent from his or her parents. Searching for one's identity is the primary role of adolescence (Box 11.4).[5,6] This period of striving for independence is characterized by peer-group pressures to fit in or conform. Subsequently, adolescents focus on the peer group (Fig. 11.3A). Adolescents' clothing, hair, and language may imitate those of other members of the peer group. Adolescents may engage in competitive games and enjoy group play and team activities. The adolescent is often more concerned with group standards rather than adult standards. Adolescents begin to show interest in town, state, and country, rather than just focusing on the family (as in childhood).[5]

Adolescence is a period of role confusion and a time of developing a sexual identity.[5,6] In general, adolescents strive to develop their own identity apart from their parents. Therefore intense variability and insecurity may occur during adolescence. Puberty occurs in early adolescence; and, with this change, adolescents demonstrate a strong desire for attention, desire for physical relationships and strengthen gender identification. They seek out support from their peers while trying to establish independence from their parents. High school graduation marks a transition point for teens as they separate from their peers and parents (Fig. 11.3B).

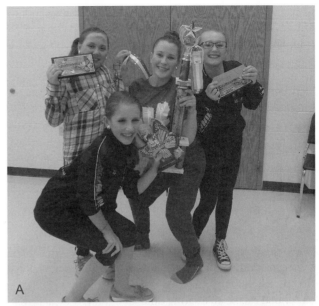

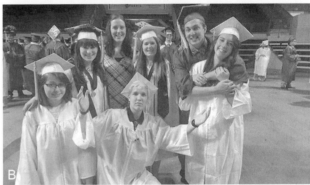

• **Fig. 11.3  A,** Teens enjoy socializing with each other and being on teams together. **B,** High school graduation marks an important milestone in adolescents' lives.

OT practitioners working with adolescents are aware of the challenges of this period of development when creating an intervention plan. OT practitioners work with adolescents who may have suffered disease, trauma, or a psychological event; they may require help to face the expected challenges of adolescence in addition to those presented by the disability.

### Developmental Tasks of Adolescence

Physically, adolescents are growing and becoming stronger.[5,6] Children going through the awkward phase of puberty may be physically self-conscious and require assistance in understanding changes in their bodies. Postural changes, awkward motor movements, and rapid growth all make movements somewhat challenging. Because the adolescent is concerned with how he or she is viewed by the peer group, the adolescent may spend more time on self-care, grooming, and hygiene issues. Girls will have to address menstruation issues. Boys will have to address the changes in their bodies as well. Furthermore, puberty is a time in which children develop a sexual identity.[4-6] Thus, parents and practitioners working

---

• **BOX 11.4    Developmental Tasks of Adolescence (12–20 Years of Age)**

- Developing identify
- Learning habits for adult roles
- Develop more mature relationships with peers
- Define social roles
- Develop sexual identification
- Select and prepare for occupation
- Seeks relationships outside of family
- Acceptance of one's physique
- Ability to use body effectively
- Set of values and ethics

with adolescents may need to address these issues. Adolescents can be self-conscious and egocentric. Safety issues may become important because an adolescent may make decisions that appear impulsive and immature. Leisure activities and social participation become very important to adolescents.

Adolescence is a period of self-identity. Adolescents start thinking about what they want to be when they grow up. Peer groups are important and influence the adolescent's dress, behavior, habits, choices, and routines.[2,6] Adolescents who experience psychological disturbances beyond those that are typical of adolescence may need intervention to develop self-concept, identity, and social skills.[2,6]

## Diagnoses and Settings

OT practitioners work with adolescents in hospitals, day treatment centers, school systems, or rehabilitation centers. Because adolescence is a time of transition, the OT practitioner may assist adolescents in transitioning to high school or with work readiness such as vocational rehabilitation. Adolescents with whom OT practitioners work require firm limits, choice, understanding, and positive role models. The OT practitioner will want to relate to the adolescent without acting like a peer. Adolescents going through puberty may have questions about sexuality, which the OT practitioner may need to address.[5,6]

Mental health issues and psychological disorders such as bipolar or borderline personality disorder[4-6] may arise during puberty. Furthermore, adolescents may exhibit signs of anorexia, bulimia, or other eating disorders. Adolescents may become conflicted. If they have difficulty coping, they may show signs of suicidal depression. Finally, adolescents who experience physical disabilities may require special attention to deal with issues of sexuality, body image, and future goals and aspirations. The OT practitioner helps adolescents with all of these issues.

The OT practitioner may interface with other professionals while intervening with adolescents, including vocational rehabilitation specialist, guidance counselor, community agencies, career planning professionals, coaches, teachers, psychologists, social workers, case managers. Adolescents who have disabilities may need help navigating insurance, policies regarding accessibility, and services in the community as they prepare for their future.

## Intervention

OT practitioners working with adolescents must set firm yet fair limits. Because adolescents typically question authority figures, the OT practitioner must be firm about expectations and consequences.[6] Generally, adolescents with whom OT practitioners work are experiencing emotional or physical trauma. This, along with the emotions associated with adolescence, may magnify feelings. Finding opportunities for the adolescent to express himself or herself appropriately (e.g., writing, reflection, small-group or individual sessions) is beneficial.[6]

Teens may push limits and question authority. However, they must learn to trust the practitioner. Practitioners gain trust by following through with tasks and checking in with the adolescent. It is helpful to give the adolescent control where possible.[6] In OT practice, this may be as simple as providing the adolescent a choice of activities.

OT practitioners consider how adolescents will interact in a group situation.[6] Sometimes, involving teens in healthy group activities provides them with the support and mentoring they need. For example, Special Olympics provides teens with disabilities a feeling of competition and team membership. Adolescents with special needs may need help in self-care, leisure, and independence. OT practitioners may lead groups to teach teens the necessary skills for grooming, hygiene, and other self-care tasks. The practitioner may use an educational approach or may have to adapt the tasks so the teen with physical problems is able to complete them. For example, providing adaptive clothing may be a good solution when a teen is unable to button or zip. However, the OT practitioner should include the teen's clothing preferences in this intervention strategy. Perhaps the teen would prefer to struggle with regular clothing so that he or she can wear a special outfit. The clinician must be aware of the client's motivations.

Other interventions target work-related activities to prepare the teen for the workplace.[6] Perhaps the teen is in need of social skills for work, refined work habits, or skills in filling out a job application. OT practitioners examine all aspects of gaining employment by analyzing what is required and by determining areas in which the client may need assistance.

Other teens may participate in few leisure activities or engage in unhealthy leisure activities. Exploring healthy leisure opportunities may open up new experiences for teens.

## Young and Middle Adulthood

*Where do you work? What do you do? Do you have a boyfriend or girlfriend?* These questions represent the challenges of young and middle adulthood. Adults assume responsibility for their own development or deterioration. **Adulthood** is generally considered a time of achievement, a time when the adult makes employment decisions. Group affiliations continue to be important (family, social, interest, civic). Adults are concerned with guiding the next generation, with creativity, and with productivity.

### Developmental Tasks of Young and Middle Adulthood

Adulthood can be separated into young (20–40 years), middle (40–65 years), and late adulthood (over 65 years). The developmental tasks may differ slightly among these stages of adulthood. In young adulthood, the developmental tasks include finding a significant relationship, securing employment, and developing a career path (Box 11.5). Adulthood includes establishing one's home—buying a home or

## Young Adulthood (20–40 Years of Age)

Independence
- Select and establish career
- Work is source of meaning
- Significant relationships
- Self-identity formed
- Establish family
- Child rearing
- Manage a home
- Balancing family, work and self

## Middle Adulthood (40–65 Years of Age)

Legacy to others
- Achieve civic and social responsibility
- Establish and maintain economic standard of living
- Develop leisure activity
- Adjust to aging parents
- Financial responsibility
- Midlife crisis - reformulate direction
- Women lose capacity to bear children
- Children leave home (empty-nest)

renting an apartment. Typically, adults have an established identity, live independently, and may choose to marry and start a family.[4,5] Families can differ in configuration. For example, a "traditional" family consists of husband, wife, and children (Fig. 11.4A and B). Today, however, families may consist of two men raising children or two women raising children. Some children are raised by grandparents or aunts and uncles. Adults make these decisions about whether and how they will raise children and what type of family configuration they wish to have.

A major focus of adulthood is selecting and establishing a career. In young adulthood, individuals may be completing educational or other work requirements for a career. Middle adulthood is generally considered a time when the adult has met the requirements for the career or job and has an established track record. However, many adults will change careers, and seeking a new career is also considered a task of middle adulthood.

Middle adulthood is a time when the adult has maintained employment, has established a satisfying lifestyle with loved ones, and is contributing to society. Successful adults may be financially secure and have friends and engage in leisure activities (Fig. 11.5).

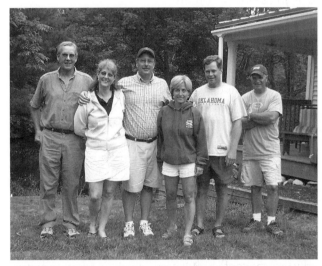

• **Fig. 11.5** Classmates enjoy spending time together during a recent reunion. The classmates (representing middle age) have established their own families and careers, and some have children entering college.

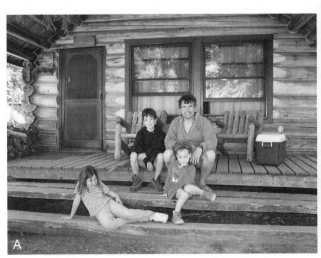
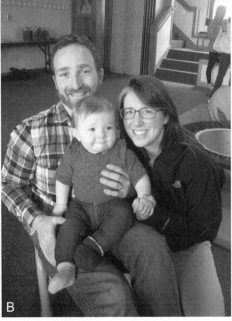

• **Fig. 11.4　A,** Adulthood is a time for raising families. This family spends vacation time together camping. **B,** These adults enjoy their new infant daughter as they balance career and family.

Interestingly, at some point many adults question decisions and examine their life progress. This is frequently referred to as the "midlife crisis." This may be a period when the adult changes jobs, goes back to school, or moves to another state. OT practitioners working with adults may encounter clients who have experienced a serious disruption due to illness, trauma, or a psychological event, and the practitioner helps the client reevaluate his or her abilities. Furthermore, later middle-aged adults must accept physical changes, such as decreased strength, decreased endurance, and signs of aging (e.g., wrinkles, weight gain, and hair loss).

Adults in this stage may be raising teenagers and adjusting to aging parents. This is sometimes referred to as the "sandwich generation" because adults may be caring for their children and their parents at the same time. Some middle-aged adults may be experiencing the "empty nest syndrome," in which their children have all moved out of the house, although it is common today that children who have left the house may return to live at home as young adults.

## Diagnoses and Settings

Adults may experience a whole range of physical illnesses affecting functioning, including heart disease, neurological impairments, orthopedic disabilities, and psychological disturbances. Schizophrenia, bipolar disorder, borderline personality, obsessive-compulsive disorder, and a wide variety of psychiatric disorders may emerge during adulthood. Furthermore, clients may have such diagnoses as obesity, substance abuse, and other unhealthy life choices, which influence their occupational performance. Adults may have experienced physical or psychological trauma that has left them ill-prepared to function in their various roles. The OT practitioner works alongside the inter-professional team to address the issues that are interfering with the adult's ability to engage in meaningful occupations. Other professionals may include physicians, specialists, psychiatrist or psychologists, life coaches, personal trainers, community agencies, financial resource specialists, dietitians, nutritionists, vendors, volunteer agencies, and family members. Practitioners remain in touch with resources and professionals who provide services for adults.

## Intervention

The goal of OT intervention with adults is to help individuals reengage in occupations that they find meaningful.[3–5] This involves examining the neuromusculoskeletal, social, psychological, and cognitive aspects of occupations within the contexts of the client's environment. OT intervention may also focus on psychological functioning and take place in psychiatric settings, group settings, day-treatment settings, or outpatient clinics. Clients with motor dysfunction may be treated at hospitals, at clinics, in rehabilitation settings, and in specialized programs. OT practitioners may also serve adults in the home or at work. Many work settings have ergonomic programs that employ occupational therapists.

## Later Adulthood

**Later adulthood** is a time of reflection and evaluation of one's life. Many physical changes occur during this period, and the older adult must adjust to physical changes. Older adults value group affiliations and may be concerned with what they will leave behind to the younger generation.

### Developmental Tasks of Later Adulthood

Later adulthood is characterized by retirement and a decrease in workload, and the emphasis shifts to community. Older adults deal with loss of spouse or peers, and this loss of others may result in depression, sadness, and prolonged grief. Some older adults have difficulty adapting to these changes; however, many healthy older adults are able to deal with loss and grief when supported by family and friends (Box 11.6).

Older individuals struggle with physical decline, although this does not have to mean a loss of independence. Physical decline common with later adulthood includes impaired hearing, poor balance and strength, and impaired vision. Adults in later adulthood may experience tactile changes or issues with poor circulation that interfere with their ability to feel changes in terrain.

Some older adults experience cognitive changes, such as difficulty with memory and attending to multiple stimuli. Remaining active physically and cognitively is important to staying independent and well. Many older adults stay active in community activities and family events (Fig. 11.6A and B).[3] Those who continue to be physically and cognitively active live longer and with fewer hospitalizations.[3] OT practitioners provide resources and supports to enable older adults to remain independent and actively engaged in meaningful occupations.

This often requires working with a variety of professionals, including physicians, therapists, social workers, case managers, and pharmacists. It may also require that the team interact with financial planners, estate planners, construction agencies (for accessibility issues) and community agencies for resources.

---

**• BOX 11.6    Developmental Tasks of Late Adulthood (Over 65 Years of Age)**

Adjustment to physical and psychosocial changes
- Decreasing physical strength and health
- Retirement and reduced income
- Loss of spouse and/or peers
- Establish affiliations with one's own age group
- Meet social obligations
- Independent living
- Adjust to decline in occupational performance
- Health changes
- Living arrangements
- Family stressors

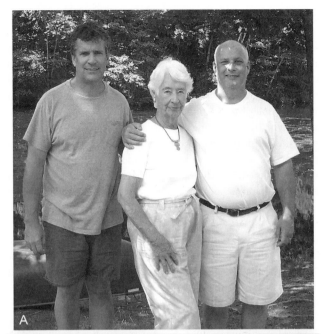

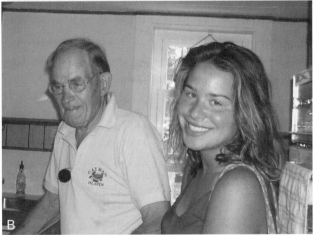

• **Fig. 11.6 A,** This mom enjoys spending time with her adult sons in the community. **B,** A grandfather enjoys spending time with his granddaughter at home.

## Diagnoses and Settings

OT practitioners working with older adults consider safety in the home and community. Wellness programs may be beneficial to older adults, such as those offered by senior citizen centers or local recreational leagues.[3–5] Clients with whom OT practitioners work may need assistance in modifying activities and help in obtaining education on the various diseases, diagnoses, and prognoses associated with them.

The **aging** process provides older adults with challenges not found in the other age levels. For example, older adults experience sensory and physical declines. Older adults may lose social supports, and they frequently lose income as a result of retirement. The OT practitioner may work with older adults who are experiencing difficulty transitioning into new roles or who have lost roles and are experiencing loss and grief. The OT practitioner working with older adults helps the client

remain active and engaged in his or her occupations, despite physical limitations. Such diagnoses as Alzheimer's disease, Parkinson's disease, stroke, cardiac conditions, rheumatoid arthritis, and diabetes may take a toll on the older adult.

Some clients with terminal illnesses may be served through **hospice,** which provides services to help the client be comfortable during the last stages of life. OT practitioners may help clients be comfortable while others are caring for them. It may be that the practitioner provides adaptive equipment (e.g., specialized lift) so that a client may be cared for more easily.

## Intervention

The OT practitioner is skilled at remediating dysfunction, compensating for lack of function, or adapting and modifying activities so that clients can be successful. Falls in the elderly and general safety issues are important concerns addressed in OT. Practitioners may be called upon to conduct a home visit to analyze the safety of the environment. Practitioners search for unsafe walking areas, which may include stairs, scatter rugs, and uneven floors. Older persons may require changes in lighting to help with safety issues. The OT practitioner evaluates whether the person is able to contact someone in case of emergency and determines whether extra precautions or accommodations need to be made in case of a fire or other home emergency.

Driving is important to older adults. Frequently, the physical changes of aging—such as delayed reaction time, slower movements, poor vision, and decreased hearing—make driving unsafe for older adults. Older adults who have suffered from cerebral vascular accidents (i.e., stroke) may have impaired physical abilities, such as decreased range of motion, causing them to have difficulty turning their heads to observe the road fully. They may have poor range of motion to depress the brake pedal adequately or a host of other issues interfering with driving ability. OT practitioners frequently analyze the numerous skills and client factors required for safe driving. The practitioner may help older adults regain skills for driving or address with the client how to use other means of transportation.

Because many older adults experience sensory changes, OT practitioners may help by providing instructions in large print and speaking loudly (although not infantilizing). Making visual accommodations, such as using contrasting materials, may be helpful to clients. Furthermore, limiting background noise, which may interfere with clarity of hearing, is beneficial to older adults. Older adults may experience difficulty maneuvering in crowded rooms with miscellaneous obstacles. Thus the OT practitioner should ensure that the physical space in which the activity occurs is not cluttered.

**Learned helplessness** refers to a phenomenon that some older adults may experience as they begin to feel and act helpless and relinquish control over things that previously held value. This occurs when others do everything for the older individual and do not allow him or her to make decisions and engage in activities. Some older persons are put into positions that do not feel comfortable to them. For example, if one spouse becomes ill, the other spouse may need to make financial and health decisions, which the spouse may not have not done before. This can cause stress on the spouse and hinder his or her health. Keeping clients active and engaged is important, and it is the foundation of OT practice. For those older adults who may not want to participate in activity, OT practitioners may ask them to help out a peer, which is frequently motivating for others. Furthermore, exploration of volunteer opportunities may prove rewarding for many older adults (e.g., reading programs, tutoring).

## Summary

OT practitioners consider the stage of life of the client when conducting evaluation and intervention. Each person enters different stages of life at different ages and for varied time periods. Clients may identify significant life events as turning points. Kielhofner suggests exploring the occupational profile of a client by examining the plots and trajectory of the person's life.[4] This provides the OT practitioner and client with a picture of a whole life to review. Understanding the developmental tasks over the life span provides important insight into the occupations associated with the period in a person's life.

## Learning Activities

1. Divide the developmental stages among members of the class. Ask each group to present the developmental tasks for the respective developmental stage in a creative and informative manner.
2. Divide the class into five groups and assign a developmental stage to each group. Ask each group to identify a variety of age-appropriate activities for the particular stage. Require each group to present the activities to the class, explaining why the activities are suited for their particular developmental stage.
3. Research the physical and psychological changes associated with a given age group. Summarize the findings in a short paper.
4. View movies such as *On Golden Pond*, *Father of the Bride*, and *The Breakfast Club*. Discuss the developmental issues displayed in each. Did the characters adjust to the tasks?
5. Develop a handout describing the expectations for each age group.

## Review Questions

1. What are the developmental tasks associated with each age group (infancy, childhood, adolescence, adulthood, later adulthood)?
2. In what settings do OT practitioners who provide services to infants work?
3. What are some of the physical changes associated with later adulthood?
4. What are some suggestions for OT practitioners working with children or adolescents?
5. What are some of the occupational concerns of children, adolescents, adults, and older adults?

## References

1. Anderson R, Boehme R, Cupps B. *Normal Development of Functional Motor Skills*. Austin, TX: Therapy Skill Builders; 1993.
1a. American Occupational Therapy Association. Specialized Knowledge and Skill for Occupational Therapy Practice in the Neonatal Intensive Care Unit. http://www.aota.org/-/media/Corporate/Files/Practice/Children/Browse/EI/Officiial-Docs/Specialized%20KS%%20NICU.pdf
2. Bundy A. Assessment of play and leisure: delineation of the problem. *Am J Occup Ther*. 1993;47:217–228.
3. Christiansen C, Baum C. *Occupational Therapy: Enabling Function and Well-Being*. 2nd ed. Thorofare, NJ: Slack Inc.; 1997.
4. Kielhofner G, ed. *A Model of Human Occupation: Theory and practice*. 4th ed. Baltimore, MD: Lippincott Williams & Wilkins; 2008.
5. Llorens L. *Application of a Developmental Theory for Health and Rehabilitation*. Rockville, MD: American Occupational Therapy Association; 1982.
6. Vroman K. Adolescent development: the journey to adulthood. In: Solomon J, O'Brien J, eds. *Pediatric Skills for Occupational Therapy Assistants*. 4th ed.St. Louis, MO: Mosby; 2016.

# 12

# Treatment Settings and Models of Health Care

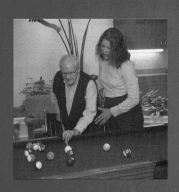

## OBJECTIVES

*After reading this chapter, the reader will be able to do the following:*

- Characterize settings in which OT practitioners are employed by types of administration, levels of care, and areas of practice.
- Identify the primary health problems addressed in different settings.
- Describe how treatment setting influences the focus of OT intervention.
- Describe workforce trends in occupational therapy.

## KEY TERMS

| | | |
|---|---|---|
| acute care | long-term care | public agencies |
| biological sphere | private for-profit agencies | sociological sphere |
| continuum of care | private not-for-profit agencies | subacute care |
| diagnosis-related groups (DRGs) | psychological sphere | |

ℯ Visit *www.evolve.elsevier.com* to access the Evolve student resources that accompany your book.

I have always been interested in why and when people choose occupational therapy as their career. I chose occupational therapy early on, but it took years for me to realize that it was, indeed, the career for me. My first love was art. However, when I was nearing the end of my sophomore year, I ran out of funds and could not continue as a contemporary crafts major at the University of Kansas. My aunt, an occupational therapist at the Menninger Foundation in Topeka, was supervising a fieldwork student from Texas Woman's University (TWU), and in her observation, there was money for OT students at TWU, and in that era OT was synonymous with crafts.

I graduated with my BS in occupational therapy from TWU 2 years later, in 1964. I set out to be an artist/craftsperson, financing my studio work by working as an occupational therapist. My next venture was graduate study in anthropology with an emphasis on American Indian textiles and textile conservation, then teaching fiber constructions in continuing education but also working as a part-time occupational therapist. The next degree was in counseling. As I moved from one discipline to another, I continued to work as a clinical occupational

therapist across the country, and then as an educator. It was somewhere around 1982, when I had returned to TWU as an instructor and was preparing to teach an occupational therapy history course, when I realized that my own personal evolution mirrored that of the profession. I didn't discover occupational therapy ... for me, it was a process—not of immediate discovery and ownership but of entering through the "back door" without much fanfare. It took some time for me to realize that occupation was the consistent thread that connected all of my interests: art, crafts, anthropology, and counseling. People and their occupations, their engagement in meaningful activities, these were the things that interested me; no matter what path I took along the way, I was an occupational therapist, or, as I prefer, an occupation-centered practitioner, and continue to be, quite happily!

**LINDA S. FAZIO, PHD, OTR/L, LPC, FAOTA**
**Professor of Clinical Occupational Therapy**
**Associate Chair of Academic and Community Program Support and Development**
**USC Chan Division of Occupational Science and Occupational Therapy**
**University of Southern California**
**Los Angeles, California**

Occupational therapy (OT) practitioners examine the biological, social, and psychological aspects of a person to determine how to help him or her engage in meaningful occupations. Consequently, OT practitioners work with clients of all ages and abilities, and in many different settings. This chapter provides an overview of the characteristics of settings, including the administration, levels of care, and areas of practice. Case examples are provided to illustrate application to practice. The chapter also provides an overview of employment trends for OT practitioners.

## Characteristic of Settings

The different types of settings in which OT practitioners are employed can be characterized according to (1) administration, (2) levels of care, and (3) areas of practice. Administration refers to the system's organization and management. Levels of care define the type of service and length of time a client receives services. Areas of practice relate to the types of conditions that the setting serves. Each of these characteristics influences the OT services provided to clients.

### Administration of Setting

Health-care agencies can be categorized as public, private not-for-profit, or private for-profit agencies. The categorization affects the agency's mission and purpose, reimbursement mechanisms, and organizational structure.

**Public agencies** are operated by federal, state, or county governments. Federal agencies include the Veterans Administration Hospitals and Clinics, Public Health Services Hospitals and Clinics, and Indian Health Services. State-run agencies may include correctional facilities, mental health centers, and medical school hospitals and their clinics. The county may operate county hospitals, clinics, and rehabilitation facilities that deliver services to clients in the same way as federal and state facilities. However, county administration follows different rules and regulations than federal and state administrations, which may affect employment or method of reimbursement.

**Private not-for-profit agencies** receive special tax exemptions and typically charge a fee for services and maintain a balanced budget to provide services. These agencies include hospitals and clinics with religious affiliations, private teaching hospitals, and organizations such as the Easter Seal Society and United Cerebral Palsy.

**Private for-profit agencies** are owned and operated by individuals or a group of investors. These agencies are in business to make a profit. Large for-profit corporations may form multifacility systems. These corporations may focus on one specific level of care (e.g., all hospitals or all skilled nursing facilities) or own multiple facilities across the continuum of care (e.g., a hospital, a skilled nursing facility, and an outpatient facility). A multifacility system is able to buy supplies and equipment in bulk at a lower rate. Because these systems provide a wider range of services, they have an advantage when it comes to developing contracts with third-party payers to provide health-care services.

### Levels of Care

Another way of characterizing health-care settings is by the level of care required by the client. Health care is provided to the consumer along a continuum, as the client's needs dictate, referred to as the **continuum of care. Acute care** is the first level on the continuum. A client at this level has a sudden and short-term need for services and is typically seen in a hospital. Services provided in the hospital are expensive because of the high cost of technology and the number of services provided.

The Prospective Payment System, introduced under Public Law 98-21 and passed in 1983, changed the way in which hospitals were paid through Medicare.[9] Under this system, a nationwide schedule defines how much Medicare reimburses hospitals. Depending on the client's diagnosis, hospitals are paid a predetermined, fixed fee, based on **diagnosis-related groups (DRGs),** regardless of the services provided.[9] The system provides an incentive for hospitals and physicians to reduce costs and to discharge clients from the hospital as soon as possible. As a result of the 1983 Prospective Payment System, the average length of a hospital stay decreased.[6,9] The move to short hospital stays and the implementation of cost-cutting measures changed rehabilitation as less funds were available for patients. The Balanced Budget Act (BBA) of 1997 and the BBA refinement (1999) were enacted to control costs. Other classification systems (i.e., Minimum Data Set—Resource Utilization Groups) and measures such as the Functional Independence Measure (FIM) were developed to better meet the needs of clients while containing costs.[6,9]

Shorter inpatient hospital stays also created a need for an interim level of care, referred to as **subacute care.** At this level, the client still needs care but does not require an intensive level or specialized service, thereby reducing hospital costs. Typically these clients require 1 to 4 weeks more of rehabilitation. Hospitals with excess acute care beds have converted beds to less expensive subacute care beds, whereas skilled nursing facilities have upgraded some beds to the subacute level. Freestanding subacute care facilities have been established to address client needs. The client typically served by a subacute care facility may have sustained a stroke or hip fracture or may have a cardiac condition or cancer. Rehabilitation services, including OT services, are a major component of subacute care.

**Long-term care** serves clients who are medically stable but who have a chronic condition requiring services over time, potentially throughout life. Persons who have developmental disabilities, history of mental illness, age-related disabilities, or injury resulting in a severe disability may require this level of care. Services provided at this level may take place in an institution, a skilled nursing or extended care facility, a residential care facility, the client's home, an outpatient clinic, or a community-based program.

## Areas of Practice

Health-care practice areas may be grouped into (1) biological (medical), (2) psychological, and (3) sociological (social). Health problems occurring in any of the areas affect a person's ability to engage in occupations. Table 12.1 provides an outline of the settings according to area of practice. OT practitioners help clients reengage in those occupations that are problematic for them because of a biological, psychological, or sociological disease, trauma, or condition.

Some settings address the **biological sphere** of health. This refers to medical problems caused by disease, disorder, or trauma. The OT practitioner working in a setting addressing biological issues targets such things as loss of capacity, diminished awareness or perception, limitation in development or growth, limitation in movement, pain, damage to body systems, and neuromuscular disorders.

Other health organizations focus on helping clients manage problems in the **psychological sphere**, such as emotional, cognitive, and affective or personality disorders. These difficulties may be caused by an inability to cope with stress, biochemical imbalance, disease, or a combination of

developmental and environmental factors. OT practitioners address psychological problems that affect thinking, memory, attention, emotional control, judgment, and self-concept. OT practitioners specifically focus on addressing issues that interfere with the client's ability to engage in desired occupations.

Health-care settings may also emphasize issues in the **sociological sphere** to help clients meet the expectations of society. Social problems may result from severe physical or cognitive disability that limits functioning, developmental delays, intellectual disability, long-term emotional problems, or a combination of problems. OT practitioners address such things as the absence of the ability to take care of one's own needs, lack or loss of life skills, poor interpersonal skills, failure to properly adapt to environmental changes, lack of capacity for independent functioning, and improper or detrimental behavior patterns. In general, these problems require long-term life adjustments. The OT practitioner addresses factors that interfere with the client's abilities to participate in social activities. The following case shows the interaction between biological, psychological, and sociological factors and how they influence occupational performance.

> Jim receives OT services to improve his work skills so he can return to work. The OT practitioner examines his work skills to determine whether his lack of skills is a result of biological (e.g., limited range of motion, loss of sensation, coordination, abnormal muscle tone), psychological (e.g., poor organization, intrusive thoughts, limited problem solving, lack of motivation), or sociological (e.g., inability to follow directions, lack of awareness of social norms, limited life skills) problems. The goals, objectives, and techniques of intervention differ with regard to the types of problems the client possesses. The practitioner prioritizes goals and addresses the areas that will allow for change by increasing the client's functioning.

OT practitioners address issues interfering with a client's ability to engage in occupations. The OT practitioner employed in a medical setting must also address psychological and sociological factors when treating a client with biological limitations. Jim's work problems may be related to his medical condition (biological) and difficulties with anxiety, organization, and concentration (psychological) or an inability to adhere to social norms in the workplace (sociological). All of these areas are important for success in the workplace. OT practitioners view clients holistically and carefully examine biopsychosocial issues affecting occupational performance.

> An OT practitioner working in a community mental health clinic is teaching life skills to adults who have intellectual disabilities as a group. The practitioner helps clients engage in community activities, use the bus system, and understand basic social interactions (e.g., "please" and "thank you"). This setting generally addresses sociological issues interfering with performance. However, the OT practitioner discovers specific upper extremity weakness in one client during a life skills group. The discovery of a weakness in the upper extremity requires further evaluation of and work on a goal that is considered biological—strengthening. Because decreased upper extremity functioning will interfere with the client's ability to complete life

**TABLE 12.1    Employment Settings**

| Areas of Practice | Settings |
|---|---|
| Biological (medical) | Hospitals (general, state and federal, specialty)<br>Clinics<br>Work sites (industry)<br>Home health<br>Skilled nursing facilities |
| Sociological (social) | Schools (public, special—visual impairment, hearing impairment, cerebral palsy)<br>Day treatment<br>Hippotherapy centers<br>Workshops<br>Special Olympics<br>Special camps (e.g., summer camps) |
| Psychological | Institutions (psychiatric, mental retardation)<br>Community mental health<br>Teen centers<br>Supervised living<br>After-school programs |
| All inclusive | Long-term care |
| Private practice | Self-defined |
| Nontraditional | Correctional facilities<br>Hospice<br>National societies |

Note: The categories do not indicate specialization. There are overlapping services in all areas; the classification highlights the setting's primary concern.
Adapted from Reed, K., & Sanderson, S. R. (1992). *Concepts in occupational therapy* (3rd ed.). Baltimore, MD: Lippincott Williams & Wilkins.

tasks, the clinician must also address this. Psychologically, the client may develop anxiety in social situations so great that she cannot participate. The OT practitioner determines that this psychological issue interferes with her social participation. The OT practitioner targets anxiety by working on relaxation techniques, role playing, and discussion.

The previous case shows how OT practitioners evaluate all areas of performance. OT practitioners evaluate biopsychosocial issues and intervene as needed to help clients perform. In the previous case, helping a client develop upper extremity strength and decrease anxiety are as important as teaching social skills to improving life skills, and therefore they are necessary components of the OT sessions.

## Settings

AOTA (2015) conducted a survey to determine the settings in which OTR and COTAs currently practice. Occupational therapists primarily work in hospitals (37%), school systems (20%) and, skilled nursing facilities (19%).[2] OTAs work primarily in skilled nursing facilities, (56%), schools (15%) and hospitals (11%).[2] Fig. 12.1 illustrate occupational therapy practice in each of these settings.

### Biological Focus

Medical facilities address biological or medical issues of clients. Intervention follows a medical model of identifying and addressing problems. These settings address clients'

medical concerns, including neurological, musculoskeletal, immunological, hematological, pulmonary, or cardiac systems. Many settings use a medical approach toward health care. Occupational therapists who work in these settings help clients perform daily occupations through remediation, restoration, rehabilitation, adaptation, or compensation techniques.

### Hospitals

Clients in hospitals receive care for acute illnesses. OT evaluation and intervention in hospitals generally focuses on medical and functional concerns. The OT practitioner evaluates feeding, dressing, bathing, and grooming, along with range of motion, muscle and perceptual functioning, problem solving, and thought processing. The practitioner may provide activities to increase strength, coordination, or self-care skills. The OT practitioner addresses concerns regarding the client's ability to return home (e.g., home equipment needs, family training, safety).

In addition to inpatient acute care, some hospitals provide rehabilitation services over a longer period of time. OT services in these specialty units occur within the general hospital. A typical rehabilitation unit provides services to clients who have sustained a disabling condition, such as stroke, head trauma, burns, or spinal cord injury. Rehabilitation services are also provided in the neonatal intensive care unit (NICU) for premature infants. The OT practitioner working in a NICU provides sensory stimulation, positioning, and feeding intervention. Training parents is also part of the intervention.

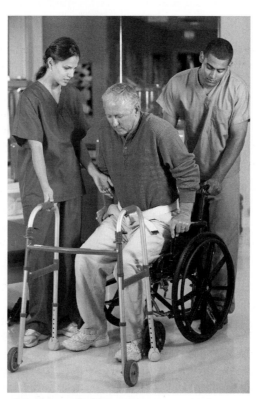

• **Fig. 12.1**  Hospital based occupational therapy practice may involve helping a client who had a stroke wash his face at bedside. © GettyImages/Creative RF/kali9.

OT practitioners are employed at rehabilitation centers to provide services to a particular group of clients, such as those with spinal cord injuries, head traumas, burns, or disorders. OT practitioners interact with a variety of medical professionals and, therefore, must understand the roles of other professionals.

## Clinics

Clinics generally serve clients with disabling conditions on an outpatient basis. These clients may have been recently discharged from a hospital setting but still need therapy services. Outpatient clinics may be affiliated with a hospital, or they may be a separate entity. The OT practitioner working in an outpatient clinic helps clients regain long-term occupational performance. Practitioners work to help clients engage in their occupations through remediation, rehabilitation, adaptation, and compensation. Rehabilitation clinics focusing on improving abilities include the Easter Seal Society, hand clinics, orthopedic clinics, cardiac rehabilitation clinics, and children's developmental clinics.

## Home Health Agencies

OT practitioners working for home health agencies provide therapy in the client's home. The practitioner works on problems related to performance in self-care, home management, work and school, or play and leisure. Because practitioners working for home health agencies travel to clients, it may be difficult to communicate with team members. Oftentimes, the practitioner maintains communication with team members through documentation.

The OT practitioner may also work in the home of a person who receives hospice care. In this case the emphasis of OT services is to maintain the person's abilities while making him or her comfortable and helping loved ones care for the client. When working with clients receiving hospice care, OT practitioners may provide modifications and compensations for decreased ability instead of trying to facilitate skill development and improve functioning.

## Settings with a Social Emphasis

Some clients experience functional limitations that impede their ability to satisfactorily interact with others. Frequently, these clients have long-term needs requiring that the OT practitioner help them improve social participation despite limitations. Interventions at settings with a social emphasis focus on social skill development rather than medical issues. Settings with a social focus may include mental health centers such as day-treatment settings or community agencies.

## Schools and Special Education

In 1975, the Education for All Handicapped Children Act, known as Public Law (PL) 94-142, passed, making public school education available to all children, regardless of handicap or disability. Related services, such as OT, physical therapy, and speech–language pathology, are included in this law, which mandates that children have the services they need to be successful in the classroom. This law allows OT practitioners to work in school systems to help children engage in education. This law has been updated to the Individuals with Disabilities Educational Act, which allows children with disabilities (physical, psychosocial, or cognitive) to receive a free public education, with services such as occupational, physical and speech therapy. IDEA also supports the use of technology and reasonable accommodations so that all children may benefit from an education. Practitioners working in school systems should become knowledgeable about the laws that support their services. OT practitioners working in school settings may work with children who are mainstreamed or in specialty schools for children with autism, visual impairment (blind or low vision), hearing impairment (deaf), and cerebral palsy (CP).

To receive federal funding, every county in every state must provide therapy services to children with disabilities in schools. OT practitioners are either hired as an employee of the school district or contracted independently to provide services.

## Day Treatment

Day-treatment facilities serve people who need daytime supervision or are able to live in the community (rather than in an institution or full-care facility) but who require some assistance. Some individuals may live at home with families whose members work, whereas others live in boarding homes but cannot plan their own activities. OT practitioners are employed in day-treatment settings to develop and provide structured programs of activities for clients. Day-treatment programs may specialize in providing intervention activities for a variety of groups, including children with behavioral disorders, persons who have mental illness, persons with Alzheimer's disease, or older persons.

## Workshops

Some communities provide special workshops for people who are not able to seek employment in a competitive job market. These workshops include sheltered workshops, training centers, and retirement workshops. Many clients in sheltered workshops have some type of developmental disability. OT practitioners may work on skill development, work hardening, environmental adaptations, or task modifications to help clients engage in the structured work.

## Settings with a Psychological Emphasis

A variety of settings focus on improving psychological functioning for occupational performance. These settings are regarded primarily as psychiatric or mental health settings but also address social difficulties.

## Institutions

Deinstitutionalization, implemented in the 1970s, refers to moving clients who have mental illnesses from institutions (such as state mental hospitals) back into the community. Some state hospitals continue to provide services for those with severe developmental or emotional disabilities. These institutions (or state hospitals) may offer traditional psychiatric OT programs wherein the practitioner plans activities (e.g., crafts, recreation, outings) for the purposes of self-care, skill development, self-awareness, leisure exploration, and social participation.

## Community Mental Health Centers

Community mental health centers emerged with the closing of institutions and are organized differently in regions and towns. Community mental health centers may offer medication clinics and counseling, crisis units, or day-treatment programs. In community mental health settings, OT practitioners work with a client or group of clients to develop life skills, encourage social participation, explore leisure opportunities, and develop abilities to engage in areas of performance.

## Supervised Living

Supervised living refers to partially or fully supervised housing for people whose problems do not warrant institutional care but who are not ready or able to manage on their own. Programming may vary from limited guidance to fully structured programs. Supervised living may include substance abuse programs (often with a specific time limit); halfway houses, which provide temporary living arrangements for someone leaving an institution before going to independent living; or group homes, which are more permanent living arrangements. In these settings, the OT practitioner may work with the client on general planning (e.g., organizing household chores), participating in social events (e.g., outings, recreational activities), and engaging in life-skills training. Older persons may live in assisted living facilities and may require OT services for physical, social, or psychological difficulties. OT practitioners may design activities for groups or individuals.

### All-Inclusive Settings

All-inclusive settings include long-term care facilities that provide OT services that address biological, psychological, and sociological functions. An all-inclusive facility (such as a skilled nursing facility) provides residence for people for long periods of time. The special skills needed by the OT practitioner in these settings depend on the nature of the facility.

### Nontraditional Settings

OT practitioners work in correctional facilities, industrial settings, hospice, and community transition settings. Practitioners may also work with therapeutic riding, aquatherapy, and in senior citizen centers. Some practitioners work with migrant workers, victims of disasters, or homeless people. The role of the practitioner varies according to the setting, but the aim is to help individuals function more fully in their lives. Practitioners may choose to work in wellness programs (such as those to help promote physical activity and nutrition for children or programs to promote healthy living in older persons).[1]

### Private Practice and Consulting

Self-employment, or private practice settings, address a variety of aspects of client functioning and include clients of all ages and diagnoses. Private practice settings in OT have increased since 1988, when the federal government, through the Health Care Financing Administration, implemented Medicare Part B coverage. This enabled OT practitioners to fully participate in Medicare programs by permitting qualified practitioners to apply for Medicare provider numbers. A provider number allows a practitioner to become an independent provider and to bill directly for services.[4,8]

OT practitioners working in private practice may take individual referrals and administer intervention in private homes or have clients come to their facilities. They may contract with agencies to spend a specific number of hours at a school or at a skilled nursing facility. Some private practice companies employ practitioners from many disciplines. Some practitioners in private practice consult with other agencies. Consultation requires highly developed professional expertise and management skills; the consultant and agency negotiate the parameters of service and set their own limits. OT practitioners also consult with organizations in areas such as ergonomics, facility design, and wellness.[1–3,8,10]

## Occupational Therapy Employment Trends

According to the Bureau of Labor Statistics (2014), OT and OTA employment opportunities are expected to grow "much faster than average" (increase 27% and 40%, respectively) between 2014 and 2024.[10] Job opportunities are good, especially for practitioners working with the elderly. Occupational therapists are taking on supervisory roles, allowing OTAs to work more closely with clients.[10] Growth in the older population, the baby-boom generation's move into middle age, and medical advances continue to increase the demand for OT.[1,10] Evidence-based research supporting the effectiveness of OT intervention continues to support therapy.[7,10]

More than half of occupational therapists (51%) are working in offices or hospitals, followed by schools and early intervention centers (12%).[2,3] Other major employers include home health services (9%) and skilled nursing care facilities (9%).[2,3,10] In May 2014, the median annual wage of occupational therapists was $78,810 and for OTAs was $56,950.[10]

According to 2014 workforce data, salaries for both occupational therapists and OTAs have risen since 2010 reports (8.2% and 9.1% increase, respectively). There was also a decline in median age for occupational therapists (39 years from 41) and OTAs (42 years from 43) and a decline in years of experience (from 12 years to 9 years).[2,3] This shows that the workforce is somewhat younger than in past reports. Of significance was the gender gap in salaries, with men making 10% more than women for both occupational therapists and OTAs.[2,3]

The 2014 data reveal that 60% of occupational therapists hold a master's degree.[2] In its examination of the academic workforce, the 2010 American Occupational Therapy (AOTA) report found that educational programs are in need of experienced faculty with earned doctoral degrees; only 48% of OT faculty held doctoral degrees.[5] Faculty are mostly between 50 and 59 years of age (40%), and more than half of program directors (62%) reported being between 50 and 69 years of age (49% fell in the 50–59 age range).[5]

Future practice areas targeted for growth include the following: broader scope in schools, bullying, childhood obesity, autism in adults, aging workforce, veterans and wounded warriors, cancer care and oncology, ergonomics, accessibility design, driver assessment and training, assisted living, technology, health and wellness, low vision, Alzheimer's, children and youth needs, and community service (see Chapter 4).[1,11]

## Summary

Settings in which OT practitioners are employed may be characterized according to (1) administration of the setting, (2) levels of care, and (3) areas of practice.

OT practitioners view the biological, sociological, and psychological functioning of clients within the context of their environment. Thus OT practitioners work in a variety of intervention settings with many types of clients who have varying abilities. As such, care is tailored to the client's needs and may take place in acute, subacute, long-term, and rehabilitation settings. OT practitioners work primarily in hospital and school settings. However, many OT practitioners are expanding services into nontraditional settings.

OT is a growing profession with many career opportunities. Practitioners may choose from a variety of settings and work with clients of all ages and disabilities. OT practitioners may elect to practice and educate future practitioners or serve in supervisory roles. Practitioners are urged to take advantage of growth opportunities.

## Learning Activities

1. Research occupational therapy employment settings in your area. Describe the types of settings, types of clients served, and the level of care provided.
2. Make salary comparisons for entry-level practitioners (occupational therapists and OTAs) in different kinds of employment settings.
3. Observe occupational therapy in two different settings. Describe the clients and the services provided. Discuss

how the practitioner worked with clients. Identify the area of practice.
4. Determine a need in your community, and define the type of services an OT practitioner could provide.
5. Review the job requirements for a particular setting that interests you. Present a brief description to the class.

## Review Questions

1. What are the levels of care provided to clients?
2. What are the types of settings in which OT practitioners work?
3. What are the three areas of practice? Provide examples of the type of OT services considered within each area.

4. What are some nontraditional settings in which OT practitioners work?

## References

1. American Occupational Therapy Association. *What Does the Future of Occupational Therapy Look Like?* Retrieved from, http://www.aota.org/Education-Careers/Advance-Career/Salary-Workforce-Survey/future-ot-occupational-therapy-look-like.aspx; 2016.
2. American Occupational Therapy Association. *2015 Salary and Workforce Survey: Executive Summary.* Retrieved from, http://www.aota.org/-/media/Corporate/Files/Secure/Educations-Careers/Salary-Survey/2015-AOTA-Workforce-Salary-Survey-LOW-RES.pdf; 2015.
3. American Occupational Therapy Association. Surveying the profession: the 2015 AOTA salary and workforce survey. *OT Practice.* 2015;20(11):7–11.
4. American Occupational Therapy Association. *Tips for Maximizing Your Clinical Documentation.* Retrieved from, http://www.aota.org/Practice/Manage/Reimb/maximize-clinical-documentation-tips.aspx; 2015.
5. American Occupational Therapy Association. *Faculty Workforce Survey.* Bethesda, MD: Author; 2010. Retrieved from, http://www.aota.org/-/media/Corporate/Files/EducationCareers/Educators/OTEdData/2010%20Faculty%20Survey%20Report.pdf.
6. American Occupational Therapy Association. *Reimbursement and Regulatory Policy Department. AOTA Guide to Medicare Local Coverage Determination;* 2007. Retrieved from, http://www.aota.org/practice/productive-aging/driving/practitioners/-/media/corporate/files/secure/advocacy/reimb/news/archives/medicare/lcds/resources/lcd%20advocacy%20packet1.pdf.
7. American Occupational Therapy Association. *AOTA Evidence-Based Practice Resources.* Retrieved from, http://www.aota.org/Practice/Researchers/EBP-Resources.aspx; 2016.
8. Reed K, Sanderson SR. *Concepts in Occupational Therapy.* 3rd ed. Baltimore, MD: Lippincott Williams & Wilkins; 1992.
9. Roberts P, Gainer F. Preparing for inpatient rehabilitation prospective payment: an introduction. *Administration & Management Special Interest Section Quarterly.* 2001;17(2):1–4.
10. U.S. Department of Labor, Bureau of Labor Statistics. *Occupational Outlook Handbook (2016–17 ed.);* 2015. Retrieved from, http://www.bls.gov/ooh/healthcare/occupational-therapist.htm.
11. Yamkovenko S. *The Emerging Niche: What's Next in Your Practice Area?* Retrieved from, http://www.aota.org/practice/manage/niche.aspx; 2016.

# 13

# Service Management Functions

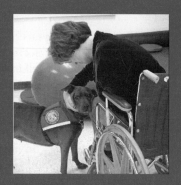

## OBJECTIVES

*After reading this chapter, the reader will be able to do the following:*

- Explain the various service management functions.
- Identify factors in a safe and efficient clinical environment.
- Describe how the spread of infection is prevented in the workplace.
- Define the three major categories of funding sources that reimburse for occupational therapy services.
- Recognize the importance of program planning and evaluation.

- Understand the purpose of documentation.
- Describe the documentation that occurs at various stages in the occupational therapy process.
- Identify the fundamental elements in a client record.
- Understand the integration of professional development and research into practice.
- State the importance of marketing and public relations as a professional responsibility.

## KEY TERMS

accreditation
diagnosis codes
documentation
electronic health records (EHR)
emergency procedures
evidence-based practice

individualized education plan
outcome measures
private funding sources
problem-oriented medical record
procedure codes
program evaluation

program process
program structure
public funding sources
service management functions
SOAP note
universal precautions

 Visit *www.evolve.elsevier.com* to access the Evolve student resources that accompany your book.

---

*On plucking thistles and planting flowers . . .*

How one lives life or chooses an occupation can be simple and straightforward or a long journey. As an undergraduate student, I wanted to be in premed—convinced that my calling was to be a physician. During undergraduate school, I explored two directions.

My first job was as a genetics technician in a university-based medical center. My days were spent centrifuging and fixing samples on slides, counting chromosomes, and photographing and creating karyotypes. When I closed my eyes each night, all I could visualize was chromosomes floating in emulsion. I would briefly meet people when they gave a sample in the laboratory, but I never got to know them or know what having the test meant to the greater scheme of their lives.

My second exploration was as a volunteer in an occupational therapy (OT) department in a psychiatric hospital. Suddenly, I was fascinated by people and their stories— intrigued by what went wrong and how their lives could

be reorganized, allowing them to return to some sense of normalcy in their day-to-day lives. OT seemed less scientific yet so very meaningful—listening while we were doing. I found that change and growth can be found through doing. I was a potential "agent of change"—the very meaning of the word therapist directed me to choose OT. The process of OT reminds me of Abraham Lincoln's words, which I have embraced: "I want it said of me by those who knew me best that I always plucked a thistle and planted a flower where I knew one would grow." I chose OT and have been plucking and planting. What a garden has grown and continues to grow each and every day!

**ANN BURKHARDT, OTD, OTR/L, BCN, FAOTA**
**Director, Division of Occupational Therapy**
**Chair & Program Director of Occupational Therapy**
**Professor**
**College of Pharmacy & Health Sciences**
**Drake University**
**Des Moines, Iowa**

Occupational therapy (OT) practitioners work with clients in a variety of environments. Along with evaluating and intervening with clients, practitioners are involved in service management functions. **Service management functions** include maintaining a safe and efficient workplace, documenting OT services, getting reimbursed for services, planning programs and evaluating them, integrating professional development activities and evidence-based practice into the workplace, and engaging in marketing and public relations. These functions are essential components of professional practice.

## Maintaining a Safe and Efficient Workplace

OT practitioners provide services to clients in an orderly and safe environment to ensure the safety of clients and efficiency of intervention and work procedures. The space in which practitioners work must accommodate clients with disabilities. For example, therapy settings must be wheelchair accessible, be free of clutter, have good lighting and ventilation, and have proper storage for equipment. The setting must be large enough to carry out intervention procedures.

Each practitioner assumes responsibility for maintaining a safe and efficient work environment. He or she is responsible for reporting problems to the OT administrator or to the maintenance department. Practitioners are directly responsible for putting away equipment and supplies that they use during a session and for cleaning the work area. The department operates more effectively and with less stress when everyone participates and cooperates in maintaining a safe and efficient work environment. The following sections describe specific factors considered in the work setting.

## Safe Environment

**Accreditation** refers to a form of regulation that determines whether an organization meets a prescribed standard. OT clinics must adhere to accreditation standards set by specific accreditation bodies. Many of these standards relate to establishing a safe work environment. For example, rehabilitation settings must meet the standards of the Commission on Accreditation of Rehabilitation Facilities (CARF).[7] Each setting develops written policies and procedures in accordance with the accreditation standards. Practitioners are responsible for following the written policies and procedures of their setting.

In general, clinical settings need to be large enough so that staff and consumers can move without bumping into equipment or objects. Equipment and furniture should be out of traffic areas. Sharp corners on cabinets should not protrude into areas where people may walk. The clinic should have nonslip floor surfaces and grab bars in bathrooms, with emergency call buttons.

The clinical setting must have proper storage for items that may potentially be a safety hazard. This may require that items be placed in locked cabinets. For example, in certain settings, scissors, knives, and other sharp objects may be considered potentially harmful and need to be monitored carefully and stored securely.

Some materials used in OT clinics may pose a health hazard. For example, some therapy clinics use toxic paints or stains, which need to be stored and used carefully. Toxic chemicals and flammable substances must be stored in a special locked cabinet for flammables. The Occupational Safety and Health Administration (OSHA) requires that manufacturers of such materials provide a safety data sheet (SDS) (formerly known as a Material Safety Data Sheet [MSDS]), which outlines information on the proper procedures for working with the material and describes procedures for storage and disposal.[15] The SDS describes the type of protective equipment required to work with the material and outlines the procedures to follow in case of a spill or accident. As of June 2015, SDS sheets must include specific information and in a specific format.[15] Practitioners should read SDSs carefully before using any hazardous material; they are kept in a readily accessible area of the clinic. All staff must be trained in the proper use of equipment and supplies that are found in the OT clinic. Practitioners may have to use protective goggles or masks when working with materials.[15]

Many OT clinics have kitchen areas, which must be maintained according to health standards.[14] Guidelines are provided for how food is handled and stored in OT clinics. Practitioners should inquire about the policies and procedures for their clinical setting, including how to ensure cleanliness of the clinic space, dishes, and materials.

OT practitioners are frequently involved in lifting and moving clients (e.g., from bed to wheelchair). It is important that practitioners use proper body mechanics to avoid injury. Employers are required to provide training on the use of proper body mechanics for lifting or transferring clients.[14]

Each setting of practice has established **emergency procedures** in the case of an injury or accident in the clinic. All staff must be aware of the emergency procedures and emergency call system. Everyone must stay aware of who is in the clinic at all times. These procedures include whom to contact and what to do. Practitioners document any injury, accident, or incident in a report (using a standard form) and submit it to the administration in accordance with OSHA procedures and the workplace policies.[14] Box 13.1 summarizes safety considerations in the OT clinic.

Workplace settings also have detailed evacuation processes in case of fire, storm, active shooter or other emergency. Employees are trained on how to respond in these emergencies and receive information on how to get information, where to go, and what to do. The evacuation plan must be reviewed with everyone so that all are prepared for emergencies. In the case of a storm or natural disaster, some personnel may be required to report to work (essential personnel) whereas other may need to stay at home. Employers conduct emergency drills to prepare employees for many situations.

• BOX 13.1 | Safety Considerations in the Occupational Therapy Setting

Sharp objects should be properly stored in a locked cabinet or drawer.
Keep flammables in a locked metal cabinet.
• Place safety data sheets (SDSs) in easy view of materials.
The clinical environment needs to be free of clutter so that staff and clients can move safely.
• Sharp corners on cabinets should not protrude into traffic areas.
• Equipment and furniture must be kept out of traffic areas.
Bathroom areas that are used by clients must have securely anchored grab bars.
• Develop a schedule for cleaning.
An emergency call system should be readily available, and all staff must understand emergency procedures.
Flooring must be nonslip.
Staff must alert others to anything that changes the floor condition (i.e., water).
All staff are required to have proper training in the safe use of equipment and supplies found in the occupational therapy clinic.
In kitchen areas, foods must be safely stored and handled.
• Label and date all food.
• Develop a schedule for cleaning the kitchen area.
Staff need to be trained in the use of proper body mechanics when lifting or moving clients, equipment, and supplies.
Staff must be aware of who is in the clinic at all times and report suspicious persons.

## Ordering and Storing Supplies

Maintaining an efficient therapy setting requires having appropriate equipment and supplies. The amount of supplies ordered and stored varies among facilities, depending on the size of the OT department and its storage capacity. Staff use an inventory system to track the supply. This responsibility is often part of the job of an occupational therapy assistant (OTA).

## Infection Control

The Centers for Disease Control and Prevention (CDC) is a federal agency that works to protect people's health and safety, provide reliable health information, and improve health through strong partnerships.[6] The CDC developed **universal precautions,** a set of guidelines designed to prevent the transmission of HIV, hepatitis B virus (HBV), and other blood-borne pathogens to health-care providers.

The CDC recommends that health-care personnel consider blood and body fluids of all clients as potentially infectious and follow universal precautions.[6,12] Universal precautions involve using protective barriers (e.g., gloves, gowns, aprons, masks, or protective eyewear) to reduce the risk of exposure to blood and other body fluids.[6,12] For example, OT practitioners following universal precautions wear protective gloves while addressing activities for daily living (ADLs), such as grooming, personal hygiene, toileting, feeding, and dressing. The practitioner changes his or her gloves and washes his or her hands after contact with

each client. In many clinical settings, a notice is placed in the client's medical record of the need for health-care workers to use precautions.[6,12] See Box 13.2 on universal precautions.

Hand washing is the most effective method for preventing the transfer of disease.[6,12] The OT practitioner washes his or her hands before and after each treatment session and before and after eating. Practitioners wash hands after using the toilet, sneezing, coughing, or coming in contact with oral and nasal areas. Procedures for hand washing are provided in Box 13.3.

Federal agencies, employers, and employees are responsible for controlling the spread of infection.[6,12] The regulations are established and monitored by the CDC and by

• BOX 13.2 | Universal Precautions

1. Wash hands before and after each session.
2. Wear gloves whenever there is the possibility of coming into contact with body fluids (i.e., saliva, blood, urine).
3. Wear full-body gowns, face masks, and eye protection when there is the possibility of blood or body fluid splashing.
4. Dispose of contaminated sharp objects in a puncture-proof container.
5. Dispose of all contaminated personal protective equipment in a biohazardous waste container.

Adapted from Siegel, J. D., Rhinehart, E., Jackson, M., Chiarello, L., & the Healthcare Infection Control Practices Advisory Committee. (2007). *2007 guideline for isolation precautions: Preventing transmission of infectious agents in healthcare settings* (pp. 66–67). Retrieved from, http://www.cdc.gov/hicpac/2007IP/2007isolationPrecautions.html

• BOX 13.3 | Techniques for Effective Hand Washing

1. Remove all jewelry, except plain band rings. Remove watch, or move it up the arm. Provide complete access to area to be washed.
2. Avoid touching the sink or nearby objects when approaching the sink.
3. Turn on the water, and adjust it to a lukewarm temperature and a moderate flow to avoid splashing.
4. Wet wrists and hands with fingers directed downward, and apply approximately 1 teaspoon of liquid soap or granules.
5. Begin to wash all areas of hands (palms, sides, backs), fingers, knuckles, and between each finger, using vigorous rubbing and circular motions. If wearing a band, slide it up or down the finger and scrub skin underneath it. Interlace fingers, and scrub between each finger.
6. Wash for at least 30 seconds, keeping hands and forearms at elbow level or below and hands pointed down. Wash longer if a patient known to have an infection was treated.
7. Rinse hands well under running water.
8. Wash hands, wrists, and forearms high toward elbow.
9. Rinse hands, wrists, and forearms under running water.
10. Thoroughly dry hands, wrists, and forearms with paper towels. Use a dry towel for each hand. Water should continue to flow from tap as hands are dried.
11. Use another dry paper towel to turn water faucet off. Discard all towels in an appropriate container.

Modified from Zakus, S. M. (1995). *Clinical procedures for medical assistants* (3rd ed.). St. Louis, MO: Mosby.

OSHA. OSHA monitors compliance of employers and fines those settings that do not follow the regulations, whereas the CDC monitors individuals' exposure to disease in the workplace.[6,14]

OSHA standards define the responsibilities of the employer to provide education on universal precautions and to provide the necessary protective barriers, hand-washing facilities, and supplies needed by employees.[6] Employers must provide employee health services to conduct mandatory annual testing for tuberculosis (TB), to provide the TB vaccine, and to maintain employee health records (i.e., tests and vaccines given and any exposure to infectious disease). Employees are responsible for attending educational programs that are offered and following universal precautions guidelines. Employees must have an annual TB test and report any exposures to the employee health services department. The employee may decide whether to take the TB vaccine or to sign a waiver.[6] Employers may also provide flu shots to employees. In some settings, employees must have a flu shot or wear protective masks while working.

## Scheduling

Each clinic maintains a schedule of appointments for each practitioner. Schedules include the time for direct service and the time to complete service management functions, attend meetings or conferences, complete paperwork, and bill for services. The schedule for each client varies, depending on the type of facility and the client's needs. For example, in some mental health outpatient programs, intervention may be performed in groups that meet once a week. Conversely, a practitioner treating hand injuries in an outpatient setting may schedule clients two to three times a week.

Third-party payers may influence the frequency and duration of scheduled sessions. For example, Medicare requires clients in acute rehabilitation settings receive therapy twice a day.[4] Clients who cannot complete two daily sessions may be transferred to a setting that provides a lower level of care (e.g., skilled nursing facility). Many health maintenance organizations (HMOs) limit the number of outpatient OT visits. This is considered when scheduling clients for intervention, along with family routines and commitments.

The supervising occupational therapist usually assigns clients to staff for scheduling. This decision-making step considers the client's needs, staff expertise, and cost-effectiveness. OT departments adhere to productivity standards to be successful. Practitioners manage and adhere to the schedule to ensure that everything is completed as planned.

## Documenting Occupational Therapy Services

Documenting provides an accurate record of service. **Documentation** provides a justification for OT intervention. The practitioner's professional judgment and clinical reasoning are reflected in documentation. Therefore documentation is used to communicate with other healthcare professionals, third-party payers, and administrators. Documentation is a record of the status of the client, techniques used, and progress the client makes in therapy. Consequently, documentation is essential to intervention planning and communication between team members. Documentation provides a chronological record of the client's status, the services provided, and the outcomes of those services. See Box 13.4.

The *evaluation or screening report* contains information on the referral source and data gathered during the evaluation process.[3] This report provides a client's occupational profile, an analysis of the client's occupational performance, factors that support or inhibit performance, and the expected outcomes of intervention. The *reevaluation* provides recommendations for changes to services, goals, frequency, and referral to other sources.

During the intervention stage, practitioners complete an intervention plan, service contacts, progress reports, and a transition plan. The *intervention plan* documents the client's goals and approaches used to reach those goals.[3] It identifies frequency and duration of service, service provider, and location of service. Documentation of *service contacts* records the specific interactions between the client and OT practitioner.[3] It is an ongoing log of therapy and includes date, length of time (units), interventions, and the client's response. Telephone contacts, interventions, and meetings with others are also documented. An example of a daily narrative note describing a service contact (intervention session) with a client is shown in Box 13.5.

A *progress report* summarizes the intervention and the client's progress toward the goals.[3] It summarizes new data and modifications to the intervention plan, and it concludes with recommendations (e.g., continue or discontinue services or be referred to another source). Progress reports vary between settings and reimbursement mechanisms. An example of a weekly progress report is shown in Box 13.6.

---

### • BOX 13.4  Purpose of Documentation

- Justification of services
- Record of services
- Description of client's journey
- Record of outcome of intervention
- Billing
- Communication

---

### • BOX 13.5  Sample Narrative Daily Note

Client actively participated in eating retraining and right upper extremity strengthening program. Client ate 75% of meal with adapted utensils and required minimal assistance for cutting meat. Established treatment plan should continue.

Modified from Early, M. B. (2006). Physical dysfunction practice skills for the occupational therapy assistant (2nd ed.). St. Louis, MO: Mosby.

---

• **BOX 13.6** **Sample Weekly Progress Note**

Client has been treated daily for eating retraining and right upper extremity functional strengthening program. Using adapted utensils, client ate 75% of meal with minimal assistance for cutting meat. Previously, client ate 50% of meal and required moderate assistance for cutting meat. Client will eat independently with no assistive devices in 1 week.

Modified from Early, M. B. (2006). Physical dysfunction practice skills for the occupational therapy assistant (2nd ed.). St. Louis, MO: Mosby.

---

• **BOX 13.7** **Sample SOAP Note**

**Problem 1: Dependence in wheelchair mobility**

S: Client stated that his hands often slip on the metal hand rims when propelling his wheelchair.

O: Friction tape was placed on rims of wheelchair to improve client's ability to grasp and propel chair. Client completed wheelchair mobility training outside over grass and on asphalt. Client participated for 30 minutes in wheelchair training with only 5-minute rest period. He experienced no difficulty propelling wheelchair over varied terrain.

A: Friction tape on rims helped improve client's ability to propel wheelchair. Client's endurance for wheelchair mobility improved since yesterday.

P: Continue occupational therapy training in wheelchair mobility. Increase time and distance for wheelchair mobility. Teach client how to maneuver wheelchair in and out of doors and up and down ramps.

---

• **BOX 13.8** **Fundamental Elements of Documentation**

Demographic information:
- Name
- Date of Birth
- Address and phone
- Identification number

Date of OT contact
Type of documentation
Setting or agency, department
Terminology and abbreviations
Clear, concise and accurate representation of contact
Signatures, with professional designation:
- OT practitioner
- Supervisor if needed (students or OTAs)

Confidentiality maintained
Storage and disposal procedures followed

---

A *transition plan* describes the client's progression from one type of setting to another within the same delivery system. For example, a transition plan must be completed when a client transfers from a rehabilitation setting to a skilled nursing facility. The transition plan provides information regarding the client's current status; the reason for the transition; a time frame for transition; and recommendations and rationale for OT services, modifications, or assistive technology.

The *discharge/discontinuation report* is completed during the outcomes stage. This report summarizes the changes in the client's ability to participate in occupations between the initial evaluation and the discontinuation of services. Recommendations for further services and follow-up are documented.

There are many types and methods of documentation. Public policy, accreditation bodies, third-party payers, and the practice setting determine documentation practices. For example, school settings funded by the federal and state governments require each child to have an **individualized education plan** (IEP) completed by a multi-disciplinary team. The problems, goals, and interventions reflect behaviors and skills necessary for the child's success in school.

There are specific documentation requirements mandated by the federal government for clients who are covered by Medicare. One common method of documentation that is used in medical settings is the **problem-oriented medical record** (POMR). This format is based on a list of problems identified by the treatment team during the assessment of the client. Subsequent progress notes relate to the problem(s) identified in the list. The format used for writing the progress note is referred to as the **SOAP note.** S stands for *subjective* (information reported by the client); O is for *objective* (clinical findings or measurable, observable data); A represents *assessment* (OT practitioner's professional judgment or opinion); and P is for *plan* (specific plan of action to be followed). See Box 13.7.

Each client receives a permanent record. The record is organized, legible, concise, accurate, complete, grammatically correct, and objective.[3] Even though the format of the documentation varies among settings, there are certain elements present in all documentation (Box 13.8). Good planning and regular documentation make record keeping easier, and, ultimately, lead to better-quality intervention.

## Electronic Health Records

The Patient Protection and Affordable Care Act (PPACA) and American Recovery and Reinvestment Act requires healthcare providers to use electronic health records (EHR) in order to receive Medicaid and Medicare funding.[5a] The use of EHR is emphasized as a way to: improve quality, safety, efficiency; reduce health disparities, engage patients and family, improve care coordination and population and public health; and maintain privacy and security of patient health information.[5a] OT practitioners will complete documentation of services through the EHR in accordance with privacy and security standards. This provides a method of communicating more effectively with other health professionals and allows practitioners to measure outcomes.

## Reimbursement for Services

To stay in business, OT departments need to produce revenue by collecting fees for services provided. Each OT practitioner is responsible for submitting accurate charges that are reflected in either units based on the amount of time spent with the client or a set fee based on services provided.[4] Determining charges involves a complex process, usually performed by the administration of the facility. Third-party payers have different amounts that they will pay in "allowable charges" for a particular client. The charges set by the facility do not reflect what is actually paid by the third-party payer for an individual client but rather for the client population as a whole.

OT services are reimbursed by a number of sources, which can be categorized into three groups: (1) public sources that include federal, state, and local government agencies; (2) private payers that include insurance companies; and (3) other sources that include service agencies and volunteer organizations.[4] Each source of payment has different regulations and guidelines that identify the services for which it will pay (number of units and equipment) and the amount of reimbursement. Because these regulations and guidelines often change, the OT practitioner must stay informed on current policies. The administration of the facility typically informs staff members of any changes in funding regulations.

## Public Funding Sources

**Public funding sources** include federal, state, and local sources, such as Medicare, the Veterans Administration, Medicaid, Maternal and Child Health programs, the Department of Education, vocational rehabilitation services, and Social Security benefits. Typically, congress authorizes funding through legislation and designates a federal agency to determine the scope and criteria for the program. An agency is designated in each state to ensure compliance with the programs mandated by the federal government.[4] The funds are then distributed to the local agencies or programs, which are responsible for ensuring that mandated services are provided. Chapter 2 discusses federal legislation that has mandated OT as a reimbursable service.

## Private Funding Sources

**Private funding sources** include health insurance, worker's compensation, casualty insurance, and disability insurance. A growing number of individuals are paying for health-care services personally because they either do not have health insurance or their plans do not provide for a specific service. Private insurance companies have a variety of plans with different benefits and restrictions. Health insurance policies stipulate whether OT services are covered and whether there are any limitations on those services (e.g., maximum number of visits, maximum amount of dollars).

Worker's compensation benefits cover expenses incurred from work-related injuries. Worker's compensation benefits are regulated by state agencies and managed by private insurance companies. For that reason, allowable OT services vary from state to state.

## Other Funding Sources

Other sources of funding of OT services or equipment include service clubs, private foundations, and volunteer organizations. (e.g., Kiwanis, Rotary Club). In some cases, private foundations, specific to a disability, will provide funding for an individual with that disability. Some volunteer agencies also provide funding. OT practitioners may need to be creative to get equipment for clients. For example, many colleges and universities require students to complete service projects that may benefit clients.

## Coding and Billing for Services

To receive payment for OT services, the provider (either a facility or individual) submits a claim form using the correct billing codes. Services provided in OT are either billed by diagnosis codes or procedure codes. **Diagnosis codes** are based on the client's medical condition or the medical justification for services. The most frequently used coding system is the *International Classification of Diseases, Tenth Revision, Clinical Modification (ICD-10-CM).*[11] Diseases are categorized in *ICD-10-CM* according to anatomical systems. Mental health providers use the *Diagnostic and Statistical Manual of Mental Disorders, Fifth Edition (DSM-5).*[5]

**Procedure codes** are based on the specific services performed by health-care providers. The most commonly used procedure coding system is the *Current Procedural Terminology (CPT)*, which is published and updated annually by the American Medical Association.[1] OT practitioners select the codes that most accurately define the services performed and bill to these codes by relative value units. Payers may limit the number and range of codes that a specialty may use to bill services; therefore, OT practitioners must be aware of the allowable codes for each insurer.

There are two types of claim forms commonly used in OT to bill third-party payers: (1) the Uniform Bill (UB-92; CMS-01450), which is used by hospitals, skilled nursing facilities, and home health agencies; and (2) the CMS-1500 claim form, used primarily by physicians or OT practitioners in private practice.[4]

OT practitioners educate third-party payers continually regarding the benefits of OT services. Practitioners advocate for including OT as a reimbursable service. It is important to keep abreast of proposed changes in state and federal legislation and regulations that have the potential to affect payment for OT services. This can be done on an individual basis and also by supporting local and national OT associations that provide lobbying efforts for the purpose of influencing legislation that may affect the profession.

## Program Planning and Evaluation

Program planning and evaluation are primarily the responsibilities of the administrator, although staff provide input into both processes. In an OT department, the administrator is involved in planning things such as space utilization, equipment needs, staff levels, effective use of staff, the annual budget, department policies and procedures, and new programs and services.

Health-care professionals conduct a **program evaluation** to determine how the program is achieving the intended goals and objectives. Program evaluation is not only important for ensuring client satisfaction, but it is also necessary for accreditation by outside agencies. As mentioned, accreditation is a form of regulation that determines whether an organization or program meets a prescribed standard. Organizations seek to be accredited so that they can be reimbursed by third-party payers. Many of the organizations in which OT practitioners are likely to work are influenced by some type of accreditation. In health care, the two most widely known accreditation bodies are the Joint Commission (formerly The Joint Commission [TJC])[8] and CARF.[7] TJC develops standards and accredits health-care organizations, including hospitals, health-care networks, and organizations that provide long-term care, behavioral care, and laboratory and ambulatory services.[8]

CARF sets standards and accredits organizations that deliver rehabilitation services. CARF's standards and guidelines are separated into three areas: behavioral health, employment and community services, and medical rehabilitation. The CARF accreditation process is aimed at improving the quality of services provided to individuals with disabilities.[7] CARF is also involved in research related to outcomes measurement and management.

Accreditation requires a detailed program evaluation, including a written report of self-study. Following the completion of the self-study, a team representing the accrediting body visits the facility. The program evaluation includes examination of program structure, program process, and outcome measures. **Program structure** refers to the system in which the services are delivered (e.g., staff levels and expertise, equipment, budget, and range of services). The **program process** refers to the stages of *referral*, *evaluation*, and *intervention*. This examines such things as how timely the evaluation was performed. **Outcome measures** refer to the results of the intervention.

OT practitioners use a number of tools to measure outcomes. One tool is the Functional Independence Measure (FIM).[13] The FIM measures an individual client's functional ability for 18 items across the domains of self-care, motor, and cognitive.[13] The person is given a separate score for each item and also a total score. The FIM scores a client at different points in the rehabilitation process (e.g., at time of referral and at discharge) and provides an objective measure of how the individual is progressing. Program evaluation looks at a compilation of client data. For example, the program could compile data over the last fiscal year that portray the average percentage of change in client scores from time of admission to time of discharge. Program evaluation is an ongoing process that helps ensure that quality services are provided by the OT program.

## Integrating Professional Development Activities and Evidence-Based Practice into the Workplace

Practitioners must maintain competence in the field through participation in educational programs and professional development activities (see Chapter 7). OT practitioners participate in educational opportunities at their workplace through in-service presentations. Another way that OT practitioners can be involved in professional development in the workplace is by supervising level I or level II fieldwork students. Occupational therapists and OTAs with a minimum of 1 year of work experience are eligible to supervise students. Clinical internships are critical to the profession. Not only is fieldwork an important component of the student's training, but it is a valuable experience for the supervisor, who learns and grows professionally from the mentoring experience.

Evidence-based practice enhances OT practice by supporting practice through research. Consumers, practitioners, and third-party payers benefit from knowing that OT is provided based on the best available evidence.[2,9,10]

**Evidence-based practice** refers to finding, appraising, and using research findings as the basis for clinical decisions.[9,10] Research evidence is used by the OT practitioner in conjunction with clinical knowledge and reasoning to determine the interventions that are effective for a particular client.[2,10] There are four steps in evidence-based practice: (1) forming a clinical question that can be researched, (2) searching the literature for the best evidence on the question, (3) appraising the evidence for validity and applicability to practice, and (4) applying the evidence to practice.[2,9] Applying research to practice does not always mean changing the intervention approach. It may mean providing clients with more specific and current information about the efficacy of the approaches used. In some situations, the research may provide information on interventions to facilitate a client's outcomes.[10]

Resources are available to assist the OT practitioner in retrieving research findings (e.g., Rehabilitation Reference Center, Cochrane Reviews). The American Occupational Therapy Association's (AOTA's) *Evidence Briefs* is a series of reviews of OT research. Each brief presents a summary of a selected article that outlines the study's key features, methods, procedures, findings, and application to practice. The *Evidence-Based Practice (EBP) Resource Directory*[2] provides information related to the use of evidence-based practice in OT. Students and practitioners are urged to use a variety of resources to critically appraise and incorporate evidence into their daily practice.

## Marketing and Public Relations

Marketing and public relations materials increase the visibility of OT. Many departments plan and implement public relations activities during the month of April, which is designated as National Occupational Therapy Month Fig. 13.1. For example, a booth set up in the facility's cafeteria that demonstrates adaptive equipment may provide good publicity for OT. AOTA is committed to increasing the visibility of OT and has materials available for members to promote the profession.

Marketing differs slightly from public relations in that it involves the development and implementation of a marketing plan. This plan requires consideration of (1) the clients served, (2) the sources who refer or have the potential to refer clients to OT, (3) the administration (or internal source of funding for the department) of the facility, and (4) the third-party payers that reimburse (or have the potential to reimburse) for OT services.

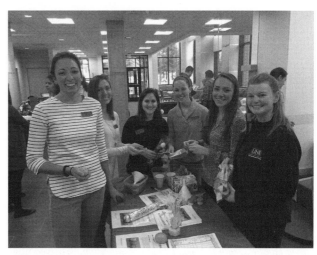

**Fig. 13.1** Students engage in OT month activities promoting health and wellness for children.

## Summary

Service management functions are activities performed by the OT practitioner outside of direct service delivery to the client. These functions include maintaining a safe and efficient workplace, documenting OT services, getting reimbursed for services, planning programs and their evaluations, integrating professional development activities and evidence-based practice into the workplace, and engaging in public relations and marketing. For an OT department to operate effectively, it is important that each practitioner take responsibility for being involved in these activities.

## Learning Activities

1. Visit an OT department. Describe the service management functions. Describe the environment of the department. Is the storage adequate? Does there appear to be an adequate amount of equipment and supplies? Does the clinic appear cluttered, or is it neat, with everything safely put away? Are there any obvious safety hazards that you noticed during your visit?
2. Interview either an OTA or an occupational therapist about the types of service management functions he or she performs. Compare notes with your classmates. Are there differences between the jobs that occupational therapists and OTAs do?
3. In a group of two or three students, develop several public relations activities to promote National Occupational Therapy Month. Conduct one activity during OT Month.
4. Visit an OT department and discuss the types of documentation used by the OT practitioners. Review examples of the different types of documentation (e.g., assessment reports, progress notes, treatment plans, and discharge summaries).

## Review Questions

1. What are the various service management functions in which the OT practitioner participates?
2. What are some factors for safety in the clinic?
3. What are universal precautions?
4. What do each of the areas of the SOAP method of documentation mean?
5. Why is research important in practice?
6. How is program evaluation used in practice?

## References

1. American Medical Association. *Current Procedural Terminology 2010*. Chicago, IL: Author; 2010.
2. American Occupational Therapy Association. *Evidence-Based Practice and Research*; 2016. Retrieved from, http://www.aota.org/ebp [must be an AOTA member for access].
3. American Occupational Therapy Association. Guidelines for documentation of occupational therapy. *Am J Occup Ther.* 2013;67:S32–S38. http://dx.doi.org/10.5014/ajot.2013.67S32.
4. American Occupational Therapy Association. *Reimbursement and Regulatory Policy Department. AOTA Guide to Medicare Local coverage Determination*; 2007. Retrieved from, http://www.aota.org/practice/productive-aging/driving/practitioners/-/media/corporate/files/secure/advocacy/reimb/news/archives/medicare/lcds/resources/lcd%20advocacy%20packet1.pdf.
5. American Psychiatric Association. *Diagnostic and Statistical Manual of Mental Disorders*. 5th ed. Arlington, VA: Author; 2013.
5a. Bisk Education. *Federal Mandates for Healthcare: Digital Record-Keeping Requirements for Public and Private Healthcare Providers.*

University of South Florida Healthcare online. http://www.usfhealthonline.com/resources/healthcare/electronic-medical-records-mandate/#.WCIrUC0rLcs; 2016, June 20.

6. Centers for Disease Control and Prevention. *Mission, Role and Pledge.* Retrieved from, http://www.cdc.gov/about/organization/mission.htm; 2014, April.

7. Commission on the Accreditation of Rehabilitation Facilities. *About CARF*; 2016. Retrieved from, http://www.carf.org/About/.

8. Joint Commission. *About the Joint Commission.* Retrieved from, http://www.jointcommission.org/about_us/about_the_joint_commission_main.aspx; 2016.

9. Law M, Baum C. Evidence-based occupational therapy. *Can J Occup Ther.* 1998;65(3):131–135.

10. Lieberman D, Scheer J. AOTA's evidence-based literature review project: an overview. *Am J Occup Ther.* 2002;56(3):344–349.

11. National Center for Health Statistics. *International Classification of Diseases, Tenth Revision, Clinical Modification.* Retrieved from, http://www.cdc.gov/nchs/icd/icd10cm.htm; 2016.

12. Siegel JD, Rhinehart E, Jackson M, Chiarello L, the Healthcare Infection Control Practices Advisory Committee, *2007 Guideline for Isolation Precautions: Preventing Transmission of Infectious Agents in Healthcare Settings*; 2007:66–67. Retrieved from, http://www.cdc.gov/hicpac/2007IP/2007isolationPrecautions.html.

13. Uniform Data System for Medical Rehabilitation. (n.d.). *FIM instrument.* Retrieved from, http://www.udsmr.org/WebModules/FIM/Fim_About.aspx.

14. U.S. Department of Labor. (n.d.). Occupational Health & Safety Administration. *Safety and healthcare.* Retrieved from, https://www.osha.gov/dsg/hazcom/enforcementmsdsrequirement.html.

15. U.S. Department of Labor. (n.d.). *Occupational Health & Safety Administration. OSHA quick card safety data sheets.* Retrieved from, https://www.osha.gov/Publications/HazComm_QuickCard_SafetyData.html.

# The Process of Occupational Therapy

# 14

# Occupational Therapy Process: Evaluation, Intervention, and Outcomes

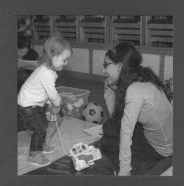

## OBJECTIVES

*After reading this chapter, the reader will be able to do the following:*

- Describe the occupational therapy referral, screening, and evaluation process.
- Identify the purpose of the occupational profile.
- Describe the occupational performance analysis and how it is used in occupational therapy.
- Discuss the steps in conducting an interview.
- Understand the importance of observation skills in the evaluation process.

- Identify the steps in the intervention process.
- Describe the five general intervention approaches used in occupational therapy.
- Characterize the roles of the occupational therapist and the occupational therapy assistant as they engage in the occupational therapy process.

## KEY TERMS

| | | |
|---|---|---|
| assessment instruments | interview | reliability |
| assessment procedures | nonstandardized tests | screening |
| consulting | normative data | standardized tests |
| discharge plan | observation | structured observation |
| education | occupational profile | test-retest reliability |
| interrater reliability | occupational therapy process | transition services |
| intervention | referral | validity |

 Visit *www.evolve.elsevier.com* to access the Evolve student resources that accompany your book.

*When I embarked upon my undergraduate studies, I did so with the intention of becoming a clinical psychologist. In my senior year, a good friend of mine, who was a physical therapy major, said that I should be an occupational therapist because I would be really good at it. At the time, I did not really know what occupational therapy (OT) was. After graduation, I was hired as a recreation therapist in a skilled* *nursing facility. It was there that I came in contact with occupational therapists. When I looked more closely at the career, I felt it would be a great fit for me. Ever since I was a child, I've enjoyed analyzing how things work and coming up with solutions. Little did I know that I was laying the foundation for occupational analysis, a key component of successful OT service delivery!*

*I applied and was accepted to Columbia University in New York City. I began my career in the public school system. After about six years, I was able to make a seamless transition to adult physical rehabilitation. I think OT is one of the only careers in which one has the flexibility to work with individuals across the life span. OT also offered me the flexibility to work part time when my children were babies. I was able to take care of their needs and keep practicing in the profession I love.*

*While supervising fieldwork students, I realized that I had a love of teaching. I explored the steps necessary to enter academia as an OT professor. After working at a community college, I had the opportunity to teach at the University of New England (UNE). Over the prior years, I'd had the privilege of working in almost every setting in which occupational therapists work: schools, hospitals, nursing homes, and so forth. Because I had such diverse experience, I was able to fill a needed role at UNE.*

*I have been practicing as an occupational therapist for almost twenty years. Since then, I have never looked back. It is a career filled with meaning. It affords endless opportunities for career growth. The opportunity to become an occupational therapist, and now contribute to the growth of the profession, has been one of the greatest gifts of my life!*

**MARY BETH PATNAUDE, MS, OTR/L**
**Assistant Clinical Professor**
**University of New England**
**Portland, Maine**

The **occupational therapy process** involves the interaction between the practitioner *and* the client. The relationship between the practitioner and the client is a collaborative one that involves problem solving to support the client's occupational performance. The process is dynamic, and the focus is on occupation and the client as an occupational being.[2] The client may be an individual, caregiver, group, or population.

The occupational therapy (OT) process can be divided into evaluation, intervention, and outcome. The evaluation process includes referral, screening, development of an occupational profile, and analysis of occupational performance. The intervention process includes intervention planning, implementation, and review. The outcomes process includes measurement of outcomes and decision making related to the future direction of intervention (i.e., continue, modify, or discontinue). In this chapter, we describe the components of each stage and delineate the roles of the occupational therapist and the occupational therapy assistant (OTA) throughout the process.

## Evaluation Process

The purpose of the evaluation process is to find out what the client wants and needs and to identify those factors that support or hinder occupational performance see Fig. 14.1.[2]

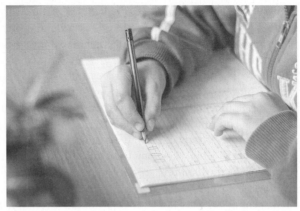

**Fig. 14.1** The practitioner may conduct a formal handwriting assessment to better understand the factors supporting or hindering the child's writing. © Getty Images/Creative RF/Kras1.

The OT practitioner develops an occupational profile of the client and analyzes the occupational performance to determine the client's skills and ability to carry out activities of daily living, instrumental activities of daily living, work, education, social participation, or sleep and rest.

The OT practitioner bases the evaluation procedures on the client's age, diagnosis, developmental level, education, socioeconomic status, cultural background, and functional abilities. The steps of the evaluation process include referral, screening, and evaluation. Observation and interviewing are essential to this process. Practitioners use a similar evaluation process to examine populations and communities.

### Referral

The OT process begins when a **referral,** a request for service for a particular client population, or community, is made.[3] The occupational therapist is responsible for accepting and responding to the referral. Referrals may come from a physician, another professional, or the client. Referrals may range from a specific prescription for a dynamic orthosis to general suggestions to improve fine motor problems. Federal, state, and local regulations and the policies of third-party payers determine the type of referral required (e.g., whether a physician's referral is necessary) and the role an OTA can have in the referral process.

### Screening

Through **screening,** the OT practitioner gathers preliminary information about the client and determines whether further evaluation and OT intervention are warranted. Screening typically involves a review of the client's records, the use of a brief screening test, an interview with the client or caregiver, observation of the client, and/or a discussion of the client with the referral source. The practitioner investigates the client's prior and current level of occupational performance and determines the client's future occupational performance needs. The practitioner communicates the screening results to the appropriate individuals, including the party who made the referral.[1,3]

The occupational therapist initiates and directs the screening process, using methods that are appropriate to the client's developmental level, gender, cultural background, and medical and functional status.[1,3] The OTA contributes to the screening process under the direction of an occupational therapist. Before screening tasks are performed by an OTA, he or she must achieve service competency in the particular tasks.

If screening suggests the client is in need of services, a comprehensive evaluation is arranged. The occupational therapist identifies a model of practice (see Chapter 15) on which the evaluation is based. The model of practice helps organize the practitioner's thinking. From the model of practice, the practitioner selects a frame of reference and chooses **assessment instruments** consistent with the frame of reference.

## Occupational Profile

The goal of this step is to gather information on the client so that an **occupational profile** can be developed. The OT practitioner obtains initial information about the client, including the client's age, gender, and reason for referral; diagnosis and medical history (including date of onset); prior living situation and level of function (e.g., independent at home or in a care home); and social, educational, and vocational background. The initial review may provide information regarding precautions that need to be adhered to during the OT process. This background information is usually recorded in the client's OT chart and on the evaluation form. Fig. 14.1 is an example of an evaluation form used in an OT setting.

An occupational profile provides the practitioner with a history of the client's background and functional performance to design intervention. The following questions from the *Occupational Therapy Practice Framework (OTPF)* help the practitioner develop the OT profile:[2]

• Who is the client (individual, caregiver, group, population)?
• Why is the client seeking service?
• What are the client's concerns?
• What are the client's current concerns relative to engaging in occupations and daily life activities?
• In which occupations is the client successful?
• In which occupations is the client experiencing difficulty? Why?
• What is the client's occupational history (i.e., life experiences, values, interests, previous patterns of engagement in occupations and in daily life activities, and the meanings associated with them)?
• What are the client's priorities and desired targeted outcomes?

## Occupational Performance Analysis

From the information gathered during the occupational profile (e.g., client's needs, problems, and priorities), the practitioner makes decisions regarding the analysis of occupational performance. This information provides direction to the practitioner as to the areas that need to be further examined. The practitioner selects specific assessment instruments to collect further information.

The OT practitioner gathers information on a client's occupational performance in regard to areas, skills, patterns, contexts, client factors, and activity demands (see Chapter 10) see Fig. 14.2.[2] The results are documented on a form similar to that shown in Fig. 14.3. This evaluation information forms the basis for the intervention plan.

Occupational performance analysis involves analyzing all aspects of the occupation to determine the client factors, patterns, contexts, skills, and behaviors required to be successful. Once the practitioner has thoroughly analyzed the occupation, the practitioner can more easily determine what is interfering with the client's ability to engage in desired occupations. Appendix A provides an activity analysis of a sampling of intervention activities.

Evaluation is an essential part of therapeutic decision-making process requiring a depth of understanding of many factors. As a result, the final responsibility of evaluation rests with the occupational therapist. The occupational therapist may delegate responsibility for certain procedures to the OTA.[3] The OTA communicates the results of all evaluation procedures to the occupational therapist. As with the screening process, service competency for tasks performed by an OTA needs to be established. The overall evaluation, or the process of compiling all of the information to form a composite picture of the client, is the responsibility of an occupational therapist.

The evaluation requires that the occupational therapist gather accurate and useful information to identify the needs and problems of the client to plan intervention.

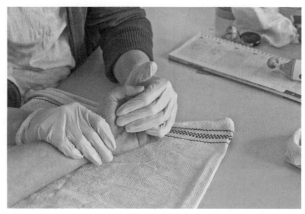

• **Fig. 14.2** Range of motion affects motor skills and is part of an occupational performance analysis. © Getty Images/Creative RF/ Meinzahn.

Occupational Therapy Initial Evaluation

Name:

DOB:

Medical Dx (ICD 10 codes):

Past Medical History:

Reason for Referral:

Occupational profile (describe the client's interests, routines, and occupations; life experiences, daily life roles):

Client's goals:

Occupational Performance:

| ADLs | Performance level | Comments |
|---|---|---|
| Bathing | | |
| Showering | | |
| Dressing | | |
| Swallowing/eating | | |
| Feeding | | |
| Functional Mobility | | |
| Personal device care | | |
| Personal hygiene/grooming | | |
| Sexual activity | | |

| IADLs | Performance level | Comments |
|---|---|---|
| Care of others | | |
| Care of Pets | | |
| Child rearing | | |
| Communication mgt. | | |
| Driving/community mobility | | |
| Financial mgt. | | |
| Health mgt. | | |
| Home establishment | | |
| Meal preparation and cleanup | | |
| Religious/spiritual activitiies | | |

• **Fig. 14.3** Sample occupational therapy evaluation form. *ADL,* Activities of daily living; *CGA,* contact guard assist; *dep,* dependent; *DOB,* date of birth; *DX,* diagnosis; *HICN,* health insurance carrier number; *IADL,* instrumental activities of daily living; *indep,* independent; *LB,* lower body; *LUE,* left upper extremity; *max,* maximum assist; *min,* minimum assist; *mod,* moderate assist; *OT,* occupational therapy; *ROM,* range of motion; *RUE,* right upper extremity; *sup,* supervised; *UB,* upper body. (From Pendeleton, H., & Schultz-Krohn, W. [Eds.]. [2012]. *Pedretti's occupational therapy practice skills for physical dysfunction* [7th ed.]. St. Louis, MO: Mosby.)

(Continued)

| Safety/emergency | | |
|---|---|---|
| Shopping | | |
| **Rest and sleep** | | |
| **Education** | | |
| **Work** | | |
| **Play/Leisure** | | |
| **Social Participation** | | |

Performance level is recorded on a spectrum regarding how much assistance the client requires:
Dependent; Maximum; Moderate; Minimum; Supervision; Independent

Client Factors:

| Mental functions (cognitive, affective, performance) | | Description of performance |
|---|---|---|
| Consicousness | | |
| Orientation | | |
| Temperament | | |
| Energy and drive | | |
| **Sensory Functions** | | |
| | Visual | |
| | Hearing | |
| | Vestibular | |
| | Taste | |
| | Smell | |
| | Proprioception | |
| | Touch | |
| | Pain | |
| | Temperature and pressure | |
| **Motor** | | |
| Structures | | |
| Joint mobility | | |
| ROM | | |
| Muscle strength | | |
| Muscle tone | | |
| Coordination | | |
| **Other** | | |

Assessment:

   Strengths

   Weaknesses

Long term goal

Short term goals

OT Intervention Plan: (include frequency and duration)

Therapist's signature     Date

• **Fig. 14.3, cont'd**

The techniques used during the evaluation process can be classified into three basic procedures: (1) interview, (2) skilled observation, and (3) formal evaluation procedures.

## Interview

The **interview** is the primary mechanism for gathering information for the occupational profile. The interview is a planned and organized way to collect pertinent information. The focus of OT is *occupations*, which include the activities in which a person engages throughout the day. Therefore the practitioner gathers information related to the individual's

occupations. The practitioner asks questions regarding the client's function in daily activities before the onset of the problem that resulted in the referral. The interview is also used as a means of developing trust and rapport with the client.

In some instances, the client is asked to fill out a checklist or questionnaire before the interview. For example, the interest checklist (Fig. 14.4) developed by Matsutsuyu[7] has served as a model for others. Interest checklists enable clients to report on hobbies and interests. The activity configuration also provides information on how a client spends the day. The client compiles a list of all the different activities in which he or she participates and classifies activities

## INTEREST CHECKLIST

| Activity | What has been your level of interest | | | | | | Do you currently participate in this activity? | | Would you like to pursue this in the future? | |
|---|---|---|---|---|---|---|---|---|---|---|
| | In the past ten years | | | In the past year | | | | | | |
| | Strong | Some | No | Strong | Some | No | Yes | No | Yes | No |
| Gardening Yardwork | | | | | | | | | | |
| Sewing/needle work | | | | | | | | | | |
| Playing card | | | | | | | | | | |
| Foreign languages | | | | | | | | | | |
| Church activities | | | | | | | | | | |
| Radio | | | | | | | | | | |
| Walking | | | | | | | | | | |
| Car repair | | | | | | | | | | |
| Writing | | | | | | | | | | |
| Dancing | | | | | | | | | | |
| Golf | | | | | | | | | | |
| Football | | | | | | | | | | |
| Listening to popular music | | | | | | | | | | |
| Puzzles | | | | | | | | | | |
| Holiday Activities | | | | | | | | | | |
| Pets/livestock | | | | | | | | | | |
| Movies | | | | | | | | | | |
| Listening to classical music | | | | | | | | | | |
| Speeches/lectures | | | | | | | | | | |
| Swimming | | | | | | | | | | |
| Bowling | | | | | | | | | | |
| Visiting | | | | | | | | | | |
| Mending | | | | | | | | | | |
| Checkers/Chess | | | | | | | | | | |
| Barbecues | | | | | | | | | | |
| Reading | | | | | | | | | | |
| Traveling | | | | | | | | | | |
| Parties | | | | | | | | | | |
| Wrestling | | | | | | | | | | |
| Housecleaning | | | | | | | | | | |
| Model building | | | | | | | | | | |
| Television | | | | | | | | | | |
| Concerts | | | | | | | | | | |
| Pottery | | | | | | | | | | |

• **Fig. 14.4** The modified interest checklist. Kielhofner & Neville (1983). The modified interest checklist. Unpublished manuscript, Model of Human Occupation Clearinghouse, Department of Occupational Therapy, College of Applied Health Sciences, University of Illinois at Chicago.

*(Continued)*

| Activity | What has been your level of interest | | | | | | Do you currently participate in this activity? | | Would you like to pursue this in the future? | |
|---|---|---|---|---|---|---|---|---|---|---|
| | In the past ten years | | | In the past year | | | | | | |
| | Strong | Some | No | Strong | Some | No | Yes | No | Yes | No |
| Camping | | | | | | | | | | |
| Laundry/Ironing | | | | | | | | | | |
| Politics | | | | | | | | | | |
| Table games | | | | | | | | | | |
| Home decorating | | | | | | | | | | |
| Clubs/Lodge | | | | | | | | | | |
| Singing | | | | | | | | | | |
| Scouting | | | | | | | | | | |
| Clothes | | | | | | | | | | |
| Handicrafts | | | | | | | | | | |
| Hairstyling | | | | | | | | | | |
| Cycling | | | | | | | | | | |
| Attending plays | | | | | | | | | | |
| Bird watching | | | | | | | | | | |
| Dating | | | | | | | | | | |
| Auto-racing | | | | | | | | | | |
| Home repairs | | | | | | | | | | |
| Exercise | | | | | | | | | | |
| Hunting | | | | | | | | | | |
| Woodworking | | | | | | | | | | |
| Pool | | | | | | | | | | |
| Driving | | | | | | | | | | |
| Child care | | | | | | | | | | |
| Tennis | | | | | | | | | | |
| Cooking/Baking | | | | | | | | | | |
| Basketball | | | | | | | | | | |
| History | | | | | | | | | | |
| Collecting | | | | | | | | | | |
| Fishing | | | | | | | | | | |
| Science | | | | | | | | | | |
| Leatherwork | | | | | | | | | | |
| Shopping | | | | | | | | | | |
| Photography | | | | | | | | | | |
| Painting/Drawing | | | | | | | | | | |

• **Fig. 14.4, cont'd**

according to the area of performance (e.g., activities of daily living, instrumental activities of daily living, education, work, play, leisure, and social participation). The client rates whether the activity is one he or she *has* to do or *wants* to do and how adequately the activity is performed. The practitioner uses the data to determine how the person spends his or her day and in what types of activities he or she is involved.

The interview takes place in a setting that is quiet and allows for privacy. Ideally, the interview should be relaxed and comfortable for both the interviewer and the client. The skill of interviewing involves blending the formal information gathering with informal person-to-person communication. The stages of an interview include initial contact, information gathering, and closure.

### Initial Contact

The skilled interviewer spends the first few minutes of the interview putting the subject at ease. Often, a person is worried and anxious at an interview. A client may experience stress related to the illness or trauma, or he or she may feel threatened by the prospect of entering into therapy.

The practitioner begins the interview by introducing him- or herself and informing the client about the clinic, the program, and standard procedures. It is important to convey general information but not burden the person with specific details that he or she may be afraid of forgetting.

Each OT practitioner develops his or her own interviewing style. Regardless, taking the time to create a relaxed and unthreatening atmosphere is beneficial to future therapy because the interview creates the "first impression" of the therapy process. The client who feels welcome will begin therapy prepared to become a partner in the therapy process.

### Information Gathering

After discussing the purpose of therapy, the OT practitioner gathers information about the client, population or community. The skilled interviewer guides the conversation in a way that yields the desired data yet keeps the flow easy and comfortable. The OT practitioner explains before beginning the interview that he or she will be taking notes. He or she asks questions conversationally, while making eye contact, and does not read directly from notes. An unskilled interviewer may spend time interviewing only to discover he or she has not collected the needed information. To ensure that the desired information is secured, the OT practitioner works from an interview outline.

### Closure

Effectively putting closure to the interview is also a learned skill. The OT practitioner guides the interview to collect needed data in a pleasant, conversational way. The interviewer signals when the interview is about to end by summarizing the information gathered and reviewing the next steps in the process. This technique avoids the discomfort of an abrupt "time is up" ending.

## Developing Observation Skills

**Observation** is the means of gathering information about a person or an environment by watching and noticing. Observation may occur through a structured series of steps introduced by the OT practitioner, or it may be intentionally left unstructured to see what takes place. The OT practitioner obtains information about the client, population, or community through observation. For example, the practitioner can observe the person's posture, dress, social skills, tone of voice, behavior, and physical abilities (e.g., use of the limbs and ambulation).

Observation is an important professional skill and can be developed through practice. Practitioners may develop observation skills by documenting findings and discussing these with an experienced practitioner. Examining skills by watching videotapes of clients is another technique to develop observational skills. Using observational questionnaires or worksheets may help guide an inexperienced practitioner and make it easier to identify important observations see Fig. 14.5.

A **structured observation** involves watching the client perform a predetermined activity. OT practitioners frequently use structured observation to gain knowledge of what the person can or cannot do in relation to the demands of the task. If, for example, the OT practitioner wishes to evaluate a self-care activity such as shaving, the client is asked to shave the way he usually does. While observing, the practitioner learns what is needed to improve function in this task. With information that identifies the extent of the lim-

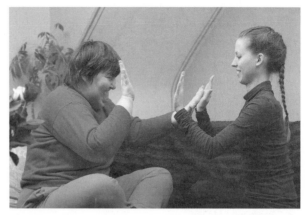

● **Fig. 14.5** The practitioner observes the client's reactions, postures, timing and sequencing during a simple game. © Getty Images/Creative RF/miriam-doerr.

itation, the OT practitioner can make a plan for correction or improvement. OT practitioners examine the quality of performance through observation of the process, not just by examining the end product. For example, the clinician may observe how the person responds to directions, approaches the activity, interacts with others, deals with frustration, and engages in the task during the activity. Box 14.1 presents a guide for observation.

## Formal Assessment Procedures

Formal assessment procedures help determine the existing performance level of the client. Formal **assessment procedures** include tests, instruments, or strategies that provide specific guidelines for administration see Fig. 14.6.[4] This informs practitioners about what is to be examined, how it is to be examined, how data are communicated, and how the information is applied in therapeutic problem solving. Formal assessment procedures have specific guidelines, and therefore they are easily duplicated and critically analyzed.[4]

A test is said to have **validity** if research testing shows it to be a true measure of what it claims to measure. Test **reliability** is a measure of how accurately the scores obtained from the test reflect the true performance of the client. There are several different types of reliability with which the OT practitioner must be familiar. **Test-retest reliability** is an indicator of the consistency of the results of a given test from one administration to another. **Interrater reliability** is an indicator of the likelihood that test scores will be the same no matter who is the examiner. OT practitioners can place more confidence in instruments that have high validity and reliability.

A **standardized test** is one that has gone through a rigorous process of scientific inquiry to determine its reliability and validity. Each standardized test has a carefully established protocol for its administration. OT practitioners follow set procedures for administering and scoring the test. Some standardized tests require that clinicians say the exact same words to each client. Standardized tests may be based on **normative data,** often called *norms*, collected from a representative sample that can then be used by the examiner to

### • BOX 14.1 | Observation Guide

1. Describe how the client performs the activity in terms of the following client factors:
   - Movement functions
   - Specific mental functions (including thought, judgment, concept formation, emotional, language, motor planning, experience of self and others)
   - Global mental functions (including consciousness, orientation, temperament, personality, energy, and drive)
2. Describe the client in terms of an overall impression during activities:
   - Physical appearance
   - Reaction to testing situation
   - Response to examiner
   - Approach to tasks
   - Quality of production
   - Communications with others
3. Gather information related to specific qualities:
   - Attentiveness
   - Independence
   - Ability to follow verbal instructions
   - Ability to follow written instructions
   - Cooperativeness
   - Initiative
   - Response to authority
   - Ability to read and write
   - Timidity or aggressiveness
   - Neatness
   - Accuracy
   - Distractibility
   - Passive or active involvement
   - Ease of movement
   - Speed of performance
   - Problem solving
   - Motor skills
   - Adaptability
   - Social skills
   - Affect
   - Interactions with others

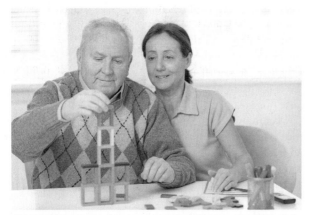

**Fig. 14.6** Formal assessments can provide additional information that may benefit clients. © Getty Images/Creative RF/FredFroese.

make comparisons with his or her subjects. Normative data are compiled by administering the test to a large sample of subjects.[4] The Jebsen Hand Test[6] and the Sensory Integration and Praxis Tests (SIPT)[5] are examples of standardized tests.

OT practitioners also use **nonstandardized tests** for measuring function. Nonstandardized tests have guidelines for administering and scoring but may not have established normative data or established reliability and validity. The administration and scoring of nonstandardized tests are more subjective and rely on the clinical skill, judgment, and experience of the therapist. For example, manual muscle testing and sensory testing are nonstandardized tests.

There is a broad range of assessment instruments available to OT practitioners. OT practitioners use frames of reference to guide the selection of a test instrument, in addition to consideration of the client's background, diagnosis, and needs.

OT practitioners administering a test instrument must be properly prepared. Before administering a test, the OT practitioner must become familiar with the procedures and know the correct way to administer items, score the test, and interpret the data. Comfort with any testing procedure is acquired through practice. Some tests even require special training or certification before they can be administered. Under the direction of an occupational therapist, an OTA may administer the test once service competency has been established.

## Intervention Process

The aim of OT is to enable the person with a disability to function more independently in his or her environment. OT may also enable populations (e.g., older adults) or communities (e.g., town or local area) to engage in occupaitons. This requires problem-solving methods to improve occupational performance. The OT intervention process requires the practitioner to develop goals for the client, population or community, select activities, direct intervention to guide the client to learn ways of engaging in occupational performance, and monitor the results of the intervention.

### Intervention Planning: Problem Identification, Solution Development, and Plan of Action

The intervention plan is based on an analysis of the information accumulated during the evaluation. The initial step in developing the intervention plan is *problem identification*. The occupational therapist reviews the results of the evaluation and identifies the client's, population's or community's strengths and deficits in performance skills, performance patterns, client factors, and contexts. From this, the occupational therapist uses clinical reasoning (also known as therapeutic reasoning) to determine the problem areas that need to be addressed through intervention. Problem identification also includes developing a hypothesis about the cause of the problem. Understanding the problem helps the OT practitioner select the most appropriate approach to treatment.

*Solution development* is the process of identifying alternatives for intervention and forming goals and objectives.

Selecting a *model of practice* and *frame of reference* from which the OT practitioner operates is an important component of solution development. Several frames of reference are used in OT practice. Each frame of reference is based on a body of knowledge that identifies principles and processes of change (see Chapter 15 for more information on models of practice and frames of reference). The frame of reference selected provides the practitioner with guidelines for clinical reasoning and intervention planning. Exploring intervention strategies based on the different frames of reference will help the practitioner develop potential solutions.

Based on the problems and the identified frame of reference along with input received from the client, the practitioner determines a *plan of action* for intervention (expected outcomes). The first step in developing a plan of action is the creation of long- and short-term goals that address the problems identified. These goals are prioritized according to the needs of the client. Next, intervention methods that will help the client achieve the goals are determined. This involves a consideration of the tools or equipment needed, any special positioning, where the activity will take place, how it will be structured and graded, and whether it is to be performed in a group or individually.[2] The intervention methods are based on the selected frame of reference. The practitioner uses his or her knowledge of the disability and the intervention to predict which methods will likely achieve the desired results as stated in the goals. Chapter 16 discusses the types of therapeutic activities used in OT.

The outcome of this intervention planning process is a written report (or intervention plan). The written plan addresses the strengths and weaknesses of the individual, interests of the client and caregivers, estimate of rehabilitation potential, and expected outcomes (short- and long-term goals), along with frequency and duration of intervention, recommended methods and media, apparent environmental and time constraints, identification of a plan for reevaluation, and discharge planning.[2] Fig. 14.7 is an example of a form used for an intervention plan. The plan is formally entered in the client's records.

The occupational therapist is responsible for analyzing and interpreting the data from the evaluation and formulating and documenting the intervention plan.[1] The OTA contributes to this process.

## Implementation of the Plan

**Intervention** involves working with the client through therapy to reach client goals. AOTA describes five intervention approaches are used in OT: create/promote; establish, restore; maintain; modify; and prevent.[2] The following examples describe how these approaches may be implemented in practice. See Appendix A for sample intervention activities.

These examples are just a few of the many intervention strategies employed by OT practitioners. Furthermore, these strategies may be used with individual clients, populations, or communities.

**Occupational Therapy Intervention Plan**

Client's Name:

DOB:

Date of Report:

Reason for referral:

Background information:

Initial level of performance:

    Strengths

    Weaknesses

Assessment (Clinical impressions):

Client's Goals:

Long Term Goals:

Short Term Goals:

Intervention: frequency and duration:

    Frame of Reference (principles and rationale)

    Space, setting requirements

Considerations:

Other

**Fig. 14.7** Modified Medicare 700 form—occupational therapy plan of treatment. (Courtesy of RehabWorks, a division of Symphony Rehabilitation, Hunt Valley, MD. From Pendleton, H., & Schultz-Krohn [Eds.]. [2012]. *Pedretti's occupational therapy practice skills for physical dysfunction* [7th ed.]. St. Louis, MO: Mosby).

*Create/promote:* The OT practitioner organizes an afternoon handwriting group for school-aged children. The practitioner recommends the group to children in his or her caseload who have difficulty with handwriting.

*Establish, restore:* The OT practitioner works with Galen, a 67-year-old man who has lost use of his right side since his cerebral vascular accident. The clinician works to help Galen return to his typical morning routine.

*Maintain:* After performing a home visit, the OT practitioner makes recommendations so 90-year-old Harry can stay at home.

*Modify:* The OT practitioner provides 35-year-old Karen, who has traumatic brain injury, with adapted feeding equipment so that she can feed herself.

*Prevent:* The OT practitioner explains proper lifting techniques to a group of workers at the blanket factory with the goal of preventing injuries.

**Consulting** is also an important part of intervention. Practitioners frequently consult with other professionals, family members, and clients regarding intervention strategies. When the OT practitioner consults with others, he or she is not directly responsible for the implementation and subsequent outcome of the intervention. For example, the practitioner may consult with a teacher on how to facilitate handwriting skills in the classroom. A practitioner may consult in a work setting about ergonomically correct lifting techniques or workspace arrangements. Consultation requires advanced knowledge, the ability to communicate clearly with others, and knowledge of the context in which the consultation occurs.

Another important aspect of intervention is **education.** OT practitioners educate the client, family, and caregivers about activities that support the intervention plan. When caregivers are responsible for implementing treatment, they need to be aware of the risks and benefits of intervention as well. Education may be formal or informal in nature. For example, the OT practitioner may provide an educational workshop to a parent group regarding a particular frame of reference. The practitioner may educate the client in a session, by providing a demonstration and handout. Education must be tailored to the client's level. The OT practitioner should speak clearly and avoid the use of jargon. OT practitioners teaching clients to reengage in occupations need to make sure that the client understands the lesson and can provide a demonstration of the targeted techniques. The OT practitioner answers any questions and follows up at the next visit.

The interaction between the practitioner and client is an essential element of therapy. A therapeutic relationship should always have the interest of the client as its central concern. The practitioner's role is to choose the interaction style that best supports the goals of the intervention plan and to help the client move toward independence. Setting the tone of interaction will be a decision based on the overall cognitive ability and attitude of the client. Chapter 17 describes in detail the development of a therapeutic relationship.

Although the implementation of the intervention plan is the responsibility of both the occupational therapist and the OTA, it is the *central* responsibility of the OTA. Educational programs are designed to ensure that OTAs develop an understanding of the philosophy and skills of OT to enable them to interpret and implement intervention plans. The OTA conducts intervention under the supervision of the occupational therapist.

## Intervention Review

As intervention is implemented, the OT practitioner reevaluates the client's progress in therapy. The practitioner continually monitors the client's, community's or population's needs, circumstances, and conditions to identify whether any permanent or temporary change in the intervention plan is required. Reevaluation may result in changing activities, retesting, writing a new plan, or making needed referrals.

The OT practitioner assesses the client each intervention session by monitoring the influence of intervention and evaluating whether the activity has the desired therapeutic effect. For example, if the activity becomes too easy for the client, the OT practitioner may increase the level of difficulty by adding resistance or by changing the demands of the activity. The OT practitioner reevaluates the plan, including how it is being carried out and the achievement of outcomes targeted for the client; modifies the plan as needed; and determines the need for continuation, discontinuation, or referral to another service.[2] Intervention services change as the needs of the client change.

## Transition Services

**Transition services** involve the coordination or facilitation of services for the purpose of preparing the client for a change. Transition services may involve a change to a new functional level, life stage, program, or environment. The OT practitioner is involved in identifying services and preparing an individualized transition plan to facilitate the client's change from one place to another.[1] In other words, the transition plan needs to be individualized to meet the goals, needs, and environmental considerations of the individual client.

The following cases provide examples of the importance of transition services.

Mr. G, a 75-year-old married man, was hospitalized for a total hip replacement. Because he is able to return home to a spouse willing to cook, clean, and assist him with self-care, he requires little outside assistance. His children, who live nearby, also will help out. His transition service plan includes training Mr. G to safely move around the house, transfer to the toilet safely, and perform basic self-care.

Mr. W, a 75-year-old single man, was also hospitalized for a total hip replacement. However, he lives alone and has no family nearby. Mr. W will require a different transition plan. His transition plan includes a daily visit by the home health nurse, meals-on-wheels services, and a home evaluation by the OT practitioner. The OT practitioner will work on mobility throughout the house, simple meal preparation, and home safety.

These two cases demonstrate the differences in transition services required. Some clients may need to be transferred to a lower level of care (e.g., a skilled nursing facility) before returning home. Careful planning is the key to preparing the client for the transition home.

## Discontinuation of Services

The last step of the intervention process is the discontinuation of the client from OT services. The client is discharged from OT when he or she has reached the goals delineated in the intervention plan, when he or she has realized the maximum benefit of OT services, or when he or she does not wish to continue services.[1,2] The **discharge plan** is developed and implemented to address the resources and supports that may be required upon discharge. The discharge plan includes recommendations for continued services (including OT, if necessary), equipment recommendations, and follow-up recommendations. In addition, the plan may include training family members and caregivers.

The occupational therapist writes a discharge summary of the client's functional level, changes that were made throughout the course of OT intervention, plans for discharge, equipment and services recommended, and follow-up needs. The occupational therapist prepares and implements the discharge plan with input from the OTA.[1]

## Outcomes Process

OT practitioners use outcome measures to determine whether goals have been met and to make decisions regarding future intervention.[2] Outcome measures provide objective feedback to the client and practitioner. Thus, selecting measures that are valid, reliable, and appropriately sensitive to change is important. OT practitioners are interested in selecting measures early and using measures that may predict future outcomes.[2] Because the broad outcome of OT is engagement in occupation to support participation, measures that evaluate this outcome should be selected. OT practitioners are also interested in measuring occupational performance, client satisfaction, adaptation, quality of life, role competence, prevention, and health and wellness.[2]

## Summary

The OT process is a dynamic, ongoing, interactive process. Generally, the process includes referral, screening, evaluation, intervention planning, implementation of the intervention plan, transition services, and discontinuation of services. Each stage requires that the OT practitioner observe carefully and listen to the client's needs.

## Learning Activities

1. Provide the class with a case study. Randomly assign students (or teams) to one of the five treatment approaches (e.g., create, establish, maintain, modify, or prevent). Ask students to provide examples of how this treatment approach would be used with the case. Compare and contrast the benefits of each in class.
2. Interview a classmate for a few minutes to determine the occupations in which he or she engages. Write a page-long summary of the interview. Submit a page-long reflection on the interview process by discussing what you could have done differently and what you did well. Ask your partner for feedback.
3. Help students improve their observation skills by having them write down everything they see while watching a fellow classmate perform a simple activity (e.g., making a cup of cocoa). After they have made a list, have them use the *Occupational Therapy Practice Framework* as a guide to examine the activity. Discuss the findings.
4. Review a journal article that examines the effectiveness of a given intervention. Summarize the intervention techniques the researchers used and the results of the study. What did you learn about OT intervention?
5. Interview an OT practitioner to find out about a particular case that the practitioner finds interesting. Find out the intervention approach and context(s) in which the intervention took place. Present this to your classmates.

## Review Questions

1. What are the five general treatment approaches used in OT practice?
2. What are some techniques for successful interviewing?
3. What are the stages of the OT process?
4. Compare and contrast the roles of the occupational therapist and the OTA in the OT process.
5. What type of information is included in an occupational profile?
6. What is included in a discharge summary?
7. What are the steps to intervention planning?

## References

1. American Occupational Therapy Association. Standards of practice for occupational therapy. *Am J Occup Ther.* 2015;69(suppl 3). Retrieved from, http://dx.doi.org/10.5014/ajot.2015.696506.
2. American Occupational Therapy Association. Occupational therapy practice framework: domain and process (3rd ed.). *Am J Occup Ther.* 2014;68(suppl 1):S1–S48.
3. American Occupational Therapy Association. Scope of practice. *Am J Occup Ther.* 2014;68(3):S34–S40.
4. Asher IE. *Occupational Therapy Assessment Tools: An Annotated Index.* 3rd ed. Bethesda, MD: American Occupational Therapy Association Press; 2007.
5. Ayres J. *Sensory Integration and Praxis Tests (SIPT).* Los Angeles, CA: Western Psychological Services; 1998.
6. Jebsen RH, Taylor N, Trieschmann RB, et al. An objective and standardized test of hand function. *Arch Phys Med Rehabil.* 1969;50(6):311–369.
7. Matsutsuyu J. The interest checklist. *Am J Occup Ther.* 1969;23:323–328.

# 15

# Models of Practice and Frames of Reference

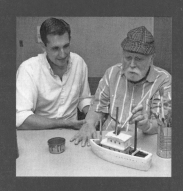

## OBJECTIVES

*After reading this chapter, the reader will be able to do the following:*

- Define theory, model of practice, and frame of reference.
- Discuss the importance of using a model of practice and frame of reference.
- Understand how research supports practice.

- Identify the components of a frame of reference.
- Summarize selected occupational therapy models of practice.
- Identify the principles guiding selected frames of reference.

## KEY TERMS

biomechanical frame of reference
brain plasticity
Canadian Model of Occupational
    Performance
cognitive disability frame of
    reference

concepts
evidence-based practice
frame of reference
Kawa model
Model of Human Occupation
model of practice

occupational adaptation
Person-Environment-Occupation-
    Performance model
principles
theory

ℯ Visit *www.evolve.elsevier.com* to access the Evolve student resources that accompany your book.

*My debut into the occupational therapy (OT) career happened by chance. After high school, I was trying to figure out what I wanted to do with my life. I was interested in studying psychology. However, in the country of Kenya, Africa, where I grew up, there was no psychology major at the time in any of the institutions of higher education. My sister had just completed her studies at the Kenya Medical Training College and had been awarded a diploma in radiography. She informed me that there was a program at the college called OT. She did not know much about the program, except that she saw occupational therapists doing much basket weaving and seemingly having lots of fun. However, she also knew that they studied a lot of psychology. So, I applied and got into the program.*

*Since graduating way back in 1985, my progress in the profession has been fortuitous. For some time, I left the profession altogether and studied, and for a while I practiced counseling psychology. However, I realized that "doing" meaningful things (meaningful occupations) with*

*clients is far more therapeutic than just talking about issues. So, I came back to the profession, hopefully much wiser and with more commitment based on insight. My experiences have led me to believe that the way to strengthen OT and ensure its survival far into the future is by therapists being very clear of their origin (which in my view is mental health) and staying true to the original principles, even while making progressive and useful innovations. That is why one of my favorites pastimes is discussing with students (future occupational therapists) OT theory and its origins, and speculating about its future development.*

**MOSES N. IKIUGU, PHD, OTR/L**
**Professor and Director of Research**
**Department of Occupational Therapy**
**University of South Dakota**
**Vermillion, South Dakota**

Occupational therapy (OT) practitioners help clients engage in occupations. They work with clients of all ages, from numerous cultures, and clients who have a variety of conditions and circumstances. Practitioners base intervention on knowledge of the underlying conditions and evidence to support the intervention techniques.

A model of practice helps organize one's thinking, whereas a **frame of reference** is a tool to guide one's intervention.[13,15] A FOR tells you what to do and how to evaluate and intervene with clients. Furthermore, FORs have research to support the principles guiding evaluation and intervention. Thus using a FOR to guide one's practice is essential to **evidence-based practice.** Evidence-based practice refers to choosing intervention techniques based on the best possible research. This chapter outlines selected OT models of practice and FORs and describes how they are applied in practice.

## Understanding Theory

A **theory** is a set of ideas that helps explain things. Research is used to support or refute theories. OT borrows theories from other disciplines, such as psychology, medicine, nursing, and social work. Theory is the analysis of a set of facts in their relation to one another.[14] There are two major structural components to theory: concepts and principles.[24,25] **Concepts** are ideas that represent something in the mind of the individual. These range from simple concrete ideas to complex, abstract ideas. Concepts are expressed through the use of symbols and language. For example, a child learns that clothing is a category that can be divided into shoes, pants, dresses, and shirts, among others. **Principles** explain the relationship between two or more concepts.[24] For instance, once the concept of color is learned, such as blue and yellow, a child learns the principle that mixing these two colors produces green.

Theory is defined as "a set of interrelated assumptions, concepts, and definitions that presents a systematic view of phenomena by specifying relationships among variables, with the purpose of explaining and predicting the phenomena."[19] Theories range in scope and complexity along a continuum. Theories may be broad in scope and attempt to cover many aspects of a discipline, or they may have a narrow focus and concern only a small portion of the field.[24] Fig. 15.1 provides an illustration of how these concepts fit together.

## Why Is It Important to Know About and Use Theory in Occupational Therapy Practice?

Some students resist theory. They prefer to "get in there and do something" rather than discuss why it is done. Not applying theory to practice is similar to taking a trip without a road map. The trip will be disorganized and lack

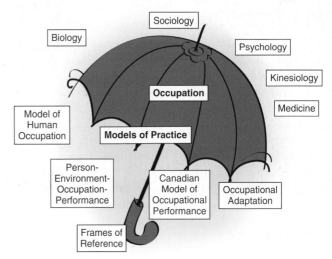

● **Fig. 15.1** The umbrella of occupation: a conceptual diagram of the relationship between theories, occupation, models of practice, and frames of reference. (From MacRae N; O'Brien J: OT 301 Foundations of occupational therapy, unpublished lecture notes, 2001, University of New England.)

structure. The traveler may eventually find a way to the final destination but may not know exactly how he or she got from point A to point B. Consequently, it is difficult to give directions to anyone else or to replicate the journey in the future. OT practitioners appreciate theory because it is required to therapeutically reason and develop effective intervention. Theory provides the basis for practice.

Parham states, "Theory is a key element in problem solving. It is a tool that enables the practitioner to 'name it and frame it.' Both language and logic are needed to identify a problem (name it) and to plan a means for altering the situation (frame it). Theory provides these by giving us words or concepts for naming what we observe and by spelling out logical relationships between concepts."[16] Theory allows the OT practitioner to structure and organize intervention.

Theory also serves to (1) validate and guide practice, (2) justify reimbursement, (3) clarify specialization issues, (4) enhance the growth of the profession and the professionalism of its members, and (5) educate competent practitioners.[24]

Theories specific to OT practice originated in science-based disciplines, such as biology, chemistry, physics, psychology, and occupational science. The practitioner may use a number of theories during intervention and combine parts of theories. To do so, the practitioner must be knowledgeable about the theories to be sure that they are compatible with one another. Theories used in OT include those developed by Mosey, Kielhofner, Ayres, Reilly, Llorens, and Fidler. It is beyond the scope of this introductory text to describe all of the various theories used. Theory is linked to clinical practice through models of practice and FORs.

## Model of Practice

The terms *model of practice, conceptual model, practice model,* and *frame of reference* have been used interchangeably. In this text, we distinguish between model of practice and FOR. However, this is just one way to organize the content.

A **model of practice** takes the philosophical base of the profession and organizes the concepts for practice. As such, OT models of practice help OT practitioners organize their thinking around occupation,[13] which is the central unifying feature of the OT profession. A model of practice provides practitioners with terms to describe practice, an overall view of the profession, tools for evaluation, and a guide for intervention.[8,13,15]

By reading and critically analyzing current literature, practitioners who use a model of practice to guide their practice find a depth of information, which allows them to better understand practice and intervention to the benefit of clients. Using a model of practice ensures a systematic examination of the client and is an important step in providing evidence-based practice.

The **Model of Human Occupation** (MOHO)[9] is the best-researched model of practice in OT. Kielhofner and colleagues have published extensively on all aspects of this model, and thus this model provides well-supported evidence to support its use in practice. The Model of Human Occupation views occupational performance in terms of volition, habituation, performance capacity, and environment. Volition refers to the person's motivation, interests, values, and belief in skill. Habituation refers to one's daily patterns of behaviors, one's roles (the rules and expectations of those positions), and one's everyday routine. Performance capacity refers to the motor, cognitive, and emotional aspects required to act upon the environment.[9] Environment refers to the physical, social, and societal surroundings in which the person is involved. Each system is divided into components with many well-researched instruments to operationalize the terms for practice.[9] Working with the assessment tools designed to operationalize the concepts of the model helps practitioners understand the concepts more fully for practice.

The **Canadian Model of Occupational Performance** (CMOP)[10,22] has also generated a wealth of research to support its design. The core of this model is spirituality, which is defined broadly as anything that motivates or inspires a person.[10,22] Person, environment (which includes institutions), and occupations are the other parts of the model. This model emphasizes client-centered care,[10,22] which refers to understanding the client's desires and wishes for intervention and outcome. Getting to know the client is crucial to this model. The *Canadian Occupational Performance Measure*[11] is a semistructured interview based on this model and provides practitioners with a tool to organize their thoughts.

The **Person-Environment-Occupation-Performance** (PEOP) model[6] developed by Christiansen and Baum provides definitions for each term and describes the interactive nature of the human being. *Person* includes the physical, social, and psychological aspects of the individual. *Environment* includes the physical and social supports and those things that interfere with the individual's performance. *Occupation* refers to the everyday things people do and in which they find meaning. *Performance* refers to the actions of occupations.[6]

**Occupational adaptation,** articulated by Schkade and Schultz, proposes that OT practitioners examine how they may change the person, environment, or task so the client may engage in occupations. In this model, occupation is viewed as the primary means for the individual to achieve adaptation. Individual adaptation is seen as both a state of being and a process that can be examined at a given time, over a specified time period, or over a lifetime.[20] This model focuses on the person, the occupational environment, and the interaction. It supports compensatory techniques if necessary.

These models provide a framework for evaluating clients and designing occupation-based interventions. Other models of practice exist in OT practice.

## Case Application

The following case examples provide an overview of the use of the different models of practice.

Raven is a 55-year-old woman who was hospitalized with a brain aneurysm, which affected her speech, right-sided movement, and cognitive abilities. Raven is unable to remain standing for long periods of time, and she needs frequent breaks during seated activities. Raven experiences difficulty with memory and poor concentration.

The occupational therapist meets with Raven on her first day on the rehabilitation unit. The following comparison describes the type of information she will collect about Raven from each model of practice.

## Model of Human Occupation

*Volition:* Raven enjoys family events, singing, and cooking. Raven lives close to her family and sees her mother, three children, and many other family members daily. Furthermore, the family attends church services on Sunday and then gathers at Raven's for a potluck supper. She is active in the church choir.

*Habituation:* Raven works 5 days a week from 8 am to 5 pm in a local grocery store, where she is the assistant manager. She attends her grandchildren's school events and periodically helps her daughters with child care and transportation. Raven attends church on Wednesday evenings and Sundays.

*Performance:* Before her aneurysm, Raven was able to complete all occupations without difficulty. Currently, she is unable to use her right side, slurs her speech, has difficulty maintaining a conversation, and becomes easily confused. Raven is unable to remain active for over 20 minutes, showing obvious signs of fatigue.

*Environment:* Raven lives in a small apartment building in the city with her husband. She has been married for 35 years. They live on the third floor. The building has elevators, but Raven is afraid to use them. Raven's family members live close by and frequently visit her. She holds many family gatherings at her house.

## Canadian Model of Occupational Performance

*Spirituality:* Raven attends church on Wednesday nights and Sundays. She is active in her church and enjoys the family camaraderie of the church. Raven sings in the choir and defines herself as a devoted Christian.
*Person:* Raven is a 55-year-old married woman who suffered an aneurysm and is in a rehabilitation hospital. She is unable to use her right side, slurs her speech, and shows poor memory and concentration.
*Environment:* Raven works for the institution of a grocery chain. As such, she must follow institutional policy and procedures. She has medical insurance. She also follows the church's institutional policies.
*Occupations:* Raven enjoys spending time with family; she is active in the church and a member of the choir. Raven works at a local grocery store. She attends her grandchildren's school events when possible.

### Person-Environment-Occupation-Performance

*Person:* Raven lives with her husband. She has been married for 35 years. She has many family members whom she sees regularly. Raven enjoys family events, singing, and cooking.
*Environment:* Raven lives in a small apartment building in the city. She lives on the third floor. Raven's family live close by.
*Occupations:* She works 5 days a week from 8 am to 5 pm in a local grocery store. Raven attends church and sees her family frequently. Raven attends her grandchildren's events.
*Performance:* Raven slurs her speech and has difficulty using her right side. She fatigues easily.

### Occupational Adaptation

*Occupation:* Raven works as an assistant manager at a grocery store. She takes care of her family and is involved in the church. She enjoys socializing with others. Currently, she is unable to engage in these occupations because of right-sided weakness, slurred speech, and fatigue.
*Adaptation:* The OT practitioner changes the demands of the occupation of socializing by allowing Raven to sit in a chair and visit with family members for short periods of time. The OT practitioner provides Raven with short projects in which she can participate with her grandchildren when they visit. This helps Raven continue her nurturing occupations while helping her gain function.

### Conclusion

The case study applications just described illustrate the subtle discrepancies among the models of practice. Although the information gathered may be similar, the focus differs. Readers should explore the complexities, definitions, and explanations of each of the terms because they provide insight into how to analyze human occupation. Furthermore, readers are encouraged to examine the available assessment tools and measures that more specifically define the concepts of the various models. For example, the Volitional Questionnaire designed under the Model of Human Occupation examines one's interests, values, and personal causation. Understanding this assessment tool helps practitioners more completely understand the concept of volition to better serve their clients.

## Frames of Reference

Williamson states that "Frames of reference are produced from the body of knowledge of the profession and address a specific aspect of the profession's domain of concern."[25] A FOR describes the process for change in the client and the principles for moving a client along a continuum from dysfunction to function. Depending on the focus of intervention, the practitioner may use several FORs at one time or use them sequentially over time.[25]

One of the most efficient and practical ways to conduct evidence-based practice is to examine FORs, which apply theory and put principles into practice. As such, FORs provide practitioners with specifics about how to treat specific clients. A FOR includes a description of the population, theory regarding change, function and dysfunction, principles of intervention, role of the practitioner, and evaluation instruments. The parts of a FOR are listed in Box 15.1 and are described in the following sections. Table 15.1 provides an overview of selected frames of reference.

### Population

The FOR identifies the types of diagnoses or population that would benefit from the intervention. It describes the age, type of condition, and type of deficit addressed in intervention. For example, clients who experience decreased strength and endurance are typically treated using the biomechanical FOR. Research supports the use of repetitive exercise in strengthening muscles. Practitioners using a biomechanical FOR do not have to conduct their own

**• BOX 15.1 Necessary Parts of a Frame of Reference**

- Population
- Continuum of function–dysfunction
- Theory regarding change
- Principles
- Role of the practitioner
- Assessment instruments

| TABLE 15.1 | **Frames of Reference** |

**Model of Human Occupation:** A dynamic frame of reference and a model of practice that examines the interactions between a person's volition, habituation, performance, and environment to design occupation-based intervention. Understanding the relationship between these components allows the therapist to intervene and promote meaningful engagement in occupations for the client.

*Principles:*

a. Occupational actions, thoughts, and emotions always arise out of the dynamic interaction of volition, habituation, performance capacity, and environmental context.

b. Change in any aspect of volition, habituation, performance capacity, and/or the environment can result in a change in thoughts, feelings, and actions.

c. Volition, habituation, and performance capacity are maintained and changed through what one does and what one thinks and feels about "doing."

d. A particular pattern of volition, habituation, and performance capacity will be maintained so long as the underlying thoughts, feelings, and actions are consistently repeated in a supporting environment.

e. Change requires that novel thoughts, feelings, and actions emerge and be sufficiently repeated in a supportive environment to coalesce into a new organized pattern. (Kielhofner, 2008)

**Developmental:** Identifies the level of motor (gross, fine, oral), social, emotional, and cognitive skills in which a child engages and targets intervention to help the client advance.

*Principles:*

a. Development occurs over time and across areas.

b. The typical developmental sequence of skills is interrupted as a result of illness, trauma, or birth condition.

c. Gaps in development can be affected by physical, social, emotional, or traumatic events.

d. Occupational therapy can help fill in those gaps.

e. Repetitive practice of developmental skills as the client is able to master them provides experiences that promote brain plasticity and learning.

f. The developmental frame of reference promotes practice of skills in a developmental sequence and at the level just above where the client is functioning. (Llorens, 1976)

**Biomechanical:** Based on concepts of kinesiology, this frame of reference evaluates and intervenes regarding range of motion (ROM), strength, and endurance. This approach focuses on the physical limitations that interfere with the client's ability to engage in occupation.

*Principles:*

a. Improving ROM through passive and active means can increase the functional mobility required for activities and movement.

   • Joint ROM influences movement. The ability to move in directions within certain degrees of motion is a result of the bony structure and the integrity of the surrounding tissues. (Trombly & Radomski, 2002)

   • Preventing or reducing contractures or deformities will enhance movement and function.

b. Increasing strength can promote stability and balance for successful engagement in activity.

   • Muscle strength refers to the ability of a muscle to produce the tension necessary for posture and movement against resistance.

c. Energy is needed for a person to produce the required intensity or rate of effort over a period of time for an activity or exercise.

   • Endurance is sustained effort of muscles.

**Sensory Integration:** The organization of sensory input to produce an adaptive response; a theoretical process and intervention approach; addresses the processing of sensory information from the environment; includes discriminating, integrating, and modulating sensory information to produce meaningful adaptive responses. (Ayres, 1979)

*Principles:*

a. Sensory input can be used systematically to elicit an adaptive response.

b. Registration of meaningful sensory input is necessary before an adaptive response can be made.

c. An adaptive response contributes to the development of sensory integration.

d. Better organization of adaptive responses enhances the client's general behavioral organization.

e. More mature and complex patterns of behavior emerge from consolidation of simpler behaviors.

f. The more inner-directed a client's activities are, the greater the potential for the activities to improve the neural organization.

**TABLE 15.1**    **Frames of Reference—cont'd**

**Motor Control/Motor Learning:** Motor control examines how one directs and regulates movement, whereas motor learning theory describes how clients' learn movements. This approach is based on dynamic system theory that many factors influence movement and must be considered in intervention. (Shumway-Cook & Woolacott, 2007; Thelen, 1995)

*Principles:*

a. The interaction among systems is essential to adaptive control of movement.

b. Motor performance results from an interaction between adaptable and flexible systems.

c. Dysfunction occurs when movement patterns lack sufficient adaptability to accommodate task demands and environmental constraints.

d. Because task characteristics influence motor requirements, practitioners modify and adapt the requirements and affordances of tasks to help clients' succeed.

e. Clients' develop improved neural pathways when they repeat meaningful, whole (occupation) tasks in the natural environment.

f. Motor learning occurs as clients' repeat motor tasks that are intrinsically motivating, meaningful, and for which they can problem solve.

**Neurodevelopmental Treatment (NDT):** Technique developed by Karel and Berta Bobath to help children with functional limitations resulting from neuropathology, primarily children with cerebral palsy. The goal of NDT is to help children perform skilled movements more efficiently so they can carry out life skills. Practitioners begin with knowledge of typical movement. Practitioners use **handling techniques** and **key points of control** to facilitate **normal postures** so that children **"feel" typical movement** patterns. (Bobath, 1975; Coker-Bolt, 2016, pp. 350–352; Schoen & Anderson, 2009)

*Principles:*

a. The goal of NDT intervention is to improve overall function in daily tasks by increased active use of the trunk and involved extremities.

b. Intervention is individualized and focused on functional outcomes.

   • The OT practitioner may attempt to normalize muscle tone before and during functional movement.

   • The OT practitioner analyzes musculoskeletal limitations interfering with movement and function.

   • The OT practitioner facilitates normal movements that are meaningful to children.

   • Intervention emphasizes quality of movement (e.g., accuracy, quickness, adaptability, and flexibility) and reproducibility of movement.

c. Experience is the driving force for children. New activities build on previous sensorimotor experiences.

d. Target postural control and movements by using key points of control. Proximal points of control (e.g., hips, trunk, pelvis) provide more support to children, whereas distal points of control (e.g., head, hands, feet) require children to perform more of the movement.

e. The OT practitioner engages children in "typical" movement and repetition using new movement patterns to develop new neural pathways.

f. Children's motivation and active problem solving is considered when developing therapy goals and intervention activities.

**Kawa model:** The Kawa model attempts to explain occupational therapy's overall purpose, strategies for interpreting a client's circumstances and clarify the rationale and application of occupational therapy within the client's particular social and cultural context (Tech & Iwama, 2016).

*Principles:*

   • The Kawa (Japanese for 'River') model uses the metaphor or image of a river as a symbolic representation of life.

   • This client-centered approach allows clients to reflect and understand the occupational therapy process, identify obstacles, and develop strategies with the practitioner.

   • Like a river where its source represents the beginning of life and its mouth meeting the sea representing the end, the Kawa Model takes into consideration the past, present and future occupational needs of the client.

   • The river metaphor becomes a vehicle of communication and mutual understanding of the service user's experience of daily life and how occupational therapy can help in a positive way (Iwama, 2016).

   • Clients use pictures or words to explain their life circumstances in terms of:

      (i) life flow and overall occupations (river)

      (ii) environments/contexts, social and physical (river banks)

      (iii) circumstances that block life flow and cause dysfunction/disability (rocks)

      (iv) personal resources that can be assets or liabilities (driftwood)

The inclusive nature of the Kawa Model allows the occupational therapy client to be considered as a collective, meaning that it can be used on individuals, families, groups and organizations.

*Continued*

| TABLE 15.1 | Frames of Reference—cont'd |
|---|---|

**References**

Ayres, JA (1979). *Sensory integration for the child.* Los Angeles, CA: Western Psychological Services.

Bobath, B (1975). Sensorimotor development, *NDT Newsletter, 7,* 1.

Coker-Bolt, P (2016). Positioning and handling: A neurodevelopmental approach. In J. Solomon & J. O'Brien (Eds.), *Pediatric skills for occupational therapy assistants* (pp. 335–352). St. Louis: Elsevier.

Kielhofner, G (2008). *A Model of Human Occupation: Theory and application* (4th ed.). Baltimore, MD: Lippincott Williams & Wilkins.

Llorens, LA (1976). *Application of a developmental theory for health and rehabilitation.* Rockville, MD: American Occupational Therapy Association.

Schoen, S, & Anderson, J (2009). Neurodevelopmental treatment frame of reference. In P. Kramer & J. Hinojosa (Eds.), *Frames of reference for pediatric occupational therapy* (3rd ed., pp. 99–186). Baltimore, MD: Lippincott Williams & Wilkins.

Shumway-Cook, A, & Woollacott, M (2007). Motor control: Theory and practical applications (3rd. ed.). Philadelphia: Lippincott, Williams & Wilkins.

Tech, JY, & Iwama, M (2016). *The Kawa Model Made Easy Manual – updated 2015.* http://www.kawamodel.com/v1/index.php/2016/08/06/the-kawa-model-made-easy-download/

Thelen, E (1995). Motor development: A new synthesis. American Psychologist (50)2, 79-95.

Trombly, CS, & Radomski, MV (2002). *Occupational therapy for physical dysfunction* (5th ed.). Philadelphia, PA: Lippincott Williams & Wilkins.

research on how to strengthen muscles; instead, they use the research from this FOR, which states that providing repetitive movements, increasing the weight, and providing gradual resistance are all techniques that improve strength see Fig. 15.1.[17,18,23]

## Continuum of Function and Dysfunction

The FOR defines characteristics and behaviors on the continuum of function and dysfunction based on available research. The therapist evaluates these behaviors, which vary according to the FOR, during the assessment process. For example, according to the biomechanical FOR, function includes strength, endurance, and range of motion (ROM) that is adequate to perform occupations. Dysfunction is measured in limitations to strength, range of motion, and endurance.[17,18,23]

Conversely, the behavioral FOR defines function as the absence of abnormal behaviors, and dysfunction is the presence of behaviors that interfere with function. According to a behavioral FOR, abnormal behaviors may be socially unacceptable behaviors or those defined by the team as interfering with function see Fig. 15.2. Research provides guidelines to determine "typical" function. Practitioners use the available research to determine whether OT services are warranted.

## Theories Regarding Change

The FOR describes the theory and hypotheses regarding change. For example, many of the neurological (e.g., neurodevelopmental theory [NDT], sensory integration [SI], motor control) are based upon the theory of **brain plasticity,** which refers to the phenomenon that the brain is capable of change, and through activity one may get improved neurological synapses, improved dendritic growth, or additional pathways. Therefore intervention is aimed at improving neuronal firing and generating improved brain activity through repetition. Understanding the theory regarding change according to the FOR is important to providing evidence-based intervention see Fig. 15.3.

## Principles

The FOR defines the underlying principles guiding evaluation and intervention. These statements relate back to the theoretical base and describe how an individual

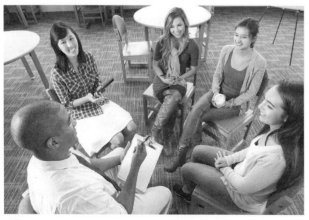

**Fig. 15.2** Clients work in an OT group to develop social behaviors. © Getty Images/Creative RF/asiseeit.

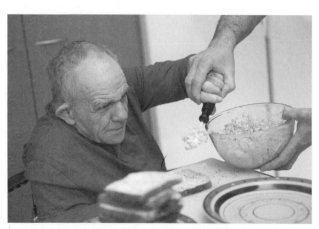

**Fig. 15.3** The client engages in the preparing lunch, which promotes motor control and motor learning and subsequent neuronal changes. © Getty Images/Creative RF/GaryRadler.

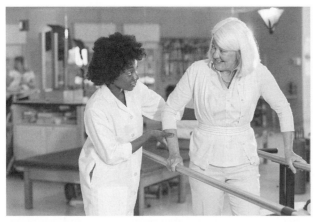

• **Fig. 15.4** The client engages in repetitive movement to increase muscle strength to complete activities of daily living. © Getty Images/Creative RF/kali9.

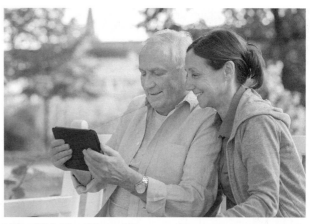

• **Fig. 15.5** The OT practitioner provides encouragement as the client finds leisure interest and activities. © Getty Images/Creative RF/FredFroese.

is aided to make changes and progress from a state of dysfunction to one of function. Understanding the principles of the FOR allows practitioners to use clinical reasoning to determine whether the FOR may benefit their client (although it may not be originally intended for that population). The principles are based on theory and research. OT practitioners critique the evidence and rationale to decide whether the FOR supports its claims. The FOR should clearly describe the principles surrounding the techniques. For example, the principle of strengthening is that by repetitive muscle contractions, more fibers are recruited and the muscle is able to lift more see Fig. 15.4.[18] Practitioners benefit from knowing that the principle behind strengthening is the recruitment of more muscle fibers.

## Role of the Practitioner

The role of the practitioner is based on the principles and theory of the FOR. These statements provide a guide as to how the practitioner will interact with the client and the environment. This is based on research evidence that supports the expectation that if a practitioner employs a certain technique the client's function will improve. Subsequently, OT practitioners can be assured when using a FOR that it worked for someone else. However, a careful analysis is still required to determine whether the technique is well founded or supported. Evidence-based practice suggests that the OT practitioner examine the rigor of the study, including the methodology, rationale, results, and design see Fig. 15.5. Examining the research of a FOR helps the practitioner fully understand the intricacies of the FOR and as such the role of the practitioner.

Importantly, the FOR describes how practitioners interact with clients. For example, practitioners using a behavioral FOR are to reward positive behaviors and ignore negative ones. The behavioral FOR provides insight into the type of cues that may be provided to clients. The neurodevelopment FOR requires that the practitioner touch the client throughout

the movement and facilitate a normal movement pattern.[4,21] Thus, knowledge and investigation into the FOR provide practitioners with a wealth of information for practice.

## Assessment Instruments

The FOR also provides the OT practitioner with a variety of instruments to operationalize the principles. For example, Allen's Cognitive Levels was designed to identify the level of cognitive functioning for clients and to be used with the cognitive disability FOR.[1,2]

The Sensory Integration and Praxis Tests, Sensory Processing Measure, Adult Sensory Profile, and clinical observations are based on SI principles and designed to assist the practitioner in determining how the client would benefit from the FOR.[3,5] The Occupational Self-Assessment, Volitional Questionnaire, and Model of Human Occupation Screening Test are some examples of the assessments designed to operationalize concepts associated with MOHO theory and practice.[9]

Numerous instruments have been developed to examine a client's functioning in relation to the principles of a specific FOR.

## Why Use a Frame of Reference?

FORs are based upon theory and research, and as such they provide OT practitioners with evidence to support intervention. OT practitioners can utilize the principles of the FOR to structure intervention sessions and organize their therapeutic reasoning. The practitioner uses previously tested strategies while considering the outcomes for the specific client. As the practitioner uses the principles and strategies, he or she can determine the client's responses and make a judgment on how the intervention session is progressing. If the client is not making the desired progress, the practitioner may revisit the theories and principles of the FOR, select a new FOR, or change his or her strategies based on the current FOR. Practitioners may also review current research related to the FOR to see if anything new has developed regarding strategies or methods for intervention. Using a FOR allows practitioners to benefit from the research that others have conducted and understand why certain intervention approaches may be more successful with specific clients.

## Application of Two Frames of Reference

Several FORs can be found in OT. For illustration purposes, two different FORs are presented using the previously described components. The first is the **biomechanical FOR**. This FOR is derived from theories in kinetics and kinematics (sciences that study the effects of forces and motion on material bodies).[23]

On the function–dysfunction continuum, the biomechanical FOR is used with individuals who have deficits in the peripheral nervous, musculoskeletal, integumentary (e.g., skin), or cardiopulmonary system. These individuals, however, have a central nervous system that is intact.[17,18,23] The deficits may cause posture and mobility problems, impairment in ROM and strength, and decreased endurance. Disabling conditions that may benefit from the biomechanical approach include rheumatoid arthritis and osteoarthritis, fractures, burns, hand traumas, amputations, and spinal cord injuries.

The practitioner evaluates the client's ROM, muscle strength, and endurance through the use of a variety of tools. Through exercise, activity, and physical agent modalities, change in the person's ROM, strength, and endurance can be demonstrated.[7]

Another FOR used for illustrative purposes is the **cognitive disability FOR** proposed by Claudia Allen. This FOR is based on the premise that cognitive disorders in those with mental health disabilities are caused by neurobiological defects or deficits related to the biologic functioning of the brain.[1,2] Its theoretical base is derived from research in neuroscience, cognitive psychology, information processing, and biologic psychiatry.[7]

Along the function–dysfunction continuum, function exists when an individual is able to process information to perform routine tasks demanded by the environment.[7] Dysfunction results when the person's ability to process information is restricted in such a way that carrying out routine tasks is impossible. Allen defines six cognitive levels, which are organized in a hierarchy along a continuum. Level 1 represents the individual who has a profound disability in information processing, whereas level 6 represents the normal ability to acquire and process information. Each cognitive level represents information-processing behaviors indicative of function–dysfunction. Two specific tools used by practitioners to evaluate an individual's level of functioning are the Allen Cognitive Level (ACL) Test and the Routine Task Inventory Test.[7] The cognitive disability FOR proposes that change occurs because of (1) the capacity of the client and (2) the environment. Change in the capacity of the client may be influenced by medical intervention, psychotropic medications, and OT intervention, which teaches the client how to perform routine tasks (cognitive levels 4 and 5). OT intervention can also produce change in the environment through modification of task procedures, amount of assistance offered, directions, and setting.[7] Environmental changes may allow the client to experience greater success in performing activities.

## Using Multiple Frames of Reference

Although organizing one's thoughts around one model of practice makes sense in OT, there are many FORs for different clientele. OT practitioners may use multiple FORs, depending on the setting and clientele. The practitioner must examine the theory, principles, and techniques used according to the FOR before deciding if the FOR would work with a given client and setting. If the practitioner is going to modify the FOR, the practitioner must be mindful of the reasons why and critically examine the rationale and research. Using a FOR in a different way may result in less dramatic changes but may be more practical in certain situations.

Sometimes, a practitioner may decide to combine FORs. For example, combining sensory integration and behavioral FORs may work with some clients. However, the OT practitioner must carefully observe how this blend is working and understand the principles behind each FOR to determine whether the blending is appropriate.

Some FORs do not fit together, and using them together may result in less progress toward the stated goals.

## Evaluating Frames of Reference

The OT practitioner is responsible for evaluating the client's progress toward his or her goals. If progress is slow or not being made, the OT practitioner reexamines the goals and the FOR. A careful examination of the techniques provided by the FOR may reveal other techniques to help the client reach the goals. Furthermore, the FOR may provide more insight into the role of the practitioner. The practitioner may change how he or she is working with the client or modify some techniques. It may be necessary to consult with a more experienced practitioner.

The practitioner explores the principles of the FOR to understand the reasoning behind the lack of progress. Could something else be going on that has been missed? The practitioner may reexamine the literature to determine whether others have found this FOR successful with the given population. If so, what techniques were used? How did the service differ from what the therapist is currently doing? It may be that the practitioner needs more time or needs to treat the client with more intensity.

When the FOR is not working, the OT practitioner may decide to change FORs. He or she considers the principles, goals, role of the therapist, and the client's motivations. Changing the FOR may provide the right momentum to spur progress.

## Case Application

George is a 34-year-old man who experienced a head trauma from a motor vehicle accident. He currently walks with a wide-based gait and shows uncoordinated movement patterns. He leans to the right and drags his left leg. George has poor lip closure (right facial droop) and difficulty chewing some foods. George has a poor right-handed grasp. He shows impaired long-term and short-term memory. Frequently, George is tearful during the session, and he has difficulty reading the cues of others.

The following examples show how the OT practitioner might view this case from different FORs.

*Behavioral:* Work on George's ability to complete activities and engage in social conversation without inappropriate affect or comments. The practitioner provides positive reinforcements when positive behavior is noted.

*Biomechanical:* Improve George's strength and endurance through repetitive activity. The OT practitioner provides George with activities that are increasingly difficult. The sessions focus on strength, endurance, and ROM.

*Cognitive-behavioral:* Help George identify his own goals and behaviors in hopes that through self-reflection he may make the changes. The OT practitioner allows George to complete an activity and discusses how it went afterward and how they would improve his behavior next time. The theory behind this FOR is that clients will make more significant changes when they are able to cognitively acknowledge them.

*Developmental:* Identify the highest level of motor, social, and cognitive skills in which George can engage, and facilitate improvements in function from that starting point. Grade activities so that he can achieve them, but is slightly challenged. Help "close the gap" in the areas in which he is unable to perform.[12]

*Model of Human Occupation:* Explore George's previous interests, motivations, routines, habits, and occupations and determine what he wants to return to doing. Consider how his environment supports or hinders his goals. Help him develop the motor skills to return to his previous occupations by remediating skills, adapting and modifying tasks along the way. Work to develop feelings of self-efficacy.

*Motor control:* Work on George's impaired motor skills through activities in the natural environment. Allow George to make mistakes and learn from them. The motor control FOR suggests that the practitioner provide verbal and physical cues as necessary. Practice should take place in short sessions with frequent breaks.

*Neurodevelopmental:* Work on George's motor skills by inhibiting abnormal muscle tone and facilitating normal movement patterns. The OT practitioner requests that George complete activities while the practitioner facilitates the movement at selected "key points of control" (i.e., hand, shoulders, and waist).

These examples provide a brief summary of how intervention differs when using selected FORs. The OT practitioner relies on therapeutic reasoning, experience, judgment, current research, and a thorough understanding of the occupational profile of the client, including the contexts in which the occupations occur. Together, this information forms the basis for the OT intervention.

## Summary

Models of practice help organize one's thinking, whereas FORs tell practitioners what to do in practice. Organizing one's practice around the concepts of occupation is central to the profession. Thus selecting a model of practice developed by occupational therapists provides the best assurance that the practitioner is "thinking" like an OT practitioner. This is helpful in educating the public, clients, and consumers about the profession.

FORs are important in ensuring that practitioners are using evidence-based practice. By critiquing the research on the effectiveness of the selected FOR, practitioners are able to fully understand the principles, intervention procedures, and techniques. This helps practitioners adapt the FOR if necessary for clients and diagnoses in which the research has not been conducted so that other clients may benefit. Practitioners with knowledge of the subtleties of the FORs are able to skillfully work with clients. Articulating the rationale behind intervention techniques is important in today's health-care environment. Furthermore, understanding the FORs helps OT practitioners better serve clients.

## Learning Activities

1. Use a selected model of practice to analyze your occupational performance. Summarize the findings in a report format.
2. Compare and contrast two models of practice in a short paper.
3. Have each member of the class present findings from at least three intervention studies on a given FOR. Discuss the effectiveness of this FOR with a selected population.
4. Select a specific FOR for a given population and provide your rationale for the choice. Use at least three research studies to justify the selection.
5. Identify the theory for change, principles, and intervention strategies for a specific FOR. Present the findings in class.
6. Visit an OT department and determine which models of practice and FORs are used at this setting. Ask to observe an OT practitioner during a treatment that implements one of the FORs.

## Review Questions

1. Explain the terms theory, model of practice, and FOR.
2. Why is it important to use a model of practice? FOR?
3. What are the parts to a FOR?
4. How does research on FOR support OT practice?
5. What are some OT models of practice? Describe them in general terms.

## References

1. Allen CK. Activity, occupational therapy's treatment method: 1987 Eleanor Clarke Slagle lecture. *Am J Occup Ther*. 1987;41(9):563–575.
2. Allen CK. *Occupational Therapy for Psychiatric Diseases: Measurement and Management of Cognitive Disabilities*. Boston, MA: Little Brown; 1985.
3. Ayres JA. *Sensory Integration for the Child*. Los Angeles, CA: Western Psychological Services; 1979.
4. Bobath B. Sensorimotor development. *NDT Newsletter*. 1975;7:1.
5. Case-Smith J, O'Brien J. *Occupational Therapy for Children and Adolescents*. 7th ed. St. Louis, MO: Mosby; 2015.
6. Christiansen CH, Baum CM, eds. *Occupational Therapy: Performance, Participation and Well-Being*. Thorofare, NJ: Slack Inc.; 2005.
7. Crepeau EB, Cohn ES, Boyt Schell BA, eds. *Willard and Spackman's Occupational Therapy*. 10th ed. Philadelphia, PA: Lippincott Williams & Wilkins; 2003.
8. Kielhofner G. *Conceptual Foundations of Occupational Therapy*. 4th ed. Philadelphia, PA: FA Davis; 2009.
9. Kielhofner G. *A Model of Human Occupation: Theory and Application*. 4th ed. Baltimore, MD: Lippincott Williams & Wilkins; 2008.
10. Law M, Cooper B, Stewart D, et al. The Person-Environment-Occupation model: a transactive approach to occupational performance. *Can J Occup Ther*. 1996;63(1):9–23.
11. Law M, Baptiste S, Carswell A, et al. *Canadian Occupational Performance Measure*. 2nd ed. Toronto: Canadian Association of Occupational Therapists Publication; 1994.
12. Llorens LA. *Application of a Developmental Theory for Health and Rehabilitation*. Rockville, MD: American Occupational Therapy Association; 1976.
13. MacRae N, O'Brien J. *OT 301: Foundations of Occupational Therapy*. Unpublished lecture notes, University of New England; 2001.
14. Mish F, ed. *Merriam-Webster's Collegiate Dictionary*. 10th ed. Springfield, MA: Merriam-Webster; 1994.
15. O'Brien J, Solomon J. Scope of practice. In: Solomon J, O'Brien J, eds. *Pediatric Skills for Occupational Therapy Assistants*. 4th ed. St. Louis, MO: Mosby; 2016.
16. Parham D. Toward professionalism: the reflective therapist. *Am J Occup Ther*. 1987;41(9):555–561.
17. Pedretti LW, Paszuinielli S. A frame of reference for occupational therapy in physical dysfunction. In: Pedretti LW, Zoltan B, eds. *Occupational Therapy: Practice Skills for Physical Dysfunction*. 3rd ed. St. Louis, MO: Mosby; 1990:1–17.
18. Pendleton H, Schultz-Krohn W, eds. *Pedretti's Occupational Therapy: Practice Skills for Physical Dysfunction*. 6th ed. St. Louis, MO: Mosby; 2006.
19. Reed KL. Understanding theory: the first step in learning about research. *Am J Occup Ther*. 1984;38(10):677–682.
20. Schkade JK, Schultz S. Occupational adaptation: toward a holistic approach in contemporary practice, Part I. *Am J Occup Ther*. 1992;46:829–837.
21. Schoen S, Anderson J. Neurodevelopmental treatment frame of reference. In: Kramer P, Hinojosa J, eds. *Frames of Reference for Pediatric Occupational Therapy*. 3rd ed. Baltimore, MD: Lippincott Williams & Wilkins; 2009:99–186.
22. Townsend E, Brintnell S, Staisey N. Developing guidelines for client-centered occupational therapy practice. *Can J Occup Ther*. 1990;57:69–76.
23. Trombly CS, Radomski MV. *Occupational Therapy for Physical Dysfunction*. 5th ed. Philadelphia, PA: Lippincott Williams & Wilkins; 2002.
24. Walker KF, Ludwig F, eds. *Perspectives on Theory for the Practice of Occupational Therapy*. 3rd ed. Austin, TX: Pro-Ed; 2004.
25. Williamson GG. A heritage of activity: development of theory. *Am J Occup Ther*. 1982;36(11):716–722.

# 16
# Intervention Modalities

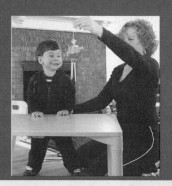

## OBJECTIVES

*After reading this chapter, the reader will be able to do the following:*

- Identify the principal tools of occupational therapy practice.
- Describe the difference between preparatory, purposeful, simulated, and occupation-based activity.
- Describe the use of consultation and education in occupational therapy practice.
- Explain the purpose of activity analysis, and describe its application to occupation.

- Understand the role of the occupational therapy practitioner in the use of physical agent modalities.
- Understand the role of the occupational therapy practitioner in orthotics and assistive technology.

## KEY TERMS

activity analysis
activity synthesis
adapting
assistive devices
grading
media

methods
modality
occupation-based activity
orthotic device
physical agent modalities
preparatory methods

purposeful activity
simulated activity
sensory input
therapeutic exercise

℮ Visit *www.evolve.elsevier.com* to access the Evolve student resources that accompany your book.

*Occupational therapy (OT) provides me with the unique opportunity to observe and to share my knowledge and my experiences to affect the well-being of another person. The potential to observe makes life interesting. It provides an opportunity to stand aside, note, and experience reality within its context, be it beautiful or painful. Observation further provides an opportunity to stand still and acknowledge. It provides the occupational therapist with an opportunity to apply performance and task analyses—the main methods of OT—to detect function or dysfunction of task performance and the client factors; but occupational performance is the focus of the human being. Observation thus allows the occupational therapist to view the human through task performance, these tasks being crucial forces responsible for shaping the human being. In other words, an occupational therapist is an observer with powerful tools: "performance analysis" and task analysis." Through*

*observation, the therapist can assess performance, set goals, guide intervention with the set goals in mind, and critically evaluate treatment effect, all by applying different forms of clinical reasoning.*

*The human being evolves around occupational performance. The human is shaped by what he or she performs, and life is meaningless without the ability and the motivation to perform, at whatever small capacity. The smallest gains can be as rewarding and worthwhile for those involved as are the bigger accomplishments or achievements for others.*

*OT has further allowed me to share my knowledge regarding occupational performance that could, in some instances, affect the quality of life of those involved. It has provided me with an opportunity to challenge limitations at different levels of performance, in a very exciting way, because some of these limitations have been at a level that I would have thought would be impossible to influence. Limitations have the potential to develop maturity in life, and many limitations not only bring about frustrations and negative aspects but also the inner beauty of the person involved and the unknown potentials that may flourish and thereby enhance maturity.*

*Occupational performance is, therefore, the force that molds the human being into an occupational being. It is a privilege to be an occupational therapist and to be involved with that powerful driving force.*

**GUÐRÚN ÁRNADÓTTIR, PHD**
**Department of Occupational Therapy Grensás**
**Landspítali, The National University Hospital of Iceland**
**Clinical Associate Professor, Faculty of Medicine**
**University of Iceland**
**Reykjavík, Iceland**

The *Occupational Therapy Practice Framework (OTPF)* (3rd ed.) identifies the four categories of intervention modalities as follows: (1) therapeutic use of self, (2) therapeutic use of occupations and activities, (3) consultation process, and (4) education process. This chapter describes the therapeutic use of occupations and activities, the consultation process, and the education process.[2] Therapeutic use of self is described in Chapter 17.

Therapeutic use of occupations and activities includes the use of preparatory, purposeful, and occupation-based activity. Occupational therapy (OT) practitioners help clients reach their goals by using specially designed activities. In using these activities therapeutically, the OT practitioner considers context, activity demands, and client factors as they relate to the goals of the client.[2] The consultation process involves working with family and other health professionals to help clients meet their goals. OT practitioners teach and educate others on a variety of topics, all designed to enable occupational participation. The educational process is used during OT intervention as a way to help clients, families, caregivers, and health-care professionals understand and meet client goals to engage in occupations.

## Therapeutic Use of Occupations and Activities

OT practitioners use a variety of modalities as tools of the trade. A **modality** includes both the method of intervention and the medium. The steps, sequences, and approaches used to activate the therapeutic effect of a medium are the **methods.**[6] The supplies and equipment used are the **media.** For example, an OT practitioner might use the medium of cooking when working on meal management. The OT practitioner may ask the person to use a variety of tools to target therapeutic goals. For example, the client may stir a mixture to work on grip strength or stand while preparing a sandwich to promote postural control. During intervention, the OT practitioner considers both the medium and the method. Practitioners become skilled at selecting and using modalities to help clients reach their goals. See Appendix A for sample intervention activities.

OT practitioners use preparatory methods in the beginning of therapy as a way to get clients ready for purposeful activity. Purposeful activity is goal-directed activity that simulates the actual occupation. The OT practitioner's goal is to help clients engage in occupation-based activity.

## Preparatory Methods

**Preparatory methods** are used in conjunction with or to prepare the client for purposeful activity and occupational performance. They include sensory input, therapeutic exercise, physical agent modalities, and orthotics/splinting.[2] These methods address the remediation and restoration of problems associated with client factors and body structure. Preparatory methods support the client's acquisition of the performance skills needed to resume his or her roles and daily occupations.

### Sensory Input

Providing **sensory input** to help a client resume functional movement is considered a preparatory activity. For example, the OT practitioner may stimulate a muscle through vibration in an attempt to activate muscle fibers for contraction and subsequent movement. Using sensory input such as deep pressure may help inhibit abnormal muscle tone so that the client can engage in purposeful movement.[10] Many of these techniques were originated by Margaret Rood, and they help clients before the actual activity. Thus, providing sensory input to change muscle tone or sensory sensitivity is considered a preparatory activity.

Sensory input may be provided as a technique to help clients relearn movements that may be lost as a result of illness, disease, or trauma. Although the goal of sensory input is improved function, the techniques do not require the client to engage in activity. Generally, the sensory input is provided to the muscle fibers directly. Therefore OT practitioners use sensory input as an adjunct to purposeful and occupation-based activity.

### Therapeutic Exercise

**Therapeutic exercise,** a modality from the biomechanical frame of reference, is the "scientific supervision of exercise for the purpose of preventing muscular atrophy, restoring joint and muscle function, and improving efficiency of cardiovascular and pulmonary function."[8] By understanding the principles of therapeutic exercise, the practitioner is able to apply biomechanical principles to purposeful activity. Therapeutic exercise is most effectively used as an intervention for lower motor neuron disorders that result in weakness and flaccidity (e.g., spinal cord injuries, poliomyelitis, Guillain–Barré syndrome) or orthopedic conditions such as arthritis.[8]

The general goals of therapeutic exercise are to (1) increase muscle strength, (2) maintain or increase joint range of motion and flexibility, (3) improve muscle endurance, (4) improve physical conditioning and cardiovascular fitness, and (5) improve coordination. The OT practitioner selects an appropriate therapeutic exercise from available options on the basis of the client's needs, goals, capabilities, and precautions related to his or her condition.[8] Although a description of each therapeutic exercise is beyond the scope of this entry-level text, Table 16.1 provides a summary of the types of therapeutic exercise used for each of the general goals.

The advantage of therapeutic exercise is that the practitioner can target specific muscle groups and motor movements by asking the client to perform particular exercises. The amount of resistance and number of repetitions can be controlled. Therapeutic exercise should not be used exclusively in OT practice, but it may be used to prepare a client for purposeful activity and occupational performance.

## Physical Agent Modalities

**Physical agent modalities** (PAMs) are also considered preparatory methods. PAMs are used to bring about a response in soft tissue and are most commonly used by OT practitioners for treating hand and arm injuries or disorders. PAMs use light, sound, water, electricity, temperature, and mechanical devices to promote changes in function.[2] Thermal modalities that involve heat transfer to an injured area (i.e., warm paraffin baths, hot packs, whirlpools, or ultrasound) are used to decrease pain and joint stiffness, increase motion, increase blood flow, reduce muscle spasms, and reduce edema.[2,4] Another thermal modality is the use of cold transfer (i.e., cold packs and ice). Cold transfer is used in the treatment of pain, inflammation, and edema. Electrical modalities include media such as transcutaneous electrical nerve stimulation (TENS), functional electrical stimulation (FES), and neuromuscular electrical stimulation devices (NMES), and these modalities are used to reduce edema, decrease pain, increase motion, and reeducate muscles.[4]

PAMs are used as an adjunct to or in preparation for intervention that ultimately enhances engagement in occupation.[1,2] The use of PAMs solely as intervention without application to occupational performance is not considered OT.[1,2] PAMs are not to be used by entry-level practitioners; rather, the practitioner needs to complete specialized postprofessional training and provide evidence that he or she has the theoretical background and technical skills needed to use PAMs. State practice acts or licensure

| TABLE 16.1 | Summary of Types of Therapeutic Exercise | |
|---|---|---|
| **General Goal** | **Type of Exercise** | **Description of Exercise** |
| Increase muscle strength | Active assisted | Client moves body part as much as he or she can and is assisted to complete movement by practitioner or therapeutic equipment. |
| | Active range of motion | Client actively moves body part through complete range of motion without assistance or resistance. |
| | Resistive | Client moves body part through available range of motion against resistance; resistance may be applied manually, by special therapeutic equipment, or through the use of weights; the amount of resistance increases as the person's strength increases. |
| Maintain or increase joint range of motion and flexibility | Passive range of motion | Client is not able to move the body part, so movement is provided by an outside force such as a practitioner or a therapeutic device (e.g., continuous passive motion device); no muscle contraction takes place. |
| | Active range of motion | Client is able to move body part without assistance through range. |
| Improve muscle endurance | Low-load, high-repetition program | Practitioner determines client's maximum capacity for a strengthening program, then reduces the maximum resistance load and increases the number of repetitions. |
| Improve physical conditioning and cardiovascular fitness | Sustained rhythmic, aerobic | Examples include jogging, bicycle riding, swimming, and walking. |
| Improve coordination | Coordination training | Repetitive activities and exercises that require smooth, controlled movement patterns (e.g., placing pegs in holes, stacking blocks, picking up marbles). |

laws may regulate the use of PAMs in occupational therapy. Practitioners must familiarize themselves with these laws and be trained properly. With proper application, the use of PAMs in OT allows the practitioner to provide a comprehensive treatment program for the client.[4]

OT practitioners must carefully review, critique and critically appraise research related to PAMs to determine the specific conditions and situations in which it may be effective. Practitioners should carefully consider outcomes and examine how and when to use PAMs in practice.

## Orthotics

Any "apparatus used to support, align, prevent, or correct deformities or to improve the function of movable parts of the body"[8] is considered an **orthotic device,** or orthosis. Orthotic devices can be prefabricated or custom made and involve assessing the client, determining the most appropriate orthotic device, designing the device, and evaluating the fit. Orthoses were previously referred to as splints; some practitioners continue to use this term, although *orthotic* is more current and accurately reflects billing codes. OT practitioners train clients in the use of the orthosis, monitor the wearing schedule, and evaluate the client's response.

Orthoses also include braces made for the lower extremities and trunk. These types of orthoses are usually made from high-temperature thermoplastic materials that are molded over a plaster model of the body part. These materials are very strong and durable, and they require special tools for cutting and shaping. Typically, orthoses made from these types of materials are fabricated by an orthotist.

Seating and positioning systems, which support, align, and help to prevent deformities, are also considered orthoses. OT practitioners may be involved with other team members in the evaluation of a client and the fabrication of a seating and positioning system. However, the subject of seating and positioning is beyond the scope of this text.

Upper extremity orthoses commonly made by OT practitioners (and previously referred to as splints) are "orthopedic devices for immobilization, restraint, or support of any part of the body."[8] They may be rigid or flexible. Three primary purposes of an orthotic device are to (1) restrict the movement of a body part, (2) immobilize a body part, or (3) mobilize a body part.[9] The OT practitioner is expected to recognize when there is a need for an orthosis, select a design that is correct for the problem, fabricate the orthosis, and educate the client in its proper use and care.

There are two main classifications of orthoses: static and dynamic. The *static orthosis* has no moving components; as the name implies, it remains in a fixed position. Static orthoses are used to protect or rest a joint, diminish pain, or prevent shortening of the muscle.[9] Fig. 16.1A shows an example of one type of static orthosis. The *dynamic orthosis* has one or more flexible components that move. The purpose of the dynamic orthosis is to increase passive motion, enhance active motion, or replace lost motion.[9] The movable components (elastic, rubber band, or spring) are attached to a static base. Fig. 16.1B shows an example of a dynamic orthosis.

Both static and dynamic orthoses can be purchased ready-made or custom fabricated by the OT practitioner. Custom-made orthoses are easily fabricated using low-temperature plastics, which become flexible and moldable when heated in hot water or with a heat gun.

The OT practitioner is responsible for evaluating the client and recommending the type of orthotic device. Either the occupational therapist or the occupational therapy assistant (OTA) may fabricate the orthosis. The OT practitioner must consider how it fits, both initially and throughout its use. The OT practitioner is responsible for assuring that the attachments that hold it in place are comfortably located and that the device keeps the body part aligned in the correct position. The client must be educated about the wearing of the orthosis—how to correctly put it on and take it off, the amount of time it should be worn, and how to keep the affected area and the orthosis clean.

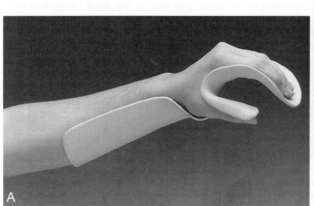
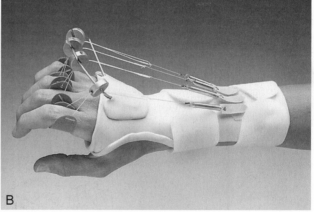

• **Fig. 16.1 A,** Static volar wrist hand orthosis. **B,** Dynamic wrist hand dorsal extension splint with four-digit outrigger. (From Pedretti, L. W. [1996]. *Occupational therapy: Practice skills for physical dysfunction* [4th ed.], St. Louis, MO: Mosby.)

At each therapy session, the practitioner looks for pressure areas and signs of distress, such as redness, swelling, or reported discomfort.

Fabricating an orthotic device requires an in-depth knowledge of body structure, motion analysis, and disability precautions, in addition to knowledge of the client. Although functional considerations are the primary concern, the practitioner must also keep in mind cosmetic and psychological factors.

Furthermore, the OT practitioner is responsible for evaluating research evidence to determine the wear schedule, type of splint, expected outcomes, and conditions for which the orthosis is intended.

## Purposeful Activity

OT practice is unique in its use of purposeful activity in intervention. **Purposeful activity** is defined as "goal-directed behaviors or tasks that make up occupations. An activity is purposeful if the individual is an active, voluntary participant and if the activity is directed toward a goal."[3,5] Purposeful activity may involve an end product. Examples of purposeful activity may include making a clay pot versus pinching clay (preparatory) or making a sandwich versus strengthening one's grip using resistive putty (preparatory).

Purposeful activity has both *inherent* and *therapeutic* goals. The inherent goal is the end product of the activity. For example, the inherent goal of a leather lacing kit may be to make a leather coin holder. The inherent goal of cooking is to prepare something to eat. The significance of this is that the client focuses on the outcome of the activity rather than the performance of individual components, such as the motor movement required to complete the activity. The result is that the client becomes absorbed in the activity itself, and performance is more automatic and natural.[2,3,5] Fig. 16.2 shows a woman making an eye glasses holder.

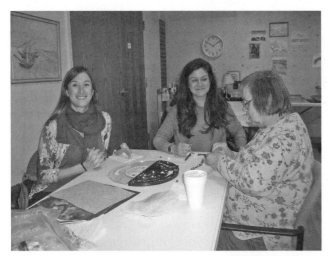

• **Fig. 16.2** Making an eye glasses holder is purposeful activity for this woman. The practitioners designed the activity to be purposeful and involve the use of fine motor skills.

The OT practitioner also has therapeutic reasons for asking the client to participate in a selected activity. For example, the practitioner may use the leather lacing activity for the therapeutic purpose of improving the individual's fine motor or sequencing skills. The therapeutic goals of the cooking activity may be to increase safety awareness, improve self-esteem, or demonstrate problem-solving skills. OT practitioners are urged to explain the therapeutic purpose of the activity to the client if it is not readily apparent.

Research suggests that clients conduct more repetitions when the activity is purposeful.[7] Purposeful activity requires client involvement and is used for prevention, maintenance, or improvement of function. Purposeful activity may include activities of daily living (ADLs), instrumental activities of daily living (IADLs), vocational activities, social activities, sports, crafts, games, or construction activities.

### Simulated or Contrived Activity

In some situations, the use of a purposeful activity is not possible or practical. The clinical environment may not have the required materials and equipment for the activity, the client may not yet have the skills or stamina needed, or there might not be enough time to complete the activity. In these instances, the practitioner uses **simulated** (or contrived) **activities.** Fisher describes contrived activities as requiring some aspect of pretending.[5] For example, a contrived activity may be imitating the movement required to spread peanut butter on a sandwich, with no actual materials. The use of clothing fastener boards that simulate dressing tasks such as buttoning or zipping and the use of manipulation boards (Fig. 16.3A) that simulate different types of hand grips for tasks such as opening a door lock, turning on a water faucet, or switching on a light are other examples of contrived activities. The inclined sanding board (Fig. 16.3B), which has a long history in OT and is used to exercise muscles of the arm, simulates sanding of wood; however, there is no actual end product.[5] There are various tabletop media used to train cognitive and perceptual skills that also fall into this category.

The use of contrived activities as a part of intervention should be carefully considered. Fig. 16.4 shows a man playing a contrived game of hockey. Contrived activities are valuable when resources are limited or when retraining motor, perceptual, and cognitive skills, but they should only be a part of a comprehensive intervention plan that also includes purposeful and occupation-based activities. They may not result in generalization. Furthermore, practitioners should be careful not to design activities that are too contrived because clients may not see the purpose of the activity.

### Occupation-Based Activity

The aim of OT services is to help clients engage in occupations.[2,3,5] See Appendix A for occupation-based intervention activities. For example, the student role may be central to one's identity. The **occupation-based activities**

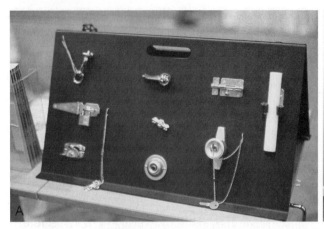
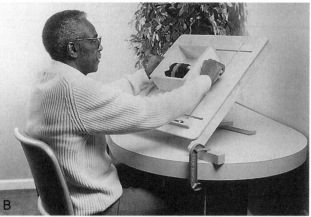

• **Fig. 16.3 A,** A manipulation board simulates the different hand grasps used in everyday activities. **B,** An inclined sanding board simulates sanding wood on an inclined plane and is used to exercise elbow and shoulder musculature. (B, Courtesy S & S Worldwide, Adaptability, 1995.)

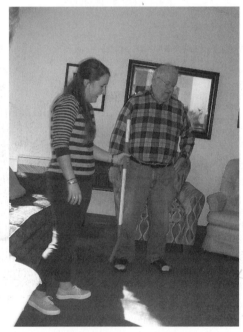

• **Fig. 16.4** The occupational therapy practitioner designed a contrived activity of playing "hockey" to engage this older man in exercise to improve postural control and balance.

the student engages in are to read literature, study for examinations, and write papers. These activities make up the occupation and therefore are necessary. For another person, being a student may not be central to his or her identity. Consider the client who attends school only because he "has to go." For this student, school is a task or activity that must be completed but is not central to his or her identity.

Although OT practitioners realize that we all engage in tasks that may not be central to our identity, finding meaningful occupations in one's life is key. Therefore the goal of OT is to help people find their meaningful occupations and return to them. Figs. 16.5A and B show people engaged in occupation-based activity. The constellation of occupations in which a person engages varies, although many of the tasks we complete are the same. It is this fine-

grained analysis of the many facets of occupations that makes the OT profession unique.

## Consultation

Consultation involves providing suggestions and intervention strategies to help clients engage in occupations. For example, practitioners use consultation to help parents care for their children or follow through with strategies in many different settings. Consultation may involve describing strategies to family members, friends, teachers, or employers. The client is always involved in the consultation; it is the client's right to know what information is being relayed to others. When providing consultation, the OT practitioner considers the personnel and their role in relationship to the client. For example, the practitioner may provide consultation to a client's teacher about the child's learning strategies. In this case consultation is focused on education. The practitioner only provides the teacher with information directly related to education and does not divulge information about the child's prognosis or medical condition. Practitioners providing consultation must be careful to provide information to benefit the client without giving away private information not related to the consultation. The practitioner considers the context and the person who will be carrying through with the recommendations when providing information. For example, the information is different if the practitioner is consulting with a spouse versus a health-care worker in a skilled nursing facility.

## Education

OT practitioners educate health professionals, clients, family members, staff, employers, and teachers on a variety of topics related to the care and follow-through of a client. Practitioners use education to help clients understand health conditions and the process of rehabilitation.

Education involves the teaching–learning process. This requires that practitioners continually teach and ask others

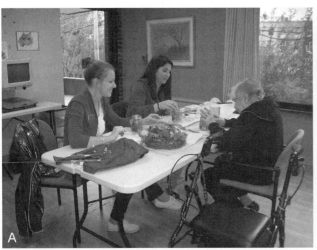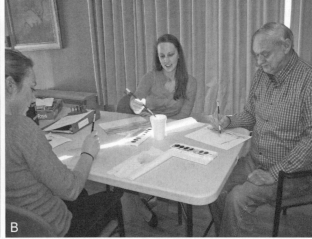

• **Fig. 16.5 A,** Decorating her room for the fall is an occupation that this woman enjoyed. She recalled many of her decorations as she engaged in this activity with the practitioners. **B,** This older man was a professional painter and still enjoys painting with watercolors. He showed the practitioners some of the lessons he learned as he created a picture.

to show that they have learned the concepts. Education begins with deciding the intended goal. For example, the practitioner may want to educate a client about work simplification techniques that may help the client be more successful. The practitioner teaches clients at their level and only provides the amount of information necessary at that time. Once the practitioner feels that the client is ready for more information, the teaching process continues. Sometimes, family members or clients request education on the progression of the condition. This education may be more appropriate for the physician or nurse to provide, but the OT practitioner often has knowledge of occupational performance as it relates to the condition.

OT practitioners frequently educate others on the occupational resources available. For example, the OT practitioner may complete a list of local leisure opportunities for clients with disabilities, such as sailing programs, adapted biking programs, wheelchair sports, or handicapped ski programs.

## Activity Analysis

To understand the many facets of occupations and how activities are selected and implemented to achieve the client's goals for occupational performance, the OT practitioner must first understand and be able to analyze activities. **Activity analysis** is the process by which the steps of an activity and its components are examined in detail to determine the demands on the client.[2,3] With experience in analyzing activities, the OT practitioner is able to quickly identify the factors required for performing an activity and assess its therapeutic value. Fig. 16.6 shows the practitioner engaging the child in play activities to facilitate play and hand skill development.

There are different ways to approach the analysis of activities. One way is to base the activity analysis on the frame of reference being used. The frame of reference identifies the areas that need to be examined. For example, when using a biomechanical frame of reference, the clinician analyzes range

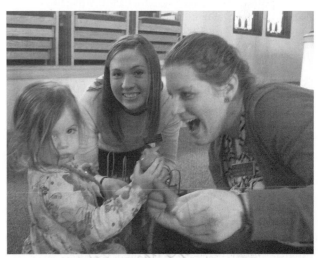

• **Fig. 16.6** The practitioner designed a fun and playful session to work on hand skills and play.

of motion, type of muscle contraction, and strength required to complete the activity.[4,10] Using a developmental frame of reference, the clinician would analyze activities to determine how they might meet age-specific developmental goals.

The practitioner may also analyze activities according to the $OTPF$[2] by determining the contexts in which the activity typically occurs and identifying what is needed to perform it (activity demands), including the physical space, tools, equipment, materials, time, cost required, and social demands. Social demands are also part of the context of the activity and include the rules of a game, number and expectations of other participants, and cultural expectations that may be associated with it.[2] Next, the practitioner divides the activity into the steps involved and describes the sequencing or timing requirements of the activity. For example, making a cake requires attention to the sequence (e.g., mix the dry ingredients before adding the wet ones). The practitioner analyzes each step of the activity to determine

---

**• BOX 16.1** | **Activity Analysis of Brushing Teeth**

<u>Name of Activity:</u> Brushing teeth
<u>Equipment:</u> Toothbrush, toothpaste, sink, water, towel
<u>Steps to activity:</u>

1. Get equipment ready.
2. Stand (or sit) at sink.
3. Pick up toothpaste while holding toothbrush in other hand, then squeeze toothpaste onto toothbrush.
4. Put paste down.
5. Turn on the water.
6. Put brush under water.
7. Open mouth and put toothbrush into mouth.
8. Move brush around to thoroughly brush teeth (approx. 3 minutes).
9. Spit and rinse.
10. Repeat.
11. Wipe face with towel.

<u>Required actions:</u> Eye–hand coordination to put paste on brush, put brush into mouth, and brush thoroughly. Grasp of materials. Bilateral hand coordination. Standing or sitting endurance.
<u>Cognitive:</u> Sequencing to do things in order. Problem solving to determine how much paste to put on brush, how long to keep under water, when to move to new section of mouth.
<u>Sensory:</u> Taste of paste in mouth. Feeling of water and brush in mouth.
<u>Body functions:</u> Ability to swallow, open mouth, close mouth, grasp and release, and move hand to mouth; postural control to sit or stand.
<u>Context:</u> Client's bathroom, which is small. Family will be nearby to assist if needed.
<u>Precautions:</u> Fall in bathroom. Client must be able to stand or sit safely.

---

the required actions, body functions, and body structures.[2] Box 16.1 provides an activity analysis example of brushing one's teeth.

Everyday activities require a number of steps and many movements and thought processes to complete. OT practitioners become skilled at analyzing the detailed steps and actions required to complete daily activities so they can help clients resume these activities within their lives. After completing an activity analysis, the practitioner develops activities to address the areas in which the client is having difficulty. The practitioner uses activity synthesis to develop a plan and design intervention.

## Activity Synthesis

After the OT practitioner has completed an occupational profile of the client to better understand the individual client's needs, the practitioner evaluates the client's strengths and weaknesses to develop an intervention plan. The intervention plan (see Chapter 14) includes the therapeutic goals and activities that will be the target of therapy. The OT practitioner completes an activity analysis to determine the steps or actions interfering with the client's performance. Intervention involves the use of therapeutic activity to assist the client in mastering a new skill, restoring a deficit, compensating for a functional disability, maintaining health, or preventing dysfunction.[3]

Once the practitioner identifies gaps in performance, he or she helps the client bridge those gaps by grading or adapting the activity or the environment to provide the "just-right" challenge for the client. This is referred to as **activity synthesis**. Activity synthesis involves deciding the activities to introduce, the timing of the activities, and how to adapt the activities for the client. Synthesis requires that the practitioner use knowledge of the client's condition, the client's individual goals and narrative, and the activity demands. An example of the use of activities to reach the client's occupational performance goals is shown in Box 16.2.

**Grading** involves changing the process, environment, tools, or materials of the activity to increase or decrease the performance demands of the client.[3] Grading an activity is used when the therapeutic goal is to improve or restore function and when the practitioner wants to challenge the client to a certain level. For example, if the practitioner thinks the client is not maximally challenged while sanding a piece of wood for a project, the sandpaper can be changed to provide greater resistance, or the wood can be positioned on an incline. When the client is experiencing difficulty performing the activity, the OT practitioner may decrease the requirements. Perhaps on a particular day, the client is feeling tired as a result of having slept poorly the night before. He does not feel capable of completing his shaving routine while standing. The practitioner may decrease the requirements of the activity by allowing him to sit while shaving or by requiring him to shave only one side of his face while the practitioner shaves the other. Table 16.2 summarizes the ways in which activities may be graded.

**Adapting** of the activity or the environment may allow the client to perform an activity at the highest possible level of function. "Adaptation is the process that changes an aspect of the activity or the environment to enable successful performance and accomplish a therapeutic goal."[3] Adaptation may involve modification of the environment and the use of assistive technologies or alternative strategies.[8,10]

**Assistive devices** range from *low-* to *high-technological devices*. Typically, devices that are considered low technology do not have electronic components. These devices, such as those designed for self-feeding, have been a part of OT for many years. High-technological devices include those with electronic components, such as augmentative communication equipment, electronic aids for daily living, and power wheelchairs. The use of devices to aid function is an integral part of the profession and can provide the necessary adaptations so that a client can achieve.

Training a client to perform an activity in an alternative way is another type of adaptation. OT practitioners educate clients daily on strategies to improve function. For example, an OT practitioner may teach a client techniques for dressing or bathing with one hand after an injury. In some situations all that is needed is training in these types of strategies, and the client can forgo assistive devices.

OT practitioners may need to make modifications to a person's environment to facilitate function. The OT practitioner evaluates the accessibility of the environment (e.g.,

## BOX 16.2 | Case Application of Activity Synthesis

Frances is a 72-year-old woman who lives with her daughter in a small ranch home in the country. Frances loves to garden and cook. She especially enjoys making cookies for her grandchildren. Frances was recently hospitalized with complications from her diabetes and heart condition. She has poor endurance now and exhibits some confusion. Frances works slowly. The occupational therapy practitioner, Leah, will be treating Frances daily while Frances remains in the rehabilitation unit.

Leah begins the evaluation by asking Frances what types of things she did before the hospitalization.

_Prior Occupations:_ Frances enjoyed gardening and cooking (cookies for her grandchildren). Her daughter made the meals. Frances dressed and bathed herself. She helped with light housekeeping, but her daughter was primarily responsible for housework. Frances enjoyed conversation with family members and spending time watching TV, playing card games, and doing puzzles. Frances did not drive.

The daughter will be home for 3 weeks after her mother is discharged and is concerned that her mother will be bored if not able to garden or cook.

The occupational therapist decides to work on helping Frances return to cooking (cookies) and gardening. Furthermore, the occupational therapist will make sure Frances is able to perform self-care activities. The following activity analysis examines the factors involved in Frances' gardening.

_Performance Pattern:_ During the summer months, Frances spends at least 1 hour a day caring for her flower garden. She waters the plants and weeds them.

_Contexts:_
- _Cultural._ Frances's mother enjoyed gardening and always had fresh flowers on the table. Frances has passed this on to her daughter. Frances likes to discuss flowers with other gardeners who share her love of this hobby.
- _Physical._ The garden is located in the country close to the house. The garden consists of many flower plants. It is situated on flat terrain with large, flat slate providing the walking path. The garden is shaded by surrounding trees.
- _Social._ Frances enjoys gardening by herself but also enjoys showing others (e.g., her neighbors and grandchildren) the beautiful flowers.
- _Personal._ Frances is a 72-year-old woman who enjoys showing others her garden and likes to be active.
- _Temporal._ Frances enjoys the summer, when she can be outside in her garden.

_Performance Skills:_
- _Motor skills._ Frances must be able to walk outside on a smooth (slate rock) path (approximately 20 feet) and bend to pick up weeds. She must be able to carry a watering can and have enough strength to dig in the dirt as needed. She must be able to get up.
- _Process skills._ Frances must be aware of the differences between plants and weeds. She must realize when the plants need water and determine how to take care of the plants.
- _Communication/interaction skills._ Frances must be able to interact with others who stop by to see her flowers. She must request assistance as needed from her daughter.

_Activity Demands:_ Gardening requires working with plants, garden tools, and the environment. One must bend and reach, pull weeds, and carry garden tools. The gardener must gather supplies, walk to the garden, and begin to care for the plants. One must identify plants from weeds and acknowledge when the job is completed.

_Client Factors:_ The occupational therapist has decided to focus on the neuromusculoskeletal and movement-related functions. Upon evaluation, the occupational therapist learned that Frances has full range of motion. Frances has difficulty maintaining her posture and fatigues quickly. She currently exhibits poor muscle strength in her arms, trunk, and legs. Endurance is limited to 20 minutes of seated activity. Frances fatigues after walking 10 feet and walks with a wide-based, unsteady gait. She is able to pick up objects with both hands but shows limited hand strength. Eye–hand coordination is adequate for fine motor tasks.

The occupational therapy practitioner may approach Frances's difficulties from many angles and design activities to meet her goal to return to gardening.

Using a biomechanical approach to address Frances's poor endurance, the occupational therapist works in the clinic on tabletop activities, including making a flower collage by tearing out pictures and pasting them on the page. The occupational therapy practitioner engages in conversation with Frances about gardening. Once Frances is able to tolerate 30 minutes of seated activity, the occupational therapy practitioner will increase the demands by engaging Frances in an indoor gardening activity, such as planting seeds in small pots or transplanting several plants. These activities can be graded so that Frances stands for the tasks as tolerated until her endurance is sufficient.

## TABLE 16.2 | Grading of Activity

| Areas of Grading | Examples of Grading |
| --- | --- |
| Strength | Increase/decrease the repetitions<br>Increase/decrease amount of resistance |
| Range of motion | Increase/decrease movement required<br>Increase/decrease assistance in moving the extremity |
| Endurance and tolerance | Increase/decrease time on task<br>Change demands of task to require less/more muscle endurance.<br>Increase/decrease number of repetitions.<br>Do activity sitting versus standing |

_Continued_

| TABLE 16.2 | Grading of Activity—cont'd | |
|---|---|
| **Areas of Grading** | **Examples of Grading** |
| Coordination | Increase/decrease the size of the objects being manipulated<br>Increase/decrease the number of objects being manipulated<br>Change the texture or properties of the object<br>Increase/decrease accuracy requirements |
| Perceptual skills | Increase/decrease the time to complete skills<br>Increase/decrease the object size (e.g., puzzle)<br>Increase/decrease the complexity<br>Increase/decrease the extraneous stimulation |
| Cognitive skills | Increase/decrease number of steps given in a task<br>Provide more or less problem solving in the task<br>Require the client do more or less of the task without asking questions<br>Increase/decrease the novelty of the task<br>Increase/decrease the familiarity of materials and directions |
| Social skills | Move from an individual activity to a group activity<br>Increase/decrease the social behaviors expected<br>Increase/decrease the familiarity with the social setting or people<br>Increase/decrease the intensity of the conversation<br>Increase/decrease the goal of the social event |

Javier was involved in a motor vehicle accident resulting in a spinal cord injury. He has lost the ability to grasp objects. The OT practitioner realizes that this deficit cannot be overcome; however, Javier wants to be able to feed himself independently. The practitioner performs an activity analysis to define the demands of self-feeding and realizes that the ability to perform hand grasp is needed to hold the utensil. Consequently, if Javier is to be independent in self-feeding, a way must be found for him to grasp. To do this, the practitioner begins by having Javier try a utensil-holding appliance cuff (called a universal cuff), which slips on his hand, thus eliminating the need to grasp the fork or spoon. Javier is able to eat using the device, although initially it is challenging for him. Javier and the OT practitioner decide that they can work together on a training program with this device to achieve the goal of self-feeding. Within a week, Javier is using the universal cuff at all of his meals to feed himself independently. This is an example of adapting the activity to compensate for lack of hand grasp.

In another treatment setting, the OT practitioner is working with Sandra, who has a mental illness. She is withdrawn and avoids social contact. The OT practitioner analyzes the available group activities to determine which may be best for the client. The practitioner uses clinical judgment and decides not to begin with a cooking group because it is a highly social activity. Instead, the practitioner chooses a craft activity that is simple, is not demanding, and can be performed in an area of the room where Sandra can be among others without interacting with them. As Sandra improves and becomes more comfortable with social interaction, the activity is graded to make it more challenging. Specifically, the OT practitioner begins by asking Sandra to work independently on a craft activity at the same table as other clients. Gradually, the OT practitioner increases the amount of interaction and sharing of supplies. The goal is that eventually Sandra will be able to participate in a group that is preparing a meal. The practitioner uses activity analysis to determine the demands of the activity, recalling Sandra's strengths (fine motor skills) and weaknesses (poor social interactions). To meet the goal, the OT practitioner grades the activity by selecting one with low social demands, gradually increasing the level of social contact until the client is able to relate to others without being threatened.

home, school, work), makes recommendations for modifications, and follows up to ensure that recommended modifications have been properly made and are effectively used by the client. Examples of environmental modifications include the installation of ramps into buildings, installation of grab bars for bathroom safety, and arrangement of furniture in the home or at work.

The following examples illustrate the process of grading and adapting.

Every OT practitioner must be able to select appropriate activities by assessing the demands of an activity on many levels, integrating the information with knowledge of the client's needs and abilities, and grading and adapting activities as needed.

## Summary

There is a wide range of therapeutic modalities used in OT to achieve the goals of the client—specifically, therapeutic use of self (see Chapter 17), therapeutic use of activities and occupations, consultation, and education. OT practitioners educate clients daily on a host of issues. For example, the OT practitioner may teach a client how to dress or bathe using one hand after an injury. Often, OT practitioners provide alternative techniques for performing occupations. Therapeutic use of activities and occupations includes the use of preparatory, purposeful, and occupation-based activity. Preparatory activities are used to prepare the client for purposeful activity or occupations and include sensory input, therapeutic exercise modalities, PAMs, and orthoses. Purposeful activity has an inherent goal in addition to the therapeutic goal. Occupation-based activity includes the performance of ADLs, IADLs, work and school tasks, play or leisure tasks, and social participation by the client, and it is the ultimate goal of OT intervention. Consultation involves discussing intervention strategies with the client and other professionals. Practitioners use education to help clients and others understand the intervention process. They also educate others on the characteristics, features, and prognosis of the disability. Activity analysis is learned through practice and becomes second nature to the experienced OT practitioner. Activity synthesis includes knowing how to grade activities and when and how to provide adaptations and assistive technology.

## Learning Activities

1. Select a simple activity and identify all of the requirements for performance of the activity. Exchange lists with classmates.
2. Find and read an article on an orthosis (with picture or design) in the *American Journal of Occupational Therapy* or another professional source. Report on the article to your class or to a small group of students from your class.
3. Gather available resources on assistive devices. This can be done in two ways:

   a. In your community, research companies that provide assistive devices and study the types of equipment and services they provide.
   b. Select one particular category of assistive devices (e.g., feeding equipment, augmentative communication devices, power wheelchairs), and search the Internet for companies that produce or sell these devices. In a report, summarize the information that you find.
4. Critique the benefits of purposeful activity in OT.
5. Develop a notebook of activities that may be used in OT.

## Review Questions

1. Define and describe preparatory, purposeful, and occupation-based activity.
2. What is the difference between purposeful and occupation-based activity?
3. What is meant by grading and adapting activities?
4. What are the roles of the occupational therapist and OTA in splinting?
5. What are PAMs, and how are they used in OT?

## References

1. American Occupational Therapy Association. Occupational therapy practice framework: domain and process (3rd ed.). *Am J Occup Ther*. 2014;68(suppl 1):S1–S48.
2. American Occupational Therapy Association. Physical agent modalities: a position paper. *Am J Occup Ther*. 2008;62(6):691–693.
3. American Occupational Therapy Association. Position paper: purposeful activity. *Am J Occup Ther*. 1993;47(12):1081.
4. Breines EB. Therapeutic occupations and modalities. In: Pendleton HM, Schultz-Krohn W, eds. *Pedretti's Occupational Therapy Practice Skills for Physical Dysfunction*. 6th ed. St. Louis, MO: Mosby; 2006:658–679.
5. Fisher AG. Uniting practice and theory in an occupational framework. *Am J Occup Ther*. 1998;52(7):509–521.
6. Hanner NK, Marsh AC, Neideffer RC. Therapeutic media: activity with purpose. In: Solomon J, O'Brien J, eds. *Pediatric Skills for Occupational Therapy Assistants*. 4th ed. St. Louis, MO: Mosby; 2016: 453–471.
7. Hseih CL, Nelson DL, Smith DA, et al. A comparison of performance in added-purpose occupations and rote exercise for dynamic standing balance in persons with hemiplegia. *Am J Occup Ther*. 1996;50:10–16.
8. O'Toole M, ed. *Mosby's Medical, Nursing, and Health Professions Dictionary*. 9th ed. St. Louis, MO: Mosby; 2013.
9. Schwartz DA. Orthoses, orthotic fabrication and elastic therapeutic taping for the pediatric population. In: Solomon J, O'Brien J, eds. *Pediatric Skills for Occupational Therapy Assistants*. 4th ed. St. Louis, MO: Mosby; 2016:543–564.
10. Trombly CS, Radomski MV. *Occupational Therapy for Physical Dysfunction*. 5th ed. Philadelphia, PA: Lippincott Williams & Wilkins; 2002.

# 17

# Therapeutic Relationships

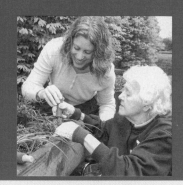

## OBJECTIVES

*After reading this chapter, the reader will be able to do the following:*

- Explain the uniqueness of the therapeutic relationship.
- Identify the stages of loss.
- Describe how "use of self" is used by practitioners.
- Understand the importance of self-awareness for effective therapeutic relationships.
- Identify the three "selves" recognized in self-awareness.

- Explain the skills needed for developing effective therapeutic relationships.
- Describe the necessary skills for leading groups.
- Define the six modes of Taylor's Intentional Relationship Model.

## KEY TERMS

| | | |
|---|---|---|
| active listening | nonverbal communication | self-awareness |
| clarification | perceived self | task groups |
| empathy | plain language | therapeutic relationship |
| group | real self | therapeutic use of self |
| group dynamics | reflection | universal stages of loss |
| ideal self | restatement | |

e Visit *www.evolve.elsevier.com* to access the Evolve student resources that accompany your book.

---

*There is a mystique in occupational therapy (OT) that is hard to put into words. When we treat a patient and affect something relevant to that person, the magic of our profession comes to light. Whether we are splinting a finger injury, demonstrating an adapted key holder, or instructing in time management, what matters is that the interaction is meaningful to the patient. We treat the entire person, not just the isolated injury or diagnosis printed on the referral form. We treat people's illness experiences, not just their illness. We probe patients' real-life needs and help them recover their abilities to participate in daily routines. We acknowledge the value of the "blissful ordinariness"\* of a day and help patients return to it. We listen as they tell us about the mundane details of their lives that are disrupted by their injury or illness. We help find ways to return to these activities, and in doing so, we validate the importance of ordinary things in their lives. And when our treatment process is successful, patients return to their "blissful ordinariness" with greater awareness of its value. The mystique of OT is not easy to articulate. What looks so simple on the*

*surface is actually very complex and powerful. Often, patients understand this intuitively. In these instances, words may not be needed.*

**CYNTHIA COOPER, MFA, MA, OTR/L, CHT**
**Cooper Hand Therapy**
**Carlsbad, CA**

\* from *The Innocent*, by Ian McEwan, Doubleday, 1990, p. 134

The interaction between an occupational therapy (OT) practitioner and a client is termed the **therapeutic relationship.** Therapeutic relationships differ from everyday relationships, in that therapeutic relationships are key for facilitating the healing and rehabilitation process. Therefore OT practitioners create therapeutic relationships to help clients achieve their desired goals. This chapter examines the uniqueness of the therapeutic relationship by describing this relationship in terms of therapeutic use of self, self-awareness, and trust. A review of the Intentional Relationship Model (IRM)[6] is provided with practice examples to illustrate its use in practice. Skills practitioners use in developing the relationship are presented, including trust, empathy, nonverbal and verbal communication, active listening, and group leadership skills. Sample cases throughout the chapter provide readers with descriptions of how therapeutic relationships are used in practice.

## Psychology of Rehabilitation

People who experience catastrophic trauma or illness, disease, or developmental disorders have emotional and physical needs. OT practitioners address both the physical and emotional needs of clients. The profession views clients holistically, meaning that practitioners treat the whole person in an individualized way. This involves understanding the client and his or her motivations, desires, and needs. To understand a client in this way, practitioners create a therapeutic relationship with each client. Through this unique relationship, the practitioner learns how to design activities that are internally motivating and meaningful to a client and best meet the client's goals.[3] Oftentimes it is the practitioner's ability to develop the therapeutic relationship that contributes to the success of the intervention.[3,6]

---

Gordon, a 75-year-old, received OT intervention after a stroke. The practitioner set up a simple task of grasping clothespins to address his poor hand skills. However, as he worked to grasp the clothespins, the practitioner sat and talked to him. Gordon valued this relationship and looked forward to attending his sessions. He felt that his time in OT was well spent and that he was improving.

In retrospect, the value of this session was not so much in the fine motor task the practitioner provided, but rather in the fact that she sat there and talked with him. In earlier years, Gordon's three daughters (who now all lived far away) frequently sat and talked to him in the same way as the practitioner did. He enjoyed this familiar occupation, and this motivated him to continue in his therapy. His wife felt assured that he was engaged in therapy when she was not there, which relieved her. This example shows the power of the therapeutic relationship.

---

Many clients receiving OT experience a sense of loss. They may lose function, health, occupations, or time. They may realize that they have a chronic illness that will require their attention. Elisabeth Kübler-Ross defined the **universal stages of loss** as *denial, anger, bargaining, depression*, and *acceptance*.[4] Clients may go through some or all of these stages during the intervention process. The process is dynamic, and clients may revisit earlier stages. The OT practitioner recognizes these stages and provides support and opportunities to help clients work through the stages.

It is essential that the practitioner not judge the client's progression through the stages because each person and family deals with experiences differently. For example, it is not helpful for the practitioner to judge how long a mother is allowed to grieve for her child's lack of development. Parents may continually grieve when their child misses milestones and may need the practitioner's support. OT practitioners who are sensitive to the emotional effects of loss are more effective in developing therapeutic relationships and helping clients progress.

## Therapeutic Relationship

Therapeutic relationships differ from friendships. In friendships, each person contributes to and receives from the relationship, whereas the goal of the therapeutic relationship is for one person (the client) to benefit. Although the practitioner often receives a "reward," in the form of helping another person, it is not the intention or design of the interaction.

In every therapy session, the OT practitioner is aware of the client's needs and uses technical and interaction skills to select responses or courses of action that benefit the client. The therapeutic relationship often makes the difference between a successful and an unsuccessful therapy experience. The practitioner continually assesses his or her interaction skills and makes judgments about how to use the skills to help the client. This process of using one's interactions for the benefit of another is referred to as the "art of relating" and termed the **therapeutic use of self.** Therapeutic use of self involves awareness of oneself, including such things as how one communicates, presents oneself, and relates with others.[1]

### Intentional Relationship Model

Taylor developed the IRM, which systematically describes therapeutic use of self and the development of modes of interacting with clients for their benefit.[6] The IRM defines six primary interpersonal modes (or styles) used in therapeutic relationships: advocating, collaborating, empathizing, encouraging, instructing, and problem solving.[6]

Taylor postulates that the intentional relationship works best when therapists are aware of their modes of interacting and are able to shift modes as needed.[6] Taylor provides techniques and exercises to develop skill and awareness in therapeutic use of self. See Box 17.1 for clinical examples of therapeutic modes. In Fig. 17.1 the OT practitioner uses the problem-solving mode to encourage participation in the activity.

### Basic Principles of Therapeutic Use of Self

Several principles are basic to therapeutic use of self. First, practitioners must possess a level of self-awareness so that they can mindfully examine their role in the intervention process. Second, practitioners learn to develop trust, provide support, actively listen, and empathize. They use genuineness, respect, self-disclosure, trust, and

| • BOX 17.1 | Therapeutic Modes and Examples |
|---|---|
| **Mode** | **Practice Example** |
| Advocating | • Justifies the need for occupational therapy services in the school system to help the child complete schoolwork<br>• Consults with employer on workplace accommodations that would allow client to return to work |
| Collaborating | • Develops goals and strategies with client<br>• Modifies intervention plan based upon client's input |
| Empathizing | • Actively listens to client's story<br>• Adjusts intervention session to meet client's needs |
| Encouraging | • Suggests that the client "do one more repetition"<br>• Provides positive reinforcement |
| Instructing | • Teaches the client to dress using one hand<br>• Reviews precautions for the condition<br>• Demonstrates use of adaptive equipment or technology |
| Problem solving | • Figures out with client how to perform daily living skills<br>• Examines with client how to access resources<br>• Modifies equipment to meet the client's needs |

Adapted from Taylor, R. R. (2008). *The Intentional relationship: Use of self and occupational therapy.* Philadelphia, PA: F.A. Davis.

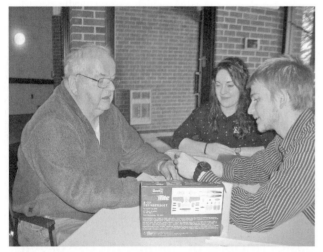

• **Fig. 17.1** The OT practitioner problem solves with the client, showing respect and acknowledging the client's abilities.

warmth when interacting with clients.[2] These qualities are useful in establishing and sustaining therapeutic relationships.

## Self-Awareness

**Self-awareness** refers to knowing one's own true nature; it is the ability to recognize one's own behavior, emotional responses, and effect created on others. OT practitioners learn to be aware of their own strengths and weaknesses so that they can better serve clients. Understanding one's own strengths and limitations allows the practitioner to focus on the other person and adapt one's behavior and interactions with others.

Becoming aware of one's self requires introspection in terms of the ideal self, the perceived self, and the real self. The **ideal self** is what an individual would like to be if free of the demands of mundane reality. This aspect is the "perfect self," with only desirable qualities and with all wants and wishes fulfilled. The ideal self is unrealistic and includes all intention, feeling, and desires. It is not well known to others, although people frequently feel the need to defend the ideal self (although perhaps subconsciously) when others do not acknowledge it.

The **perceived self** is the aspect of self that others see without the benefit of knowing a person's intentions, motivations, and limitations (i.e., as defined only by outward behavior). Therefore the perceived self is not the true self. Many times the perceived self is different from the ideal self's perceptions.

The **real self** is a blending of the internal and external worlds involving intention and action, plus environmental awareness. The real self includes the feelings, strengths, and limitations of the person, in addition to the reality in which the person exists (his or her environment).

A lack of self-awareness may result in distorted self-perceptions that are destructive to "real" relationships. People who are busy defending the ideal self and denying the perceived self do not allow the real self to emerge and consequently have superficial or misunderstood relationships, whereas a self-aware person is able to realistically acknowledge his or her own strengths and limitations and adapt and modify behaviors to help others or engage in healthy relationships. Practitioners with self-awareness are able to help clients who are struggling with new identities and crises. Practitioners may engage in a variety of exercises to develop self-awareness of therapeutic use of self.

## Self-Awareness Exercises

• Keep a journal and write down feelings and reactions to life events.
• Participate in group activities. Ask for feedback to better understand your strengths and weaknesses.
• Ask for specific feedback (e.g., communication style, body position, listening, interactions while providing intervention).
• Videotape yourself having a conversation or providing intervention. Reflect on your performance by describing those things you liked about your interactions and also those things you would like to improve.

- Giving feedback to others may help you become more aware of how others may view you.
- Complete some activities from the IRM[6] textbook.
- Describe your style and what is unique about how you interact with others. Ask people who know you well to comment.
  - Reflect on how this style can work in a therapeutic relationship.
  - Reflect on areas wherein your style may interfere with the therapeutic relationship.

## Skills for Effective Therapeutic Relationships

Health-care professionals work with clients from a variety of cultures and environments. The ability to develop an effective therapeutic relationship requires self-awareness and a variety of skills. These skills and techniques can be refined with practice so that the practitioner is able to work effectively with a variety of clients. Practitioners may need to adjust their techniques and skills to work with clients from other cultures who may perceive things differently from the practitioner. In general, developing and sustaining therapeutic relationships involves the ability to develop trust, demonstrate empathy, understand verbal and nonverbal communication, and use active listening.[1,2,6]

### Developing Trust

Health-care professionals first develop a rapport with each client. Once the client trusts the practitioner, he or she will feel comfortable sharing personal information that may shape the intervention process. Trust between a client and practitioner develops as an honest and open relationship evolves. In a therapeutic relationship, the practitioner is honest and professional about the situation, process of therapy, and knowledge of the issues. The practitioner relays concern while honestly addressing the client's issues. The practitioner develops trust by being sincere, following through with plans, and listening to the client. The practitioner develops trust to learn from the client and direct intervention. Fig. 17.2 shows a practitioner demonstrating a warm and trusting interaction while interviewing a parent.

Practitioners may find that in relating to a client they divulge personal information. Although this may be beneficial to the intervention process, practitioners are careful to remember that the therapeutic relationship is about the client, not the practitioner.[2] Self-disclosure should never be offered when the client is in the middle of a crisis or expressing thoughts.[2] The amount and type of information disclosed must be considered; the practitioner does not give his or her address or phone number to a client. A variety of techniques may help practitioners earn trust from clients, which benefits the therapeutic relationship.

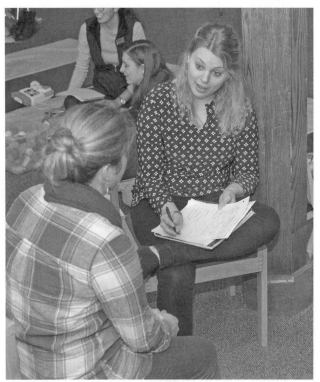

• **Fig. 17.2** The practitioner makes clear eye contact, is attentive, and asks clear questions during the initial interview. The OT practitioner establishes a trusting relationship with this parent by listening carefully.

## Techniques to Develop Trust

- Follow through with plans.
- Be on time to appointments with clients.
- Be honest with clients.
- Do not overpromise things you cannot deliver.
- Be cautious when disclosing personal information.
- Discuss clients' progress and intervention plans in private.
- Always involve the client in decisions.
- Be direct with decisions.
- Use clear language so the client understands.
- Address any issues or problems that develop in the therapeutic relationship.
- Remember to put the client first.
- Respect the client by being on time and prepared for the session.

### Developing Empathy

**Empathy** is the ability to place oneself in another person's position and understand the other's experience. The empathetic practitioner understands and is sensitive to the thoughts, feelings, and experiences of the client without losing objectivity. Empathy is important to the development of trust in the therapeutic relationship and helps clients communicate and participate in treatment.[2] Fig. 17.3 shows a

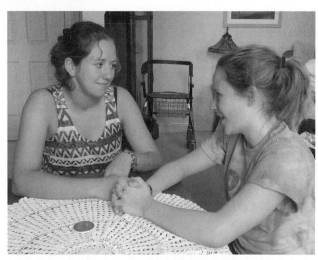

● **Fig. 17.3** Listening to a parent allows the therapist to empathize and better understand the child's needs, which results in a better intervention plan.

therapist and a mother discussing intervention goals for the child. As the therapist learns more about the issues, she empathizes with the parent.

Empathy is not to be confused with pity or identification. To express pity for the client is to feel sympathy with condescension. Pity is demeaning to the individual and conveys the attitude that the practitioner is better than the client. Identification is a term that describes the event of the OT practitioner feeling at one with a client and, as a result, losing sight of the differences. In identifying with a client, the practitioner may forget that the individual has different values and feelings; the values and needs of the practitioner may become confused with those of the client in such a way that they become less important to the therapy process.[1] Understanding clients and being empathetic is central to developing occupation-based intervention. Therefore OT practitioners may utilize a variety of techniques to develop empathy.

## Techniques to Develop Empathy

- Read stories about others who have undergone significant life events.
- Participate in activities of other cultures.
- Interview others and try to understand their life views.
- Watch movies depicting stories of people who may have experienced trauma, disease, disability, or health conditions, and discuss the characters' stories.
- Reflect on the stories of clients and peers.
- Reflect in writing how you felt after viewing a movie or reading a story about a person with a disability, trauma, or condition.
- Experience a condition by spending a day in a wheelchair, not using your hand for your morning routine, wearing glasses that make it difficult to see, and so forth. Discuss how the experiences made you feel and what you learned.

- Spend time socially with a person who has a disability to understand his or her life view.
- Attend a support group meeting to better understand the issues clients face.
- Talk with clients in a waiting room (be sure to get permission first).
- Try to imagine conditions, disability, or trauma from the family and client's point of view.

## Communication

Communication is an essential component of the therapeutic relationship. Practitioners use both verbal and nonverbal communication to express themselves to clients. Communication is key to gathering information, developing the intervention plan, and following up with plans. Consequently, practitioners develop communication skills and continually examine how effective their skills and abilities in communication are with different clients.

Clients communicate with practitioners using verbal and nonverbal communication skills. Practitioners who listen or watch carefully for communication from clients are more effective in developing therapeutic relationships.

### Verbal Communication

Perhaps the most obvious form of communication, verbal communication involves speaking to others. Therapeutic relationships may be formed through verbal communication. Practitioners use verbal communication to convey thoughts and ask questions to develop intervention plans. Therefore practitioners who are clear, concise, and speak in "plain language" are most easily understood by clients, who may not be familiar with the health-care environment. **Plain language** refers to language that is understood by "laypeople" (e.g., those not familiar with or educated in health-care environments). Typically, professionals suggest using a sixth-grade level of language to communicate with others. This allows the person hearing the information to process the questions or responses. Practitioners use plain language to better communicate to clients, considering that the client may be experiencing stress, discomfort, or difficulty with the many life changes occurring. Practitioners should consider that the information is new to the client and not use professional "jargon," which may be confusing.

Practitioners also consider the quality of the verbal communication they provide. For example, talking too fast, loudly, or in a rushed fashion suggests that the practitioner is too hurried or consumed with something else to listen and may make the client feel unimportant. This does not build a trusting therapeutic relationship. Practitioners speaking confidently and clearly help clients trust them as opposed to practitioners who speak timidly and mumble. Because OT practitioners work with clients from many cultures, it is essential that practitioners continually examine and develop communication skills.

## Techniques to Develop Communication Skills

- Practice interacting with a variety of people in a variety of circumstances.
- Reflect on your communication skills.
- Seek and listen to feedback from others.
- Review videotaped sessions to observe strengths and weaknesses.
- Practice using different techniques.
- Identify communication skills in others that you may use.
- Become familiar with your own style of communicating.
- Observe others' style of communication and reflect on those aspects that are beneficial.
- Engage in a difficult conversation and reflect on your performance.

## Nonverbal Communication

**Nonverbal communication** includes facial expressions, eye contact, tone of voice, touch, and body language. Practitioners are aware of their own nonverbal communication expression. For example, crossing one's arms during an interview may make a client feel like the practitioner is not listening or is angry. Sighing or avoiding eye contact may indicate disinterest in what the person is saying. Practitioners pay attention to how the client might perceive them and use nonverbal communication to support clients. For example, a practitioner may smile and nod to provide positive support for a client's progress. The practitioner may decide to gently touch the client on the shoulder to show he or she understands how difficult therapy may be. Sometimes eye contact alone is enough to show understanding.

Interest and support can be demonstrated by nonverbal behaviors such as smiling, touching, leaning toward the client, and making eye contact. Fig. 17.4 shows a practitioner using nonverbal communication (facial expressions) to interact with a child. The OT practitioner uses body language carefully and matches it to the particular needs of the client.[2] Obviously, it is not appropriate to smile when the individual is sharing feelings of how life has changed for the worse while touching a person may indicate that the practitioner cares and is there to help some people may be uncomfortable being touched.[2] The OT practitioner needs to be alert and sensitive to these possibilities and respect individual differences.

The effective practitioner is sensitive to and watchful for nonverbal forms of communication from clients as well. The nature of the client's disability may make it difficult for him or her to verbally communicate or understand verbal communication. In these situations, both the OT practitioner and client rely on nonverbal forms of communication, such as being aware of the client's facial expressions and body language. Clients may verbally express one thought while communicating an entirely different message with facial expressions or body language. Practitioners use knowledge of nonverbal communication to better understand clients.

For example, Mr. Bertrand is working to increase his shoulder range of motion after an injury. The OT practitioner moves Mr. Bertrand's arm through its available range of motion and asks him if it hurts. Mr. Bertrand responds "No." However, the OT practitioner observes him wince as he responds. The practitioner feels Mr. Bertrand is experiencing pain. The practitioner requires Mr. Bertrand to stop the movement and she documents the pain. She notes that Mr. Bertrand is impatient about getting better and works very hard in therapy. The practitioner reinforces to him that it is important that he not push himself too hard despite his verbal response.

Following are some exercises that may help practitioners develop nonverbal communication skills.

## Exercises to Develop Nonverbal Communication

- Observe an intervention session and identify nonverbal communication used.
- Observe how others use nonverbal communication in a variety of settings:
  - Eye contact
  - Body language (leaning, position of hands, body position)
  - Touch
  - Facial expressions
- Communicate with a peer without talking.
- Practice expressing your emotions without talking.
- Observe how you use nonverbal communication by having someone videotape you interviewing another person. Reflect on strategies that you used and identify strategies you would like to try at another time.
- Play charades as a way to tune in to nonverbal communication.

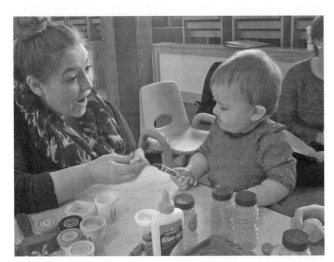

**Fig. 17.4** The OT practitioner makes eye contact and shows nonverbal expression to interact with this child. She is encouraging the child through her playful nature.

## Using Active Listening

A critical skill for maintaining an effective therapeutic relationship is **active listening.** The practitioner actively listens to the client without making judgments, jumping in with advice, or providing defensive replies. With active listening, the receiver paraphrases the speaker's words to ensure that he or she understands the intended meaning.

Davis describes active listening as having three processes: restatement, reflection, and clarification.[1] When using **restatement,** the receiver of the message (the practitioner) repeats the words of the speaker (the client) as they are heard. For example, the client says, "I am angry that I had this stroke. I just retired, and my wife and I planned to travel and see the world." The practitioner may respond with the restatement, "You are angry because your stroke may prevent you from traveling with your wife." Restatement is used only in the initial phases of active listening; its primary purpose is to encourage the person to continue talking.[1]

**Reflection** is a response wherein the purpose is to "express in words the feelings and attitudes sensed behind the words of the sender."[1] The OT practitioner using reflection verbalizes both the content *and* the feelings that are implied by the client. For example, the client says, "I've been trying to dress myself for weeks now; I just can't do it." The practitioner may reflect and state back, "You're frustrated and feeling defeated because you can't dress yourself." Using reflection, the OT practitioner demonstrates to the client that he or she is hearing the emotions behind the words, not just the words.[1] If the practitioner has not correctly identified the emotions, reflection is posed as a question, which gives the client an opportunity to express what he or she is really feeling.

During **clarification,** the client's thoughts and feelings are summarized or simplified.[1] For example, the client may say, "When my doctor referred me to OT, I thought you would be the person who would help me get the use of my arm back. I've been coming to therapy for weeks now, and I still don't have full functioning in my arm. What am I supposed to do? Will I ever be able to use my hand again?" The practitioner may use clarification by stating, "When you came to OT, you expected to immediately get the function back in your arm. Now you realize that the return of arm and hand function is going to take longer than expected and is more than a matter of someone just fixing it." Clarification helps the client look closer at the thoughts and feelings experienced. The following techniques may improve active listening skills.

## Techniques to Improve Active Listening

- Practice using restatement, reflection, and clarification.
- Role-play a variety of interviews.
- Interview others and ask for feedback. Try to summarize what they told you.
- Receive feedback from peers.
- Record (or videotape) conversations to review how you listened.
- Identify strengths and weaknesses.
- Develop techniques to improve listening skills by setting goals.
- Observe others and identify active listening techniques they used.

## Application of Therapeutic Use of Self to Occupational Therapy

The therapeutic process is complicated and involves identifying goals and objectives, developing an intervention plan, and using one's interactions to help clients achieve their desired goals. Following are more examples of the therapeutic process.

---

Jack is an OT practitioner in a public school setting who has an easygoing and cheerful personality. Although his approach serves many children, successful interaction with the following two clients requires a style change.

Amanda is an overly indulged child who acts out her feelings. Jack is aware of the use of self as a therapeutic tool and of the importance of building a therapeutic relationship with each client. He quickly realizes that his usual easygoing, cheerful manner may be detrimental to therapy with Amanda. She may view him as a "pushover" for her manipulative behavior. He elects to employ a firm, no-nonsense approach. His plan for Amanda involves clearly defined expectations with rewards and consequences.

In the first session, Amanda "tests" him with a tantrum. He calmly allows the behavior to run its course and then unemotionally repeats his expectations of her. By using this approach, Jack convinces the child that she must follow the rules and that he will not be influenced by her manipulations. Once this relationship is established, he gradually relaxes and resumes his usual approach yet remains prepared to return to the no-nonsense approach if needed.

---

Nicole is a child who is fearful, shy, and compliant. As Jack works with Nicole, he again considers the child's personality and assesses her needs. He concludes that Nicole needs to have fun and exercise choice-making. He presents her with several alternative activities and lets Nicole plan the games. Jack uses a playful and easygoing approach with Nicole.

---

These two examples illustrate how a practitioner effectively works one-on-one, builds therapeutic relationships, and uses interaction as a tool to promote progress toward meeting the client's goals. The effective OT practitioner applies the therapeutic use of self to address the client's needs.

---

The OT practitioner, Jennifer, is intent, serious, and competent; she makes good technical intervention choices in a matter-of-fact and informative way.

Mr. Butler is 40 years old. He agrees to his therapy plans, but he never quite finishes the activities. He talks throughout the sessions but appears to be "unmotivated."

Mr. Butler has had several OT practitioners and has developed a reputation for being difficult and "unmotivated." The practitioner realizes that her typical direct, informative, and matter-of-fact approach may not be effective with Mr. Butler. She spends the first session getting to know Mr. Butler and identifying his interests, motivations, and goals. She schedules 1-hour, individual intervention sessions with Mr. Butler. During the hour, she also schedules two other clients, both men his age, to overlap each end of the hour, leaving him as her "only" client for approximately 10 minutes, 20 minutes into the hour. She provides him with projects (based on his stated interests) that can be completed within the time frame and that he can take home.

Jennifer meets with him, speaks in a friendly manner, and explains that she is aware that he works slowly and has allowed more time for treatment and that she has scheduled others at the same time. She hopes that Mr. Butler will talk with these other clients and that they may support one another.

As the intervention is implemented, Jennifer regularly checks in on the client. After 20 minutes, she remains with him only when he has completed most of the activities, in which case she uses the remaining 10 minutes to pleasantly talk about nontherapeutic topics. Mr. Butler begins to share his frustrations with the projects, allowing Jennifer the opportunity to reinforce his progress (and to find projects in which he can be successful). She begins to understand his motivations even more clearly.

Because Jennifer took the time to actively listen to Mr. Butler, she was able to design activities that were meaningful to him. Spending the time explaining the process with him allowed Mr. Butler to feel a part of the process and gave him some control of his situation. Jennifer realized that although she empathized with Mr. Butler, she could not relate in the same way as his peers, and this may be beneficial to him. Thus, providing a small group of men the chance to interact proved beneficial. Mr. Butler was proud to bring things home that he had completed, and he enjoyed talking with the two other men (who were close to his age). The men looked forward to seeing each other each week. Mr. Butler was no longer viewed as "unmotivated." Importantly, he made progress on his goals.

---

Mr. Viejo is a young adult who is sullen and angry. He is the same age as his therapist, Jennifer. He was in an automobile accident that left him in a wheelchair. In therapy, he refuses to cooperate. Jennifer uses a different approach with Mr. Viejo. She schedules individual sessions and plans activities in which Mr. Viejo can be successful. She exerts no pressure on him to accept the plan or engage in the activities, but rather grades the activities depending on his mood. They discuss his past interests, and she integrates these into therapy sessions. She encourages him to talk about what he is experiencing inside, but she is careful not to say that she understands how he feels. Instead, Jennifer asks the client to describe what it is like to have his life changed so drastically, using active listening techniques to restate, reflect, and clarify what he says. She also asks him what he would like to accomplish in therapy and agrees to revise the plan to include his goals for treatment. While Jennifer is talking with Mr. Viejo, she engages him in simple daily activities to help him reengage in typical living. Jennifer uses the fact that they share similar taste in music to relate. She frequently has this music playing in the background during the sessions.

Mr. Viejo became more invested in therapy as he began to feel that Jennifer was listening to him as a young adult and not judging him. They shared a common interest in music, and Jennifer used music to keep Mr. Viejo invested. Mr. Viejo felt he could regain past experiences and relate to a same-aged peer. As he made progress, Jennifer helped him redefine his new identity and realize that he could establish new relationships and interests.

---

In each of these cases, the OT practitioner considers the needs of the client. Mr. Butler needed structure and support. He was not "unmotivated," but rather the activities and sessions were not viewed as valuable to him. Once Jennifer actively listened to him and incorporated his interests into the sessions, Mr. Butler was able to progress. Having same-aged peers to talk to gave him an outlet for his anxiety. Realizing that he was not alone allowed him to focus on therapy goals.

Mr. Viejo is dealing with the beginning stages of loss, denial, and anger as a result of becoming paralyzed at a young age. In response, the OT practitioner gives the client her full attention—making no demands. Initially, Jennifer develops simple goals for Mr. Viejo, so that they can develop trust and he can be successful. As therapy progresses, Jennifer incorporates their mutual interest in music into therapy as a way to relate to the client and help him be comfortable with his new physical self. She discusses past interests and signals a willingness to discuss any aspect of the trauma the client desires. The client believes he has lost control of his life; therefore, the OT practitioner does not take more of his sense of control by forcing him into therapy for which he is not ready. She accepts his hostility and anger by simply being there. She is aware that often a person needs the patience of another who is willing to wait and listen.

## Group Leadership Skills

OT practitioners often conduct intervention in groups. As people interact in groups around shared concerns or tasks, patterns of behavior emerge. The awareness and understanding of these patterns allow the OT practitioner to guide and direct interactions in positive, goal-oriented directions. It is important for OT practitioners to understand how to run groups, lead members, and address individual goals in groups.

OT practitioners generally lead **tasks groups,** which can be categorized as therapeutic, peer support, focus, and consultation and supervision. See Table 17.1 for a description of these groups. Before leading a **group,** the practitioner determines the individual goals of the members. The next step is to determine the group goal and decide how to meet individual needs within a group task. For example, when working with clients in a psychosocial setting, the practitioner may lead a cooking group with individual members' goals ranging from socialization, to sharing, to following the steps of a recipe. Although all members are working on the same task, each member is addressing his or her goal. The practitioner skillfully sets up the environment to address each goal. This involves delegating responsibilities to certain clients based on their therapeutic needs.

Group activities may include cooking, arts and crafts, exercise, activities of daily living, leisure participation, and reality orientation. OT practitioners may lead groups to help clients become more aware of community resources or develop self-esteem. When developing group activities, the practitioner considers such factors as the size of the group and composition of group members, client population,

| TABLE 17.1 | Types of Small Task Groups Used in Occupational Therapy | |
|---|---|
| **Type of Group** | **Description** |
| Consultation and supervision groups | Use of group format for peer support, consultation, and supervision of OTAs, aides, and caregivers; seen as an increasing need as large OT departments diminish and more practitioners work independently in private and community-based practices. |
| Focus groups | Objective of these small groups is to find out about the attitudes and opinions of the members; gaining popularity in OT as a means of investigating a theme to generate research hypotheses or organizing a discussion around a specific topic. |
| Functional groups | Group is created to accomplish specific goals, such as a fundraising group or publicity group. |
| Interest groups | Group formed around common interests, such as a support group for parents, exercise group, teen support group, or veterans group. |
| Peer support groups | Primary purpose is to provide support for individuals who have a diagnosis, medical-related problem, or disability in common; group may also involve the partners, families, and caregivers of the individuals; involvement of the OT practitioner varies from active involvement as leader to consultative role as facilitator. Group size can be large or small, depending on the format. |
| Task groups | Specific outcomes and tasks to be accomplished. Members may have common needs, such as learning to cook low-cost meals, how to get around in the community, or leisure exploration. |
| Therapeutic groups | Primary aim of group is individual change; OT practitioner uses therapeutic tasks that are designed to restore or develop functioning in occupational performance areas and client factors; other purposes may include prevention and support of existing strengths. Group size is typically 6–10 individuals. |

*OTA, occupational therapy assistant; *OT, occupational therapy.

**References**

O'Brien, J (2013). Occupational analysis and group process. In J. O'Brien & J. Solomon (Eds.), *Occupational analysis and group process* (pp. 1–15). St. Louis, MO: Mosby.

Scaffa, M (2014). Group process and group intervention. In B. Boyt-Schell, G. Gillen, M. Scaffa, & E. Cohn (Eds.), *Willard and Spackman's occupational therapy* (12th ed., pp. 437–452). Philadelphia, PA: Lippincott, Williams & Wilkins.

frame of reference, and the setting, duration, and frequency of group meetings.[5]

Once the practitioner has determined the group goals, he or she organizes the activity by analyzing the steps involved. The practitioner defines how many participants will be involved in the activity and the setting, timing, and materials needed. A thorough analysis of the activity demands and structure of the group is required to be sure that all group members are working toward their goals during the group process. After preparing the group, the OT practitioner uses therapeutic use of self skills to lead the members in the activity.

Leading a group of clients in an activity involves using therapeutic use of self and awareness of group dynamics.[5] The practitioner must be continually aware of how group members are working together. A skillful practitioner is aware of all members' individual goals and helps each member meet those goals. This can be accomplished by adapting and changing tasks, delegating responsibility, and intervening where needed. For example, the practitioner may help a member who is working to improve right-hand use by placing objects closer to the member. The practitioner may suggest to another member that he should ask for the supplies or walk to the other end of the table to help get the supplies. The key to working in groups is addressing group and individual group goals through a common task. Fig. 17.5 shows a practitioner leading a group of women in playing a game to increase socialization and memory.

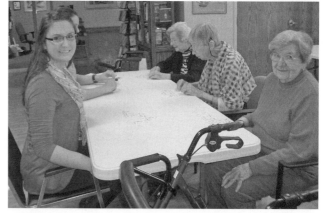

• **Fig. 17.5** The practitioner leads a women's group in a game of Scrabble. This therapeutic group is aimed at facilitating memory and social participation.

**Group dynamics** refers to the interactions between members based on personalities and relationships.[5] Groups work differently together, and members behave in certain patterns. The OT practitioner observes the group in session to facilitate positive group dynamics and intervene when the dynamics of the group are detrimental to the progress of the members. This may involve setting limitations on certain individuals who may take over the group. For example, the practitioner may require that the client sit away from another member to allow the other member space to interact with others. The practitioner may decide to meet individually with members who are disrupting the group as a way to help them work more effectively with others or to help them gain awareness of their presence in the group. The practitioner may collaborate with clients on group goals that improve the group dynamics.[5] In other settings, the practitioner may allow the group to address the work of the group. Members may need to address one another directly to help one another meet goals.

Developing group leadership skills is essential to helping clients reach their goals in therapy. Leaders convey knowledge to the members, structure and carry out organizational tasks, and guide members' performance. The leader informs members of their task assignments, reinforces active listening, and facilitates the group process. If a group experiences difficulty, the leader may be called on to make decisions on how to proceed. In OT groups, many times the leader allows the group to problem solve through difficulties because this helps clients in therapy. Overall, the group leader needs to convey confidence and clarity in the goals and structure of the activity. Leadership may shift in the group, but the OT practitioner is ultimately responsible for the structure and form of the group. Box 17.2 provides guidelines for exercising leadership in group formation.

Group leaders are responsible for introducing the group theme or goals, structuring the tasks, delegating responsibility, supervising the activity, concluding the group, and making sure that the area is cleaned up. The leader documents the members' progress and decides on the course of action for future groups. Many times OT practitioners work with the members to determine future activities. The group leader is ultimately responsible for making sure that all materials are available and that all members are safe. In

---

**• BOX 17.2  Taking Charge of a Group**

1. Plan and practice or rehearse the activity to know what is needed.
2. Anticipate! Think how people might interpret the instructions.
3. Carry a written list of all of the points to remember.
4. Stand to address the group.
5. Get everyone's attention before talking (expect it, and it will happen).
6. Regulate voice appropriately (loud and clear, as needed).
7. Tell in sequence. Keep words to a minimum, and demonstrate "first," "next," and so on.
8. Tell the group what to do when the task is complete.
9. Indicate the end of instructions and the beginning of the activity.

---

the case of emergency, the group leader follows emergency procedures as outlined by the facility. The OT practitioner is responsible for informing new members of the rules and expectations of the group. These expectations may be determined in collaboration with group members.

## Summary

Therapeutic use of self is key to OT practice because it is the essence of the therapeutic relationship. Self-awareness, empathy, verbal and nonverbal communication, trust, and active listening are needed to work with clients of varying abilities. OT practitioners engage in a variety of exercises to enhance their skills for developing therapeutic relationships. Practitioners frequently lead group activities to help clients meet their goals. This requires that practitioners understand and practice group dynamics and leadership. OT practitioners seek to provide a supportive atmosphere through the therapeutic use of self to help clients improve their functioning.

## Learning Activities

1. Make a list of desirable qualities for use in therapeutic relationships. Seek out a written description for each quality. Write a one- or two-sentence description for each, and make a self-rating scale.
2. Working with a partner, agree to monitor each other's communication (verbal and nonverbal) in a specific situation (e.g., class discussion, visit to a clinic, at lunch table). Each person is to keep a "personal reaction log" on the events and a "report log" of the other's behavior. At the end of the monitored time, share the logs and compare the personal reactions against the reported behavior.
3. Watch videotapes of people with impairments, disabilities, or problem behaviors. Write a description of the therapeutic relationship you would develop in each case, should that person become your client. Include a rationale for your choice of therapeutic relationship.
4. Select a partner. Each person is to write four to five verbal messages that a client may say to an OT practitioner. Switch your messages with those of your partner. On a separate piece of paper, each person is to write an appropriate active listening response to each message. When finished, ask your partner to read his or her messages one at a time as you give your response. Share feedback to the responses with each other (e.g., How did it feel getting the response from your partner? Did the response demonstrate active listening?).
5. Practice taking charge of a group. The object is to "own" the activity and demonstrate leadership. This can be accomplished in small groups of 6 to 10 in the following manner:
   - On slips of paper equal in number to the people, write simple activities (e.g., write a word on the board, form a line and walk around the desk).
   - Each member should draw one slip and not let the others know the content.
   - Given planning time, each member then leads the group in the identified activity.
   - After the activity, provide written feedback about leadership qualities displayed.
6. Lead an activity for three to five classmates and reflect on your group process and therapeutic interactions.

## Review Questions

1. What are the characteristics of a therapeutic relationship?
2. What are Kübler-Ross's stages of loss?
3. What is meant by the ideal self, the perceived self, and the real self?
4. What are the six modes of interacting in Taylor's Intentional Relationship Model?
5. How can an OT practitioner develop trust with a client?
6. What is empathy, and how can it be developed?
7. What are some verbal and nonverbal communication strategies used in therapeutic relationships?
8. How can practitioners actively listen to clients?
9. What is required to lead therapeutic groups effectively?

## References

1. Davis CM. *Patient–Practitioner Interaction: An Experiential Manual for Developing the Art of Health Care*. 3rd ed. Thorofare, NJ: Slack; 1998.
2. Early MB. *Mental Health Concepts and Techniques for the Occupational Therapy Assistant*. 3rd ed. Philadelphia, PA: Lippincott Williams & Wilkins; 2001.
3. Kielhofner G. *Model of Human Occupation: Theory and Application*. 4th ed. Baltimore, MD: Lippincott Williams & Wilkins; 2008.
4. Kübler-Ross E. *On Death and Dying*. New York, NY: Macmillan; 1969.
5. O'Brien J. Occupational analysis and group process. In: O'Brien J, Solomon J, eds. *Occupational Analysis and Group Process*. St. Louis, MO: Mosby; 2013:1–15.
6. Taylor RR. *The Intentional Relationship: Use of Self and Occupational Therapy*. Philadelphia, PA: F.A. Davis; 2008.

# 18

# Therapeutic Reasoning

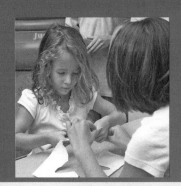

## OBJECTIVES

*After reading this chapter, the reader will be able to do the following:*

- Explain the nature of therapeutic reasoning.
- Describe the three elements of therapeutic reasoning.
- Describe the thought processes and strategies of therapeutic reasoning that are used by occupational therapy practitioners.

- Compare the therapeutic reasoning skills of the novice with those of the expert.
- Identify ways the occupational therapy practitioner can develop therapeutic reasoning skills.

## KEY TERMS

advanced beginner
artistic element
competent practitioner
conditional reasoning
clinical reasoning

ethical element
expert
interactive reasoning
narrative reasoning
novice

pragmatic reasoning
procedural reasoning
proficient practitioner
scientific element
therapeutic reasoning

 Visit *www.evolve.elsevier.com* to access the Evolve student resources that accompany your book.

*I found out about occupational therapy (OT) when I was 13 years of age, and it immediately appealed to me. I learned that OT helps people perform activities that make life worth living—cooking a good dinner, eating food, playing a game with friends, or completing a project. What could be more important? I was right; OT is about the power of engagement in occupations. It is one of the best-kept secrets of our American health-care system. Over the years, I have found working directly with clients tremendously rewarding—and challenging—but it is also extremely gratifying to plan programs, educate student therapists, and conduct research. I have been an OT for 31 years; at this stage in my career, I find that I help shape the future of the profession by contributing to our knowledge base through research, a particularly rewarding and fun part of being a practitioner. I keep coming back to the insight I had when I was 13 years of age—occupations have a powerful influence on who we are as individuals and who we will become as we grow older. What could be more fascinating than exploring how occupation works? What could be more exciting than working with a group of people who share the commitment to understand*

*occupation and how it can be used to help people lead healthy, fulfilling lives?*

**L. DIANE PARHAM, PHD, OTR, FAOTA**
**Professor**
**Occupational Therapy Graduate Program**
**School of Medicine**
**University of New Mexico**
**Albuquerque, New Mexico**

Zach is a 2-year-old boy with developmental delays. Corinne, the occupational therapist, is scheduled to see him for an evaluation and intervention planning session. What does she know about this child's diagnosis? What are his strengths and weaknesses? How will she determine the type of therapy he needs? How will she choose a frame of reference? What types of activities will be most useful? How will she measure his success? What are the issues the family is experiencing? How will she organize the information?

There are many questions to contemplate when working with a client. Figuring out how to address client issues and intervene requires **therapeutic reasoning,** which is the thought process that therapists use to evaluate clients and design and carry out intervention. Therapeutic reasoning may also be referred to as **clinical reasoning**. However, many occupational therapy (OT) practitioners work in settings other than clinics, so the term *therapeutic reasoning* is inclusive of all settings and will be used throughout this chapter. Therapeutic reasoning involves complex cognitive and affective skills; that is, it involves both thinking and feeling. All OT practitioners use therapeutic reasoning throughout each step of the OT process. Knowledge of therapeutic reasoning helps practitioners better serve their clients.

OT practitioners use therapeutic reasoning to make decisions.[12] Consumers and employers search for practice that is based on evidence (i.e., supported through research). OT practitioners use therapeutic reasoning to critically analyze research, make decisions regarding services, and work with individual clients. This chapter provides an overview of the therapeutic reasoning process and provides strategies to help students develop these skills.

## Elements of Therapeutic Reasoning

Therapeutic reasoning may be characterized into three elements: scientific, ethical, and artistic.[12] The **scientific element** addresses the question, "What are the possible things that can be done for this client?" The answer to this question is found in the evaluation and assessment procedures used to determine the strengths and weaknesses of the client, the writing of a plan to guide and direct the change process, and the selection of therapeutic modalities that result in successful occupational performance outcomes. The scientific element demands careful and accurate assessment, analysis, and recording.

Aiko is a 7-year-old girl diagnosed with Williams syndrome. Marie, the occupational therapist working in the school system, investigates this syndrome and reviews literature on the issues that children with Williams syndrome face. She decides that she needs to evaluate Aiko's muscle tone, musculoskeletal functions, endurance, visual-motor integration skills, and fine motor abilities, and she believes that she will be able to work with Aiko on improving her ability to function in the classroom by providing modifications.

By determining the child's strengths and weaknesses in light of the medical condition, Marie used scientific reasoning to plan the child's intervention. Frequently, clinicians start the therapeutic reasoning process using scientific reasoning because this type of reasoning follows the medical model. Scientific reasoning helps practitioners understand the client's process and story. Thus it makes a good starting point.

The **ethical element** addresses questions such as, "What *should* be done for this client?" and "What is the right and fair path to take?" The answer takes into account the client's perspective and his or her goals for intervention. Each individual has different views on health, what is important in life, and how things are accomplished. When the OT practitioner understands and respects the client's perspective, an intervention plan that preserves the client's values can be developed.[12] The OT practitioner consults with the client so that he or she can participate in making decisions regarding intervention goals

and methods. The OT practitioner considers all of the scientific and ethical information in relation to the individual's needs, goals, culture, environment, and lifestyle.[12]

Mark, a 79-year-old man, wants to return home after his cerebral vascular accident (stroke). The team does not feel this would be the best solution for him because he lives far from others and he has no one to care for him. Mark refuses to discuss options of living elsewhere. The team feels he would not be safe alone. The OT practitioner conducts a home evaluation. The OT practitioner provides a list of suggestions and home modifications so the team may explore other options. The OT practitioner must decide whether to support Mark's choice to return home. The OT discusses her role with the client and explains that she will try to support his choice if at all possible.

This example illustrates one of many ethical dilemmas OT practitioners may face. The practitioner must consider the right of the client and decide based on the ethical principles of practice (see Chapter 8). The practitioner uses therapeutic reasoning to examine all of the alternatives, predict future success, and investigate the client's needs. In this case the clinician uses therapeutic reasoning to investigate all areas that might interfere with Mark's living alone. This information can help the team develop alternative ethical solutions. Ethically, she is contributing to the desires of the client without letting the team down.

The **artistic element** of therapeutic reasoning is evident in the skill used by the OT practitioner to guide the treatment process and select the "right action" in the face of uncertainties inherent in the therapeutic process.[12] The therapeutic process involves integrating and blending many areas, such as deficiencies to be addressed, the client's interests and wishes, the medium or activity to be used, and the interpersonal climate that is to support the therapy process. The therapeutic relationship and the way in which the OT practitioner interacts with the client play a major role in the artistic element. The artistic element involves using creativity to skillfully design intervention specific to a client. This requires the practitioner to modify activities, use humor or coaching, and read the cues of the client when interacting.

Missy, the occupational therapy assistant (OTA), jokes in therapy with Brian, a 77-year-old veteran who had his right leg amputated just below the knee. Brian does not want to come to OT today, and Missy looks him gently in the eyes, smiles, and jokes, "Brian, you say that every day. Come on, let's go." Missy does not take no from him, and Brian smiles as he follows her to therapy.

Missy has developed a rapport with Brian, and the art of this interaction is evident as Missy reads Brian's words as joking. Missy knows she has connected with Brian and can afford to joke with him. This same scenario may be interpreted as refusal of therapy and handled differently for another client. The art of therapy involves reading the client's cues within the context of the setting and the client–therapist relationship. Artistic reasoning requires skill in the therapeutic relationship, creativity, reflection, and self-awareness (see Chapter 17).

## Thought Process During Therapeutic Reasoning

Therapeutic reasoning is a cognitive thought process in which many diverse bits of information are gathered together (evaluation), many outside factors are considered (e.g., life space, prognosis, and desires), the demands of activities are analyzed (activity analysis), time investment choices are made (plan), and identifiable goals are organized (intervention). Therapeutic reasoning used throughout the therapy process requires analysis of data, use of specific knowledge bases, and synthesis of the process and information. The OT practitioner must actively think about and process information from multiple sources. Fig. 18.1 shows OT students working through a case to develop therapeutic reasoning skills.

Rogers and Holm[13] describe the steps in the thought process of therapeutic reasoning that is used during the OT evaluation and intervention process. During each step, the OT practitioner gathers, organizes, analyzes, and synthesizes information.[13] See Box 18.1.

In the first step, the OT practitioner forms a *preassessment image* of the client, an initial outline that will be used for further assessment of the client. The practitioner considers the client's diagnosis, age, and contexts (e.g., time in life). The OT practitioner seeks to find out information related to the diagnosis, client's life roles, and functional status before the injury or trauma. At this stage, the practitioner is forming a general picture of the person.

The OT practitioner uses the preassessment image to begin the *cue acquisition* step. This step involves gathering the data regarding the client's current functional status, occupational roles, and past experiences. The purpose of this stage is to gather data, or *cues,* to inform the intervention planning. Fig. 18.2 shows an OT practitioner gathering information by observing a child playing.

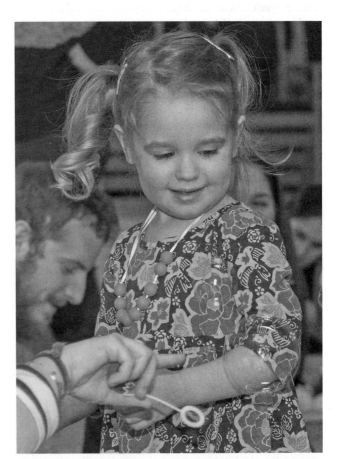

• **Fig. 18.2** The occupational therapy practitioner can observe posture, balance, motor planning, playfulness, and hand skills during play. This provides information to develop hypotheses for intervention planning.

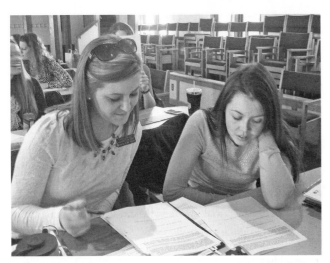

• **Fig. 18.1** Occupational therapy students use the steps of therapeutic reasoning to analyze the many factors of a case example in class.

The practitioner generates a *hypothesis* using the cues regarding the client's needs. The practitioner organizes the data that have been gathered and makes tentative assumptions, which serve as the basis for therapeutic action. The hypotheses generated are based on all available data, knowledge of models or practice and frames of reference, and the practitioner's experience.

> In evaluating a female client's ability to feed herself, the OT practitioner notices that the client is having difficulty and does not eat all of the food on her plate. The food spills out of her mouth. The client is unable to use her left hand. The practitioner's hypothesis is that the difficulty is the result of poor oral motor skills caused by the client's stroke. The practitioner could also hypothesize that the client's difficulty results from the fact that she must use her nondominant hand to feed herself, which makes it hard to get the food on the utensil and tires her out easily.

The process continues with step 4, *cue interpretation*, where the practitioner continues the search for data based on the hypothesis being considered. During this stage, the practitioner may conduct intervention on a given hypothesis and collect more data to verify the relevancy. This leads to the *hypothesis evaluation*, in which the practitioner interprets whether the cues confirm the hypothesis, do not confirm the hypothesis, or do not contribute in either way to the hypothesis.[12] The hypothesis with the most supporting evidence forms the basis for intervention. Fig. 18.3 shows a team of students interviewing a patient actor as a way to help students develop therapeutic reasoning.

This therapeutic reasoning process leads to an assessment of the client's OT performance deficits and an intervention plan based on available data. The process considers the cause of the deficit, the signs and symptoms, knowledge of the condition, and a definition of the problems.[13] OT practitioners use therapeutic reasoning during all aspects of the OT process. They select from a variety of intervention approaches and make decisions on goals, modalities, and activity selection. They use therapeutic reasoning to evaluate the effectiveness of intervention.

The practitioner closely monitors and evaluates the intervention to determine whether the modalities that were selected achieve the intended goal(s). Importantly, the OT practitioner collaborates with the client throughout the process to confirm that therapy is proceeding on a track that is meaningful to the client. The process of therapeutic reasoning is a dynamic process.

## Therapeutic Reasoning Strategies

Therapists who understand and employ a range of therapeutic reasoning strategies are able to adapt their interventions to meet individuals' needs. Several types of therapeutic reasoning strategies are described in Table 18.1.

Mattingly and Fleming discovered that OT practitioners used three distinct strategies, or tracks, for therapeutic reasoning: procedural, interactive, and conditional tracks.[3,8] Practitioners shift easily and frequently among the three tracks, depending on what they are addressing in therapy with a specific client.

**Procedural reasoning** is a strategy used by the OT practitioner when he or she focuses on the client's disease or disability and determines what will be the most appropriate modalities to use to improve functional performance. Central tasks for the OT practitioner during procedural reasoning are problem identification, goal setting, and treatment planning.[3] This track is similar to the scientific element of therapeutic reasoning.

> The OT practitioner working with a new client examines the diagnosis, etiology, characteristics, prognosis, and suggested interventions. The practitioner determines the most commonly used approach for clients with this diagnosis and begins intervention based on this knowledge. The practitioner is engaged in procedural reasoning.

**Interactive reasoning** is a strategy used by the OT practitioner to understand the client as a person. This type of reasoning takes place during face-to-face interactions between the practitioner and the client. OT practitioners use interactive reasoning strategies to (1) understand the disability from the client's point of view, (2) engage the client in treatment, (3) individualize the intervention setting by matching goals and procedures to the particular client and his or her life experiences and disability, (4) impart a sense of trust and acceptance to the client, (5) relieve tension by using humor, (6) develop a common language of actions and meanings, and (7) determine whether the intervention is working.[3]

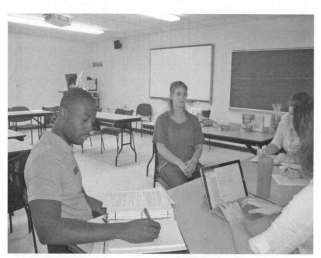

• **Fig. 18.3** A team of occupational therapy students interviews a patient actor to develop hypotheses regarding an intervention plan. Working with simulated clients is one way to facilitate therapeutic reasoning skills.

| TABLE 18.1 | Strategies Used by Occupational Therapy Practitioners in Therapeutic Reasoning | |
|---|---|
| **Strategy** | **Description** |
| Procedural reasoning | Strategy used by the OT* practitioner to focus on the client's disease or disability and determine what will be the most appropriate modalities to use to improve the client's functional performance. Central tasks include problem identification, goal setting, and treatment planning. |
| Interactive reasoning | Strategy used by the OT practitioner when he or she wants to understand the client as a person; takes place during face-to-face interactions between the practitioner and the client. |
| Conditional reasoning | Involves consideration by the practitioner of the client's condition as a whole, including the disease or disability and what it means to the person, the physical context, and the social context; consideration of how the client's condition may change, depending on level of participation in treatment. |
| Narrative reasoning | Use of storytelling wherein practitioners tell "stories" about clients to one another. Use of story creation, wherein the practitioner envisions how the future may be for the client so that he or she may guide the intervention process. |
| Pragmatic reasoning | The practitioner takes into account how factors in the context of the practice setting and his or her personal context might affect intervention. Factors in the practice setting relate to the availability of resources (i.e., reimbursement or availability of equipment). Factors in the personal context of the practitioner might include repertoire of therapeutic skills and personal motivation. |

*OT, occupational therapy.
Adapted from Mattingly, C., & Fleming, M. (1994). *Therapeutic reasoning: Forms of inquiry in a therapeutic practice.* Philadelphia, PA: F.A. Davis; Neistadt, M. E. (1996). Teaching strategies for the development of therapeutic reasoning. *American Journal of Occupational Therapy, 50,* 676–684; Rogers J. C., & Holm, M. B. (1991). Occupational therapy diagnostic reasoning: A component of therapeutic reasoning. *American Journal of Occupational Therapy, 45,* 1045–1053; and Schell, B. A., & Cervero, R. M. (1993). Therapeutic reasoning in occupational therapy: An integrative review. *American Journal of Occupational Therapy, 47,* 605–610.

The OT practitioner learns that the client lives at home with his wife of 20 years and three teenage children. The client hopes to return to his job as a certified public accountant (CPA); he enjoys biking with his family and hiking in the country. The OT practitioner uses this information along with the information about the diagnosis, prognosis, etiology, and intervention strategies when designing the intervention plan.

Anna, the OT practitioner, evaluates Sam's progress in therapy and decides to change the focus of intervention from remediation to compensation. Anna believes that Sam has worked hard in therapy, but based on the severity of his condition and the progress to date, Anna decides that compensation techniques will enable Sam to return to his occupations earlier.

Interactive reasoning takes into account the client's identity, goals, and environment. Although OT practitioners use procedural reasoning to form a foundation for intervention, they personalize the intervention through interactive reasoning.

The third type of strategy used by OT practitioners is **conditional reasoning.** Conditional reasoning has several aspects.[3] The practitioner considers the client's condition as a whole, including the disease or disability and what it means to the person—the physical context and the social context. The practitioner motivates the client to participate in intervention by sharing the same vision for the outcome of intervention.[3] With these images in mind, the practitioner implements intervention and compares changes observed in the client with the client's future goals.[3] The practitioner using conditional reasoning examines all aspects of the client's circumstances. In particular, the practitioner evaluates the context of the intervention in relation to the client's goals and desires.

Anna used conditional reasoning to change the focus of the intervention and to allow Sam to return to his occupations. She analyzed multiple factors contributing to Sam's

progress and reasoned that changing the intervention may allow him to return to his occupational goals faster.

Another therapeutic reasoning strategy described in the literature is called **narrative reasoning.** Mattingly describes two different ways in which OT practitioners use narrative reasoning: storytelling and story creation.[7] In storytelling, OT practitioners tell stories about clients to other practitioners to better understand and reason through concepts. This type of storytelling may be observed during case-study presentations. Mattingly states, "Narratives make sense of reality by linking the outward world of actions and events to the inner world of human intention and motivation."[7]

Clients also use storytelling to reframe their own narratives and make sense of events. Telling one's story about one's past is a helpful way to create a future story. Thus storytelling can be therapeutic for clients and families. For example, a young athlete who sustained a spinal cord injury may tell stories about his past successes as an athlete. As he progresses through therapy, he may develop new stories about successes and reinvent his athlete image by engaging in adapted sport activities, such as wheelchair races, adapted sailing programs, or wheelchair basketball. He may use storytelling to redefine who he is in his current body. Storytelling can help clients understand their occupational performance and develop a new identity.

**Pragmatic reasoning** takes into consideration such factors as the context of the practice setting and the personal context of the OT practitioner that may inhibit or facilitate intervention. Factors related to the context of the practice setting include reimbursement and the availability of equipment and space.[14] For example, a practitioner considers reimbursement and available resources when developing an intervention plan. The OT practitioner must also consider personal factors, including his or her repertoire of therapeutic skills, knowledge, and experience. Other pragmatic factors include time/habits, costs, resources, environment, setting, and personnel.

Nick, the OT practitioner, is treating Carlos, a 63-year-old client who has had a stroke. Nick and Carlos are working toward improving movement in Carlos's affected arm and hand so that he can return to his occupation as a car mechanic. Carlos creates a vision for his future by explaining to the therapist the many tasks he performs at work and identifying the pride he receives from his co-workers and family. Nick explains that the projects he completes in OT require concentration, design, problem solving, and fine motor skills, which are also skills Carlos needs when working as a mechanic. Together, Nick helps Carlos understand that he has heard his story and will help him return to his job as car mechanic.

## From Novice to Expert: Development of Therapeutic Reasoning Skills

Therapeutic reasoning develops over time with practical experience. Generally, authors describe five different stages of career development: novice, advanced beginner, competent, proficient, and expert[15] (Table 18.2).

The focus of the **novice** practitioner is on learning procedural skills (e.g., assessment, diagnostic, and treatment planning procedures) necessary to practice.[3,15] The novice practitioner feels most comfortable performing and refining the techniques and procedures learned in school. Novice practitioners do not feel comfortable using interactive reasoning strategies. The **advanced beginner** recognizes additional cues and begins to view the client as an individual.[15] However, the advanced beginner still does not see the whole picture.

The **competent practitioner** sees more facts and determines the importance of these facts and observations.[15] At this stage, practitioners have a broader understanding of the client's problems and are more likely to individualize treatment. However, flexibility and creativity are still lacking. The **proficient practitioner** views situations as a whole instead of as isolated parts.[15] Practical experience allows him or her to develop a direction and vision of where the client should be going. If the initial plans do not work, the proficient therapist is easily able to modify them.

**Expert** practitioners recognize and understand rules of practice; however, for this group of practitioners, the rules shift to the background.[15] The expert practitioner often uses intuition to know what to do next. "This intuitive judgment is based on correct identification of relevant cues at a particular time in the patient's therapy and a variety of medical, physical, and psychosocial factors."[15] Expert practitioners use procedural, interactive, and conditional skills without difficulty.[3] They rely on past therapeutic situations to process imagined outcomes for the client.

## Techniques to Develop Therapeutic Reasoning Skills

OT educators realize the importance of facilitating and fostering therapeutic reasoning skills in students and clinicians. Problem-based learning is one technique used by

| TABLE 18.2 | Development of Therapeutic Reasoning Skills | |
|---|---|---|
| **Stage of Development** | **Name** | **Type of Functioning** |
| 1 | Novice | Uses procedural or scientific reasoning, knowledge from coursework |
| 2 | Advanced beginner | Recognizes additional cues and begins to see client as an individual |
| 3 | Competent | Sees more facts, understands client's problems, individualizes treatment, may lack creativity and flexibility |
| 4 | Proficient | Views situations as whole instead of in isolated parts, able to develop a vision of where the client should go, able to modify easily |
| 5 | Expert | Recognizes and understands rules of practice, uses intuition to know what to do next, uses conditional reasoning |

Adapted from Dreyfus, H. L., & Dreyfus, S. E. (1986). *Mind over machine, the power of human intuition and expertise in the era of the computer* (pp. 101–121). New York, NY: The Free Press; Neistadt, M. E., & Atkins, A, (1996). Analysis of the orthopedic content in an occupational therapy curriculum from a therapeutic reasoning perspective. *American Journal of Occupational Therapy, 50,* 669–675; and Benner, P. E. (1994). *From novice to expert: Excellence and power in therapeutic nursing practice.* Menlo Park, CA: Addison-Wesley.

educational programs to encourage therapeutic reasoning skills. Other closely related techniques include case-based integration courses and assignments requiring students to complete evaluation and intervention protocols in a simulated manner. Figs. 18.4A–C show students engaged in a case-based integration course to facilitate therapeutic reasoning. The intent of these courses and assignments is to help the students participate in therapeutic reasoning, reflect on their learning, and advance in their ability to consider multiple factors. In a comparison of therapeutic reasoning skills in OT students in the United States and Scotland, McCannon et al. found that the predominant form of therapeutic reasoning by students in a problem-based learning course was procedural.[9] Vroman and MacRae reported similar findings in their work.[18] Educational programs provide students with the tools to engage in therapeutic reasoning by providing authentic experiences for students.[5] Bailey and Cohn suggest that faculty help students learn from clients.[1] They provided students opportunities to interview clients with disabilities and discuss the process. Reflection and introspection are key factors in developing therapeutic reasoning. Students and practitioners must be able to seek and receive feedback.

In her study of expert and novice practitioners, Unsworth suggested that novice practitioners could benefit from more time reflecting on the therapy process and discussing their therapy with expert clinicians.[17] Interestingly, she found, as did Taylor[16] and Mattingly,[6] that expert clinicians were able to self-critique their work and showed willingness to change. Liu et al. found that more experienced therapists used conditional reasoning, whereas junior therapists relied on procedural reasoning.[5]

Novice practitioners and students gather information using individual cues, whereas experts use chunking to sort and record information. Chunking is a strategy that is used to remember several units of information. For example, it is easier to remember a phone number if it is divided into chunks (e.g., 501-555-9487) instead of trying to remember individual numbers (e.g., 5015559487). Expert practitioners use the technique of chunking to categorize information about clients and apply it to practice.[12]

The student or novice practitioner can enhance his or her therapeutic reasoning skills through coaching, reflecting, analyzing, and role modeling.[2,10,15] Reading and reflecting on the personal experiences of individuals with disabilities can help a practitioner develop therapeutic reasoning skills.[10] The student can analyze case studies to develop reasoning. The novice practitioner can observe expert practitioners and examine the therapeutic reasoning processes and strategies that the experts use. Furthermore, discussions and systematic analysis of fieldwork experiences may help novice practitioners develop therapeutic reasoning skills.

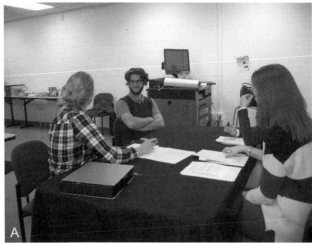

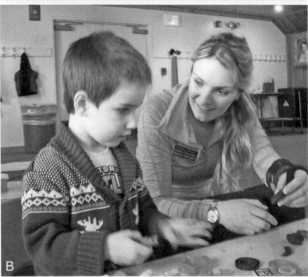

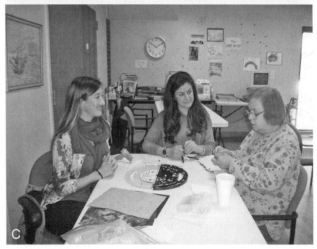

• **Fig. 18.4 A,** Occupational therapy students interview a patient actor as a way to develop therapeutic reasoning skills. **B,** Occupational therapy students engage a child in a developmental assessment, interview the parents, and complete the therapeutic reasoning required for an evaluation. **C,** Occupational therapy students use therapeutic reasoning skills to engage an older adult in a therapeutic activity.

Students trying to advance their therapeutic reasoning abilities benefit by exploring the literature, critically analyzing data, and reflecting on their own performance. Requesting feedback from more advanced practitioners helps the novice understand approaches and reasoning. Practitioners develop skills by discussing specific cases and problem solving through the therapeutic reasoning process.

Practitioners are encouraged to seek education and knowledge and remain reflective of their own practice. Therapeutic reasoning skills may be further developed through new knowledge and careful analysis of one's practice skills and thinking. Practitioners may improve therapeutic reasoning skills by seeking feedback from others on intervention approaches and reasoning. Reflective writing and self-assessment will help practitioners develop therapeutic reasoning. Practitioners may benefit from examining their abilities by observing videos of their work. Using the Self-Assessment of Clinical Reflection and Reasoning (SACRR)[13a] may provide insight into one's therapeutic reasoning.

Conducting research through case-study analysis may enhance a practitioner's therapeutic reasoning skills because this requires a careful examination of the intervention process. Following a specific frame of reference can help practitioners develop therapeutic reasoning skills. For example, in separate studies, O'Brien et al.[11] and Keponen and Launiainen[4] examined the therapeutic reasoning process using the Model of Human Occupation. Finally, remaining current and critically examining available research enhances a practitioner's therapeutic reasoning skills and abilities, thereby benefiting clients.

## Summary

Therapeutic reasoning provides the foundation for making choices and helping improve clients' ability to function and engage in occupations. The elements of science, ethics, and art are combined in the therapy process. OT practitioners skillfully design intervention to make a difference in the lives of the clients they serve. Knowledge of science provides data on the condition, diagnosis, prognosis, and client factors that may be involved. The art of therapy involves designing creative intervention to address occupational performance deficits. The art of therapy involves the therapeutic use of self and refers to how practitioners relate to clients. Finally, ethical considerations may influence the course of the intervention and outcomes.

OT practitioners use a variety of strategies to effectively integrate the scientific, artistic, and ethical elements into intervention plans. These reasoning strategies include procedural, interactive, conditional, narrative, and pragmatic reasoning. The strategies are seldom used in isolation, and, in fact, expert practitioners intertwine the strategies to provide the most effective and intuitive intervention. Novice practitioners may be limited in the strategies they use.

Practice, reflection, education, supervision, research, and critical analysis of practice provide excellent techniques for increasing a practitioner's ability to use therapeutic reasoning. OT practitioners must always remain mindful of the therapeutic reasoning strategies they are employing so that intervention remains beneficial to clients.

## Learning Activities

1. Provide students with a case study. Provide examples of the type of therapeutic reasoning strategies based on the specific client. Share examples in class.
2. View a videotape of a case study of a client in a therapy session. Analyze the therapeutic reasoning strategies used by the practitioner. Were the strategies effective? What would you have done differently?
3. Write a short story about someone who has a disability. Report how this individual's past and present may reflect on his or her possible future.
4. Read a literary work about an individual who has experienced a disabling condition. Using the narrative reasoning strategy, analyze the person's experiences. Describe the person's story. (Your instructor can provide suggestions for books to read.)
5. Use therapeutic reasoning strategies to develop an intervention plan for a given case study, in which the only information available is the client's age, diagnosis, and living situation. Discuss the findings in class. What would be the next step in the process?

## Review Questions

1. What is therapeutic reasoning?
2. What is the therapeutic reasoning thought process?
3. Provide an example of the scientific, ethical, and artistic elements of therapeutic reasoning.
4. What are the three types of therapeutic reasoning as described by Mattingly and Fleming?
5. What are the stages of therapeutic reasoning? Provide a description of each.

## References

1. Bailey DM, Cohn ES. Understanding others: a course to learn interactive therapeutic reasoning. *Occup Ther Health Care.* 2001;15(1/2):31–46.
2. Benamy BC. *Developing Therapeutic Reasoning Skills: Strategies for the Occupational Therapist.* San Antonio, TX: Therapy Skill Builders; 1996.
3. Fleming MH. The therapist with the three-track mind. *Am J Occup Ther.* 1991;45:1007–1014.
4. Keponen R, Launiainen H. Using the model of human occupation to nurture an occupational focus in the therapeutic reasoning of experienced therapists. *Occup Ther Health Care.* 2008;22(2/3):95–104.

5. Liu KPY, Chan CCH, Hui-Chan CWY. Therapeutic reasoning and the occupational therapy curriculum. *Occup Ther Int.* 2000;7(3):173–183.

6. Mattingly C, Fleming M. *Therapeutic Reasoning: Forms of Inquiry in a Therapeutic Practice.* Philadelphia, PA: F.A. Davis; 1994.

7. Mattingly C. The narrative nature of therapeutic reasoning. *Am J Occup Ther.* 1991;45:998.

8. Mattingly C. What is therapeutic reasoning? *Am J Occup Ther.* 1991;45:979.

9. McCannon R, Robertson D, Caldwell J, et al. Comparison of therapeutic reasoning skills in occupational therapy students in the USA and Scotland. *Occup Ther Int.* 2004;11(3):160–176.

10. Neistadt ME. Teaching strategies for the development of therapeutic reasoning. *Am J Occup Ther.* 1996;50:676–684.

11. O'Brien J, Asselin L, Fortier K, et al. Using therapeutic reasoning to apply the model of human occupation in pediatric occupational therapy practice. *J Occup Ther Sch Early Interv.* 2010;3(4):348–365.

12. Rogers JC. Therapeutic reasoning: the ethics, science and art. *Am J Occup Ther.* 1983;37:601–616.

13. Rogers JC, Holm MB. Occupational therapy diagnostic reasoning: a component of therapeutic reasoning. *Am J Occup Ther.* 1991;45:1045–1053.

13a. Royees CB, Mu K, Barrett K, et al. Pilot investigation: Evaluation of clinical reflection and reasoning before and after workshop intervention. In: Crist P, ed. *Innovation in Occupational Therapy Education.* Bethesda, MD: AOTA; 2001:107–114.

14. Schell BA, Cervero RM. Therapeutic reasoning in occupational therapy: an integrative review. *Am J Occup Ther.* 1993;47:605–610.

15. Slater DY, Cohn ES. Staff development through analysis of practice. *Am J Occup Ther.* 1991;45:1038–1044.

16. Taylor RR. *The Intentional Relationship: Use of Self and Occupational Therapy.* Philadelphia, PA: F.A. Davis; 2008.

17. Unsworth G. The therapeutic reasoning of novice and expert occupational therapists. *Scand J Occup Ther.* 2001;8:163–173.

18. Vroman KE, MacRae N. How should the effectiveness of problem-based learning in occupational therapy education be examined? *Am J Occup Ther.* 1999;53:533–536.

# Appendix A

# Sample Intervention Activities

OT practitioners develop activities to facilitate engagement in occupations. They analyze the client factors and skills needed to perform activities, and consider how to create opportunities for clients to succeed while working towards a specific goal. The following activities offer students ideas of how to create intervention activities.

## Activity of Daily Living: Feeding

### Activity: Lunch Sampler

*Goals:*

1. Client will eat three different textured foods with a 30-minute session.
2. Given meal set up, client will eat lunch within 30 minutes.
3. Client will drink 4 ounces of liquid from adapted cup independently.
4. Client will chew a cookie and swallow it independently.

*Materials:*

Food of various textures:
- Pudding or yogurt (soft)
- Crackers or cookies (crunchy)
- Raisins or Fruit Roll-Ups (chewy)
- Juice or milk (liquid)
- Apple or orange (hard)
- Cheese (spread or sliced)
- Bread

*Sequence:*

1. Have client choose items for lunch from each group.
2. Prepare foods in a creative way. For example, cut bread and cheese using cookie cutters. Place pudding or yogurt in decorated cupcake tin (Fig. A.1).
3. Once meal is prepared, have client sit down and enjoy the snacks with at least one other person.
4. Engage client in light conversation to facilitate a positive experience.

*Population:*

Children and up.

*Body functions targeted:*

- Oral motor control required to feed oneself.

- Fine motor skills to pick up utensils or food.
- Sitting posture to remain upright.
- Bilateral hand skills to hold food (i.e., bread) while spreading cheese with other hand.
- Coordination to chew and swallow.

*Considerations:*

- Dietary needs
- Food allergies
- Ability to swallow

*Therapeutic techniques:*

- For clients who have sensory issues related to textures, the OT practitioner may want to begin by having the client rub or brush his/her face. Washing one's face with a rough cloth may help the person prepare for feeding.
- Proper positioning promotes success in feeding. Clients should be sitting upright with head slightly flexed (to promote swallow) and feet on the floor.
- Placing food at midline promotes proper body position and will not elicit muscle tone fluctuations.
- Speaking to clients in conversational voice is calming as is neutral warmth, dim lights and quiet.

## Activity of Daily Living: Dressing

### Activity: Dress Up

*Goals:*

1. Dress self completely with verbal cues.
2. Undress self independently.
3. Button large buttons.
4. Use both hands to don and doff clothing.

*Materials:*

- A variety of brightly colored clothes, costumes, and accessories (e.g., hats, hair pieces, pocketbooks, swords, badges, masks)
- Mirror
- Materials can be grouped by themes such as prince/princesses, superheroes, cowboys, monsters (getting Halloween costumes), or grown up people (Fig. A.2).

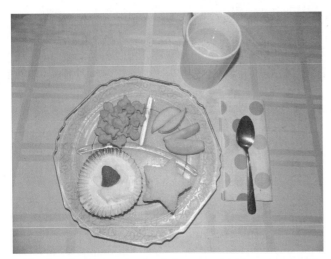

**• Fig. A.1** Presenting the lunch in a special way may promote engagement in the activity.

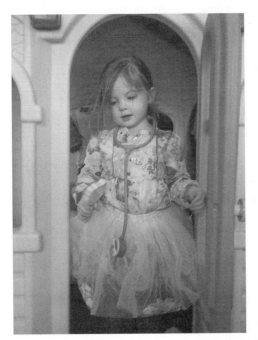

**• Fig. A.2** This young girl enjoys dressing up as a "princess doctor."

## Sequence:

Develop a dress-up theme and invite the children to dress up. Assist children if they need help buttoning or arranging clothes. Encourage them to do as much as possible. They may want to put on some make-up or wear a hat. Once they are satisfied with their new look, they can show it to others. They may want to pretend to be the character, demonstrate the walk of a fashion show, or play a game in the dress up. Once completed, the children will have to take the clothes off and put them away.

## Population:

Children (but can be adapted for teens and adults).

## Body functions targeted:

- Bilateral hand use to hold and fasten clothing.
- Motor planning to put arms through sleeves and legs into pants.
- Balance to raise leg and put on pants.
- Hand skills (pincer grasp) and hand strength to zip.
- Fine motor coordination to tie.

## Mental functions targeted:

- Cognitive processing to imagine and "pretend."
- Visual perceptual skills to put the clothing on correctly.
- Experience of self in new clothing.
- Awareness of self even though "pretending."

## Considerations:

- Visual perceptual skills
- Size of clothing
- Degree of difficulty of snaps, buttons, zippers

## Therapeutic techniques:

Children enjoy playing dress up. Having a variety of interesting clothing makes the activity fun and motivating. Some children may have difficulty with too many choices, so the activity may have to be structured more carefully. The therapist may need to provide hand-over-hand assistance or help the child adapt the task (for example, sit down to put on one's pants). Dress up games can be more fun by singing songs, having a parade, performing a skit or dancing. Taking photos and sending them home may provide the child with a nice memory and may reinforce dressing skills.

## Helpful Hints:

Second hand stores, garage sales, and after holiday sales are inexpensive ways to get "dress-up" clothes.

# Activity of Daily Living: Grooming/Hygiene

## Activity: Make-Over Monday

### Goals:

1. Client will brush hair.
2. Client will complete morning grooming routine.
3. Client will apply make-up.
4. Client will brush teeth.

### Materials:

- Make-up (cover-up, blush, mascara, eye shadow, lipstick)
- Soap and water
- Wash cloth
- Facial cream
- Toothbrush, toothpaste, mouthwash
- Brush, curling iron, comb, hairdryer
- Mirror
- Sink

*Sequence:*

1. Take "before" photo.
2. Wash face and hands.
3. Brush teeth. Use mouthwash.
4. Dry hair (if wet).
5. Style hair.
6. Apply facial cream and make-up.
7. Take "after" photo.

*Population:*

All ages (especially good for teens; Figs. A.3A and A.3B).

*Body functions targeted:*

- Fine motor skills for applying make-up and brushing teeth.
- Hand strength for holding hair dryer.
- Upper extremity range of motion to reach back and top of head for hair styling.
- Visual perceptual skills for applying make-up and styling hair.
- Grasp towel for washing face and holding soap.
- Pincer grasp to remove cap off toothpaste and make-up.

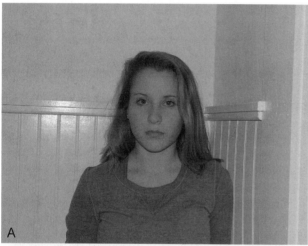

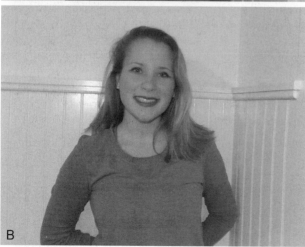

• **Fig. A.3 A,** "Before" photo of teen without make-up or styling hair. **B,** "After" photo where teen can show off her make-up, hair styling, and self-expression.

*Mental functions targeted:*

- Self-concept by taking care of self.
- Cognitive processes of sequencing and timing.
- Orientation to person, place and time for morning routine.
- Memory to complete sequence.

*Considerations:*

- Personal preferences for make-up
- Temperature of water.
- Allergic reactions to soap and make-up.

*Therapeutic techniques:*

The OT practitioner may adapt the activity by providing a picture sequence. See Fig. A.4 for an example. Some clients may benefit from a mirror that magnifies or built up handles on make-up brushes. Some clients may need a hair dryer that is stable so they do not have to hold it.

The OT practitioner should encourage the client to do as much as possible. Hand-over-hand support or adaptations to the materials may help the client succeed.

Variation: Have clients dress themselves and walk down the "runway." This activity may help clients develop a positive sense of self.

## Instrumental Activities of Daily Living: Care of pets

### Activity: Goldfish Bowl

*Goals:*

1. Provide care to goldfish.
2. Arrange materials to consistently care for goldfish.
3. Develop care routine to care for pet.
4. Develop memory strategies to care for pet.
5. Develop fine motor skills to care for pet.

*Materials: (Fig. A.5A shows sample materials)*

- Goldfish
- Goldfish food
- Glass bowl
- Small fish net scooper
- Rocks
- Water
- Colorful stickers, paint—for outside decorations
- Paint brush
- Paper (to write down sequence of care instructions)

*Sequence:*

1. Decorate a glass bowl using stickers and/or paints.
2. Place crushed rocks into bowl.
3. Add water so that bowl is ¾ full.
4. Gently add in goldfish (Fig. A.5B shows sample of completed decorated bowl).
5. Add a pinch of food.

| Morning Routine | | Monday | Tuesday | Wednesday | Thursday | Friday | Saturday | Sunday |
|---|---|---|---|---|---|---|---|---|
| 1. Wash face | 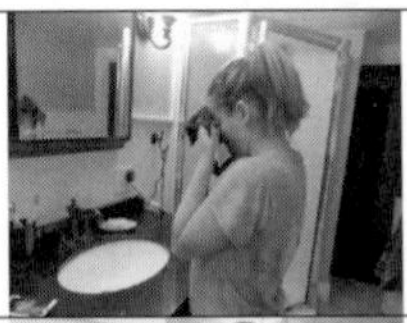 | | | | | | | |
| 2. Brush Teeth | 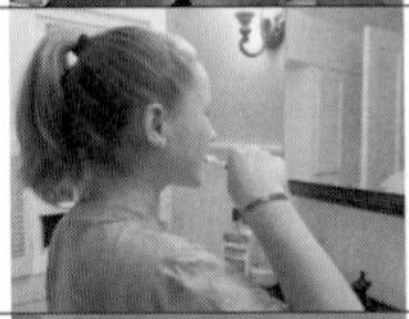 | | | | | | | |
| 3. Comb hair | 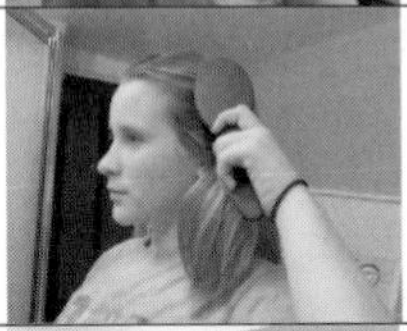 | | | | | | | |
| 4. Style hair | 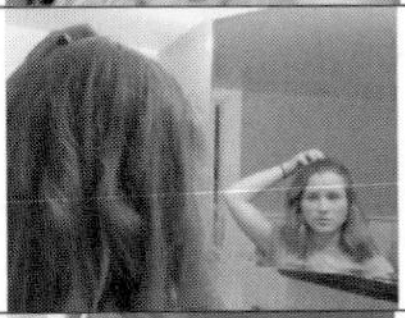 | | | | | | | |
| 5. Put on make-up | 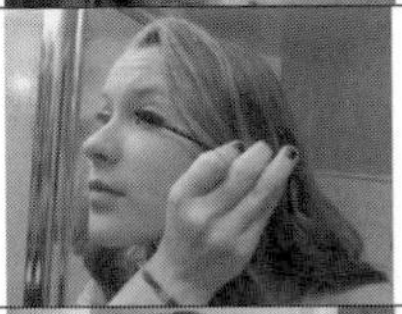 | | | | | | | |
| 6. Get dressed | 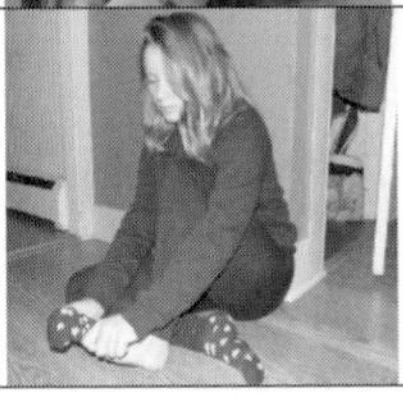 | | | | | | | |

**Fig. A.4** Sample sequence chart for grooming/hygiene.

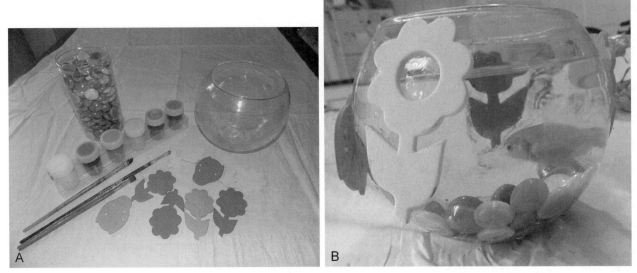

**Fig. A.5  A,** Materials required for goldfish bowl. **B,** Decorated goldfish bowl.

6. Write down a schedule to feed fish daily and a weekly schedule to clean out the fish bowl.
7. Review plan to care for pet, including how to clean out the bowl.

### Population:

Children (may need more supervision) to older adults.

### Body functions targeted:

- Fine motor skills for holding paintbrush and decorating bowl.

### Mental functions targeted:

- Visual functions to place rocks in container and decorate bowl.
- Memory to feed fish daily and clean bowl weekly.
- Visual perception to identify how much food is a "pinch."
- Judgment (higher-level cognitive) to identify when the bowl must be cleaned.
- Emotional to show care for pet.

### Considerations:

- Be sure that the family members or caregivers are okay with the client having a pet fish.
- Pet food should not be eaten and should be out of reach of children.
- Goldfish may not survive long, so practitioners should consider the client's emotional responses.

### Therapeutic techniques:

The OT practitioner may provide client with written instructions or ask the client to write them out. The practitioner may add to the activity by asking the client to discuss pets he or she has owned, describe stories about fish (e.g., Finding Nemo), or name the fish.

## Instrumental Activities of Daily Living: Financial Management

### Activity: Budgeting for Success

### Goals:

1. Develop a monthly budget.
2. Pay bills on time.
3. Save $500 over the year.
4. Use an ATM for cash withdrawals.

### Materials:

- Budget form (Fig. A.6)
- ATM card
- Calculator (can be done on computer, IPad, or phone as well)
- Journal

### Sequence:

1. Have client record all expenses for 1 week (or 1 month) prior to activity in journal.
2. Record all income (weekly or monthly).
3. Brainstorm all expenses; record on budget form.
4. Calculate remaining funds.
5. Discuss financial goals (such as saving $500 annually) and determine how this could be done.
6. Review steps to an ATM withdrawal.

Budget Form

Keep track of income and expenses by writing down all transactions for one week using this form. Make adjustments as needed each week to establish a workable budget. Revise headings as needed.

| | Income | Expenses (actually spent) | total |
|---|---|---|---|
| Weekly Income | | | |
| Other allowance | | | |
| | | | |
| Rent | | | |
| Heat, electricity, water | | | |
| Cable | | | |
| Phone | | | |
| Food | | | |
| Health/medications | | | |
| Transportation (car payment, registration) | | | |
| Insurance | | | |
| Memberships | | | |
| Credit card bills | | | |
| Clothing | | | |
| Entertainment | | | |
| Savings | | | |
| Other | | | |
| | | | |
| Net Total (Income–Expenses) | | | |

• **Fig. A.6** Budget form.

7. Go to ATM and assist client with withdrawal (once he or she is ready).
8. Teach client how to record all expenses.
9. Follow-up weekly or monthly to make adjustments if needed.

### Population:

Teens and older.

### Motor skills targeted:

- Hand and finger strength to grip writing utensil to record expenses and income.
- Fine motor coordination to manipulate ATM card and align ATM card at machine.

### Process skills targeted:

- Attends to task at hand without interruptions.
- Complies with assignment to complete budget and ATM withdrawal.
- Balance to maintain upright posture if using walk-up ATM.
- Uses ATM card and other materials (budget, writing utensils) as they are intended.
- Inquires when needs assistance.
- Sequences the steps in a logical order.
- Benefits: Prevents problems with ATM or budget from recurring.

### Specific mental functions targeted:

- Higher-level cognitive—Discusses and works through income and expense discussion. Develop strategies to save money.
- Exhibits memory for guidelines established so that he/she can stay within established budget.
- Thinks through financial decisions in a logical manner and follows established budget.
- Shows self-control and impulse control over budget decisions.

### Considerations:

The client's age and situation will influence financial management. The OT practitioner may want to involve other people (e.g., parents, caregiver) in the discussion.

### Therapeutic techniques:

The practitioner could teach the basics of financial management with a "sample" budget or even with "pretend" money. Recording income and expenses is an effective way to manage money. This activity will require follow-up and adjustments over time.

## Instrumental Activities of Daily Living: Meal Preparation and Cleanup

### Activity: Two for Lunch

#### Goals:

1. Client will plan and prepare a well-balanced lunch for two people.
2. Client will cleanup food and materials after meal.

3. Client will eat lunch with a friend or peer.
4. Client will complete a shopping list of items needed.

### Materials:

- Food: Client will be asked to develop a shopping list of food items that fit within the five food groups, including: meat/protein, fruit, dairy, vegetable, bread/pasta.
- Plates, silverware, napkins, cups
- Serving dishes

### Sequence:

1. Invite a peer or friend to lunch. Ask if they have any dietary restrictions.
2. Client to develop a menu and shopping list.
3. Client to go shopping (with OT practitioner, if necessary) for food items.
4. Client to prepare lunch (Fig. A.7).
5. Client and peer/friend eat lunch together.
6. Client cleans up.

### Population:

Children and up (excellent activity for adults and older adults).

### Motor skills targeted:

- Stabilizes bowl when stirs or cooks.
- Positions self in relation to cutting board.
- Reaches for food, plates, bowls, and silverware.
- Bends down to get containers in lower cabinets.
- Grips utensils (spoons, knife) and food items.
- Coordinates to hold and stir, hold and cut, etc.
- Lifts food and walks to preparation area.
- Walks around kitchen and in grocery store.

### Process skills targeted:

- Attends to tasks of cleaning and preparing food.
- Follows through to complete lunch preparation, set-up, and cleanup.
- Chooses appropriate bowls, knifes and utensils.
- Handles materials in the intended manner.
- Inquires when needs help with directions.

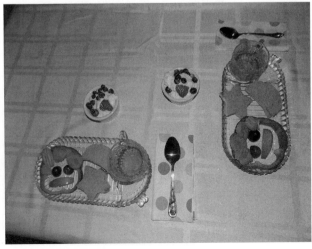

● **Fig. A.7** Set-up for lunch for two.

- Initiates preparing the meal.
- Continues with actions and steps until completion.
- Sequences actions in a logical manner (e.g., cleans salad before preparing it).
- Terminates actions with cleanup.
- Searches for dishes, silverware, napkins, in kitchen cabinets.
- Gathers materials and equipment for tasks.
- Organizes kitchen space and lunch table.
- Navigates through the environment without bumping into anything.

### Considerations:

Children will need much more supervision. Diet and food texture restrictions must be considered.

### Therapeutic techniques:

Clients may have specific meals that bring up memories or hold special significance. The OT practitioner may want to begin this activity with a discussion of favorite foods, meaningful dishes, cultural meals, or family memories around mealtimes. Adding some fun napkins or a homemade centerpiece may add some more meaning to the lunch.

## Rest and Sleep: Sleep Preparation

### Activity: Good Night Moon

### Goals:

1. Develop a sleep routine for health and well-being.
2. Prepare the environment for bedtime.
3. Follow a scheduled bedtime routine for 5 days.

### Materials:

- Soft music (variety of choices)
- Pillows (variety)
- Bedtime books
- Warm liquid of choice (tea or warm milk can be relaxing)
- Variety of pictures (bedtime rituals) to allow client to sequence activities on bedtime schedule. (See Fig. A.8 for examples.)

### Sequence:

1. Discuss the importance of a bedtime routine with client.
2. Using the pictures, ask client to sequence activities for bedtime.
3. Select pillows, books, music that appeals to client.
   - Client may want to decorate his/her own pillow and include a scent (lavender is relaxing).
   - Soft music or sounds of nature may be soothing.
   - Dim lights prior to bedtime.
   - Provide client with choice of pajama.
4. Once client has identified a routine, walk him/her through it.
5. Prepare a written schedule based on client's choices. (See Fig. A.9 for an example.)
6. Ask client to follow routine for 5 days before next visit.
7. Revise schedule and routine and require client record progress in a journal.

### Population: Children to adults

- Parents will have to be involved in the routine for children.

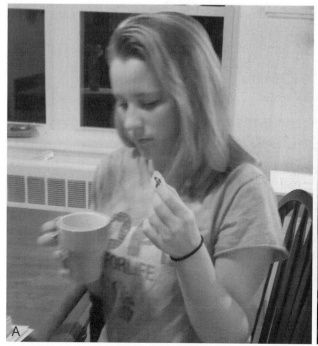
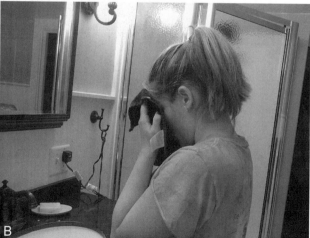

• **Fig. A.8** Sample bedtime routine pictures to be used in the schedule. **A,** Have a cup of soothing tea. **B,** Wash face with warm water.

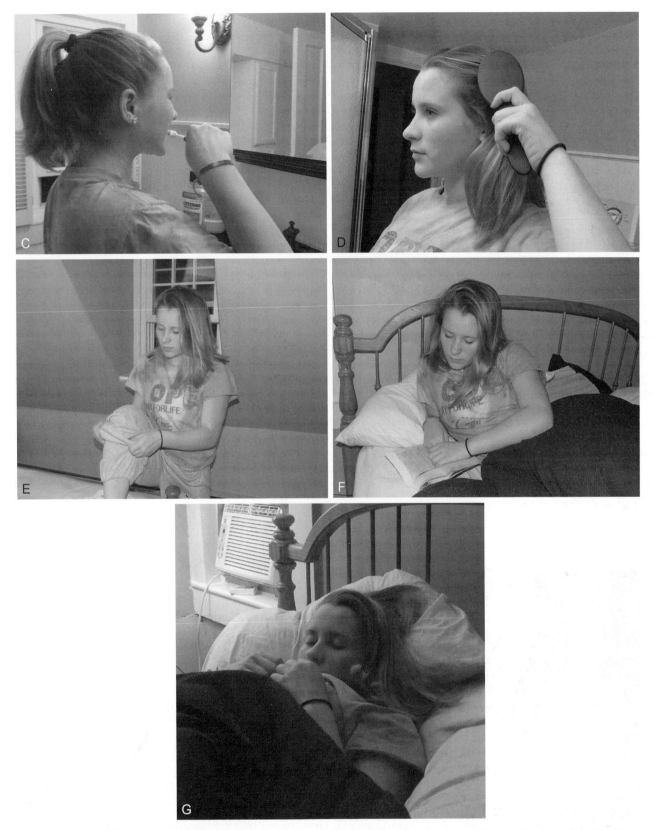

• **Fig. A.8, cont'd  C,** Brush teeth. **D,** Comb hair. **E,** Put on pajamas. **F,** Read a book (30 minutes). **G,** Turn off lights and go to sleep.

Name: _____

Goal: To go to bed by 8:00 pm every night  Monday through Friday.

| | | Time | Mon | Tues | Wed | Thur | Fri |
|---|---|---|---|---|---|---|---|
| 1. Night time snack<br>• Warm liquid<br>• Light snack | | 7:00 pm | | | | | |
| 2. Night time hygiene<br>• Brush teeth<br>• Comb hair<br>• Wash face and hands | | 7:15 pm | | | | | |
| 3. Put on pajamas | | | | | | | |
| 4. Read for 30 minutes | | 7:30 pm | | | | | |
| 5. Turn off the lights | | 8:00 pm | | | | | |

• **Fig. A.9** Sample bedtime schedule.

## Body functions targeted:

- Control of voluntary movement required to complete bedtime routines.

## Mental functions targeted:

- Experience of self and time to understand the bedtime routine.
- Perceiving sensory stimulation as calming.
- Regulating one's emotions to calm and relax for bedtime.

## Sensory functions targeted:

- Hearing calming noises.
- Noticing the dimmer lights.
- Proprioception as heavy pillow calms client.

## Considerations:

Bedtime routines are individualized. Therefore, family cultures should be considered.

## Therapeutic techniques:

Educate client on the importance of bedtime routines. Include the client's choices in the routine. It helps to customize pillows, pajamas, and sensory stimulation. It may take a few sessions to find the objects and routine best for the client. The OT practitioner reinforces the bedtime routine through a schedule (picture schedule may be used for children). Keeping track of one's bedtime routine may help reinforce the pattern.

## Education

### Activity: Hand Skills for School

#### Goals:

1. Develop bilateral upper extremity hand skills for academics.
2. Hold crayon in one hand while holding paper down with other.
3. Copy simple shapes.
4. Write name on the paper.

#### Materials: (Fig. A.10A)

- Crayons (thin and thick)
- Paper (cardstock)
- Sandpaper
- Craft materials (glue, paint, Popsicle sticks)

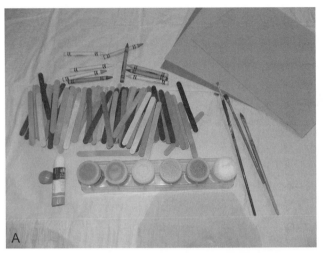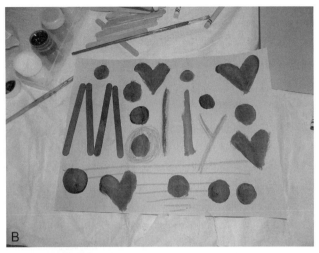

• **Fig. A.10  A,** Materials for hand skill name project. **B,** Sample completed project.

## Sequence:

1. Pick out color of cardstock.
2. Use Popsicle sticks to make the first letter of the child's name.
3. Glue onto cardstock.
4. Draw a picture or color around the Popsicle sticks.
5. Sign drawing (or copy name). (Fig. A.10B shows sample completed project.)

## Population:

Pre-school or elementary school children.

## Body functions targeted:

• Bilateral fine motor skills to manipulate crayon, glue, color.
• Hand coordination to place Popsicle sticks on paper.
• Sitting posture to remain upright throughout task.
• Grip strength to hold crayon and materials.

## Mental functions targeted:

• Attention to details and the task.
• Visual perception to recognize shapes and color.
• Cognition to identify letters and shapes.
• Awareness of one's identity (name).
• Memory to recall letters in the alphabet.

## Considerations:

May want to include some curved cardboard shapes that are round to make letters requiring it (such as O, G, J).

## Therapeutic techniques:

Having a completed product available allows children to see what is expected. The OT practitioner may have to provide one-step instructions and structure the activity by presenting materials for each step. Providing wide crayons may make it easier for some children to grasp. Conversely, thin crayons may be more challenging as they require more hand control. Adding more details to the drawing will increase the complexity.

# Work: Employment seeking and acquisition

## Activity: Job Search (this may take several intervention sessions)

### Goals:

1. Client will complete two job applications.
2. Client will interview for one potential job.
3. Client will follow up with interview.

### Materials:

1. Computer, newspaper ads
2. Clothing for interview
3. Sample interview questions
4. Rubric for job interview performance (Fig. A.11).

### Sequence:

1. Find several possible jobs through search of Internet, newspapers, and word of mouth.
2. Complete application forms.
3. Prepare for interview by selecting interview clothing.
4. Discuss sample questions and practice responses.
5. Engage in "mock interview" with therapist.
6. Discuss and review performance using rubric.
7. Determine the next steps.

### Population:

Teen to adult.

### Body functions targeted:

• Functional mobility to get to interview.
• Postural control to remain sitting throughout interview.

### Mental functions targeted:

• Attention to interviewer and conversation.
• Memory to recall job related tasks and work history.
• Self-awareness of body position and one's identity.
• Higher level cognitive thought to respond to questions with good judgment and insight.
• Ability to link experiences to job responsibilities.

Sample Rubric for evaluating client's performance in a mock job interview.

This rubric provides a format to discuss the client's strengths and weaknesses. The OT practitioner may want to begin by focusing on only a few items.

Name: _____

| Observation/skill | Excellent | Good | Needs Improvement | Comments |
|---|---|---|---|---|
| On time (at least 15 minutes early) for interview | | | | |
| Dressed/groomed appropriately for job | | | | |
| Shakes interviewer's hand firmly | | | | |
| Maintains professional space throughout interview | | | | |
| Makes eye contact | | | | |
| Attends to speaker | | | | |
| Answers questions confidently | | | | |
| Provides thoughtful answers to questions | | | | |
| Asks questions pertinent to job | | | | |
| Highlights why interviewer should select him/her | | | | |
| Demonstrates knowledge of job | | | | |
| Shows interest in job | | | | |
| Respectful to speaker | | | | |
| Positive throughout interview | | | | |
| Flexible to interruptions | | | | |
| Concludes interview | | | | |
| Other observations | | | | |

**Fig. A.11** Sample rubric for job interview.

*Considerations:*

The client's strengths and weaknesses should be considered to find a job that best matches the client's strengths. Safety must be considered. Consideration for the type of employment, setting, and travel is required.

*Therapeutic techniques:*

The OT practitioner assists the client in working through the entire process (which may take several sessions). It may be helpful to include vocational rehabilitation personnel or social workers who know the area's opportunities. Reviewing interviewing skills with other personnel may provide additional training. Reflecting upon performance and selecting jobs that match a client's strengths is necessary.

## Play Participation

### Activity: Themed Play Boxes

*Goals:*

1. Play with a peer for 20 minutes.
2. Share toys with a peer.
3. Engage in play session for 30 minutes.
4. Use an object in an unconventional way during a 30-minute play session.
5. Use bilateral upper extremities to play.

*Materials: (Fig. A.12A)*

- Large cardboard boxes
- Paint, paper, stickers to decorate box
- Pretend clothing

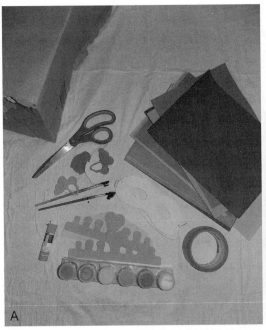
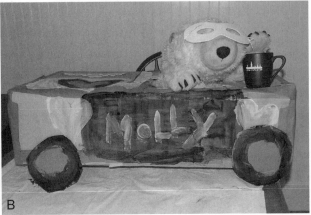

● **Fig. A.12  A,** Materials for themed play boxes. **B,** Sample of box created for play. This child's favorite stuffed animal (polar bear) takes a ride in the decorated car.

### Sequence:

1. Decide on a theme for the play session (animals, super-heroes, space).
2. Decorate box with the theme (e.g., cave for animals, super-hero home, and space ship). (See Fig. A.12B for example.)
3. Dress up to match theme.
4. Play a game using materials and home. For example, go out into the woods and find the other animals and bring them home. Hide animals that can be made from paper or stuffed animals.

### Population:

Children (4 to 12 years).

### Body functions targeted:

- Fine motor skills to paint and manipulate objects in play.
- Muscle strength to pick up objects, walk, and run.
- Control of voluntary movements to engage in eye-hand and eye-foot activity.
- Postural control for sitting, standing, and walking.

### Mental functions targeted:

- Higher level cognition to negotiate play and move body around objects.
- Attention to the play scenario.
- Memory of the theme and how to act it out.
- Visual perception to imagine the box as a "home."
- Awareness of one's self in time and understanding one's identity.
- Responding to peer's cues.
- Sharing materials with others.

### Considerations:

Play sessions can focus on the goal of improving play or they can be used to improve client factors (e.g., upper extremity functioning). The OT practitioner considers the client's needs and focusses on that during the session.

### Therapeutic techniques:

Provide a variety of choices. Be flexible and spontaneous to promote play. The OT practitioner models playful behaviors and encourages the client to engage in play. The session should be enjoyable for the client.

## Leisure exploration

### Activity: What's New in Town?

#### Goals:

1. Identify 10 leisure opportunities in the area.
2. Participate in two new leisure activities.
3. Compare and contrast interest level for new activities.

#### Materials:

- Computer, local papers, newsletters, tourist brochures
- Clothing and additional funds (if needed) to engage in leisure interests
- Camera

#### Sequence:

1. Brainstorm 10 leisure activities by looking through local newsletters, paper, or computer.
2. Select three activities that are most interesting.

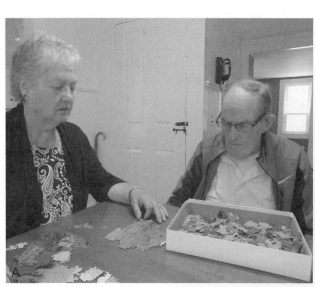
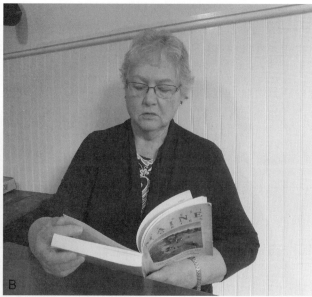
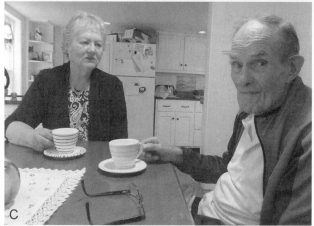

• **Fig. A.13  A,** Putting together a puzzle. **B,** Reading a book. **C,** Enjoying a cup of tea.

3. Discuss cost, setting, skills, and transportation to see if they are possible opportunities.
4. Participate in each activity (this may take several weeks). Take pictures while engaged in the activity. (See Figs. A.13A, A.13B. and A.13C for examples of leisure activities.)
5. Compare and contrast each activity to determine future interest in the activity. Use pictures to remember event and for conversation.

### Population:

Adult or older adults.

### Body functions targeted:

- Gait patterns to get to and engage in the activity.
- Endurance to engage in activity.
- Muscle strength for walking or lifting.

### Sensory functions targeted:

- Visual acuity to be aware of environment and participate in activity.
- Hearing directions or conversation.
- Taste and smell (for some activities).

- Proprioceptive—being aware of one's body position.
- Vestibular—being aware of one's balance, position and movement.

### Mental functions targeted:

- Higher level cognitive: Judgment to make decisions during activity.
- Showing insight into self and activity choices.
- Cognitive flexibility to problem solve during activity.
- Memory to recall decisions and event.
- Regulating emotions when frustrated or unsure.
- Being aware of one's identity and the environment.
- Thinking through things logically.

### Considerations:

This may be more fun in pairs. Clients may be able to engage in the leisure activity outside of OT intervention session. However, the OT practitioner may support clients by attending the activity with them. Safety considerations include safety with transportation, physical demands of activity, and dietary requirements. The physical environment (outside versus inside) and duration (endurance requirements) must be considered.

## Therapeutic techniques:

OT practitioners may have resources to promote leisure exploration for clients who have experienced disability. For example, many states have skiing, sailing, baseball, basketball, dance, horseback riding, camps, and other opportunities for persons with disabilities. There may be support groups, lunch meetings, or conferences that may benefit clients. Sometimes students from occupational therapy programs may even host events to benefit the community. Clients may enjoy being interviewed by students as a way to give back.

# Social Participation

## Activity: Family Game Night

### Goals:

1. Engage in positive family activities.
2. Develop social skills in a family setting.
3. Become more adept at interpreting non-verbal and verbal social cues during a family social event.
4. Read other people's cues during a family social event.

### Materials:

- Board games (Monopoly, Life, cards, Pictionary)
- Puzzles
- Charades

### Sequence:

- Teach client to play a specific game.
- Model social interaction such as maintaining appropriate personal space, reading other people's non-verbal cues, and taking turns.
- Ask open-ended questions during the "practice" and wait for response.
- Review and discuss social cues, taking turns, maintaining appropriate personal space, and participating in conversation.
- Once client is ready, have client plan family game night time place and day.
- Review performance after event.

### Population:

Any age, but games will have to be adapted based on age level and number of participants.

### Movement-related functions targeted:

- Postural control to sit (or stand) during activity.
- Hand skills to hold objects as needed.
- Muscle endurance to engage in light activity for 1 hour.
- Voluntary movement control to complete gross and fine motor movements.

### Mental functions targeted:

- Higher-level cognition to use judgment for conversation, humor, and planning.
- Attention to the task.
- Memory to recall game rules.
- Perception to discriminate between senses.
  - Perceive where sound is coming from.
  - Determine how far people are from you.
  - Integrate sense of balance changes.
- Regulate emotions in relation to conversation and game.
- Be aware of one's identity.

### Sensory Functions targeted:

- Visual to see objects and discriminate between objects at a distance.
- Determine the distance of sounds and identifying who is speaking in a crowded room.
- Vestibular—being aware of balance, position and movement.
- Awareness of body position in space (proprioception).

### Social skills targeted:

- Approaches or initiates interactions with family member.
- Effectively ends conversation and says goodbye.
- Speaks so others can understand.
- Uses gestures appropriately.
- Speaks fluently.
- Turns towards the person speaking.
- Looks at others.
- Maintains appropriate body personal boundaries.
- Regulates social interactions so that others can speak.
- Expresses a range of emotion that fits the situation.
- Disagrees in a way that is socially appropriate.
- Thanks and acknowledges others.
- Handles transitions between activities appropriately.
- Takes turn when playing game.
- Clarifies when necessary.
- Encourages others during game.

### Considerations:

The ages of the family members must be considered when developing games. The practitioner also considers any cultural preferences.

### Therapeutic techniques:

The OT practitioner may want to focus only a few social skills at a time. Practicing in a safe setting (such as the OT clinic) may help the client develop skills. Self-reflection and discussion can reinforce behaviors. Starting the activity with a small group of family members (even one other person) in the clinic may help the client succeed at home.

# Resources

## Professional Organizations, Foundations, and Certification

American Occupational Therapy Association, Inc. (AOTA)
4720 Montgomery Lane
PO Box 31220
Bethesda, MD 20814-3449
Phone: 301-652-6651
TDD: 1-800-729-2682
Fax: 301-652-7711
Website: www.aota.org

American Occupational Therapy Foundation (AOTF)
4720 Montgomery Lane, Suite 202
PO Box 31220
Bethesda, MD 20814
Phone: 240-929-1079
Fax: 240-346-6138
E-mail: aotf@aotf.org
Website: www.aotf.org

Australian Association of Occupational Therapists
OT Australia National
6/340 Gorest
Fitzroy, UIC 3065
Phone: 03941 15 2955
Toll-free: 13006 82 878
E-mail: info@otaus.com.au
Website: www.otaus.com.au

Canadian Association of Occupational Therapists (CAOT)
100-34 Colonnade Road
Ottawa, ON K2E 7J6
Canada
Phone: 613-523-CAOT (2268)
Toll-free: 800-434-CAOT (2268)
Fax: 613-523-2552
Website: www.caot.ca

National Board for Certification in Occupational Therapy, Inc. (NBCOT)
12 South Summit Avenue, Suite 100
Gaithersburg, MD 20877
Phone: 301-990-7979
Fax: 301-869-8492
E-mail: NBCOTatinfo@nbcot.org
Website: www.nbcot.org

World Federation of Occupational Therapists (WFOT)
PO Box 30
Forrestfield, Western Australia
Australia 6058
Fax: 61 8 9453 9746
E-mail: admin@wfot.org.au
Website: www.wfot.org

## Research and Education

American Association of Retired Persons (AARP)
601 E Street NW
Washington, DC 20049
Phone: 1-888-687-2277
Website: www.aarp.org

Centers for Disease Control and Prevention (CDC)
1600 Clifton Road, NE
Atlanta, GA 30329-4027
Phone: 800-232-4636
E-mail: cdc_info@cdc.gov
Website: www.cdc.gov

Centers for Medicare & Medicaid Services (CMS)
7500 Security Boulevard
Baltimore, MD 21244
Website: www.cms.gov

United States Department of Education
400 Maryland Avenue, SW
Washington, DC 20202
Toll-free: 1-800-872-5327
Website: www.ed.gov

United States Department of Health and Human Services
200 Independence Avenue, SW
Washington, DC 20201
Toll-free: 1-877-696-6775
Website: www.hhs.gov

# Glossary

## A

**Accreditation** A form of regulation that determines whether an organization or program meets a prescribed standard

**Accreditation Council for Occupational Therapy Education (ACOTE)** The national organization that regulates entry-level education for occupational therapists and for occupational therapy assistants

**Active being** The view of humans as actively involved in controlling and determining their own behavior

**Active listening** A manner of communication in which the receiver paraphrases the speaker's words to ensure that he or she understands the intended meaning

**Activities of daily living (ADL)** Activities involved in taking care of one's own body, including such things as dressing, bathing, grooming, eating, feeding, personal device care, toileting, sexual activity, and sleep/rest

**Activity** State or condition of being involved (participant); a general class of goal-directed human actions

**Activity analysis** The process in which the steps of an activity and its components are examined to determine the demands on the client

**Activity demands** The aspects of an activity needed to carry out that activity, such as objects used and their properties, space demands, social demands, sequencing and timing, required actions, required body functions, and required body structures

**Activity director** The practitioner responsible for planning, implementing, and documenting an ongoing program of activities that meet the needs of the residents

**Activity synthesis** The process of identifying gaps in performance and bridging those gaps by grading or adapting the activity or the environment in order to provide the "just right challenge" for the client

**Acute care** The first level on the continuum of care in which a client has a sudden and short-term need for services and is typically seen in a hospital

**Adaptation** A change in function that promotes survival and self-actualization

**Adolescence** The period of development between 12 and 20 years of age

**Adolf Meyer** A Swiss physician committed to a holistic perspective; developed the psychobiological approach to mental illness

**Adulthood** The period of development after 20 years of age; broken into a young stage (20–40 years of age), middle (40–65 years of age), and late (over 65 years of age)

**Advanced beginner** A practitioner who is learning to recognize additional cues and beginning to see the client as an individual; still does not see the whole picture

**Advanced-level practitioner** The **advanced-level practitioner** is considered an expert or a resource in the respective role. Advanced-level practitioners gain knowledge and expertise through practice and education. They reflect and develop skills through feedback.

**Affordable Care Act** The Affordable Care Act of 2010 seeks to reduce healthcare spending while increasing quality of care. It addresses the need for efficiency by rewarding settings that prevent hospital acquired conditions (such as falls), prevent hospital re-admission, and provide quality care in which patients are satisfied.

**Aging** The unique changes that occur over time, such as sensory and physical declines

**Aging in place** The trend of more elderly people staying at home and living independently or with minimal assistance

**Altruism** The unselfish concern for the welfare of others

**American Journal of Occupational Therapy (AJOT)** The American Occupational Therapy Association's (AOTA's) official publication that traditionally has served as the main source of research and resource information for the profession

**American Occupational Therapy Association (AOTA)** Formerly called the National Society for the Promotion of Occupational Therapy; the nationally recognized professional association for occupational therapy practitioners

**American Occupational Therapy Foundation (AOTF)** A national organization designed to advance the science of occupational therapy and to increase public understanding of the value of occupational therapy

**American Occupational Therapy Political Action Committee (AOTPAC)** The organization that furthers the legislative aims of the profession by attempting to influence the selection, nomination, election, or appointment of persons to public office

**American Student Committee of the Occupational Therapy Association (ASCOTA)** Student representatives from all accredited schools who participate in the American Occupational Therapy Association by meeting regularly and providing feedback to the organization

**Americans with Disabilities Act of 1990** Legislation that provides civil rights to all individuals with disabilities

**Areas of occupation** Various life activities, including activities of daily living (ADLs), instrumental activities of daily living (IADLs), education, work, play, leisure, and social participation

**Artistic element** The element of clinical reasoning in which the occupational therapy practitioner guides the treatment process and selects the "right action" in the face of uncertainties inherent in the clinical process

**Arts and crafts movement** A late-19th-century movement born in reaction to the Industrial Revolution; emphasized craftsmanship and design

**Assessment instruments** Standardized or non-standardized measurements used to obtain information about clients

**Assessment procedures** The clinical techniques and instruments used to determine the strengths and weaknesses of a client for therapeutic purposes

**Assistive devices** Low- or high-technology aids to improve a person's function

**Assistive technology** Devices that aid a person in his or her daily life as necessary

**Autonomy** The freedom to decide and the freedom to act

**Axiology** The part of philosophy that is concerned with the study of values

## B

**Balanced Budget Act (BBA) of 1997** Legislation intended to reduce Medicare spending, create incentives for development of managed care plans, encourage enrollment in managed care plans, and limit fee-for-service payment and programs

**Beneficence** A principle that requires that the occupational therapy practitioner contribute to the good health and welfare of the client

**Benjamin Rush** An American Quaker who was the first physician to institute moral treatment practices

**Biological sphere** Sphere of practice in which clients have medical problems caused by disease, disorder, or trauma

**Biomechanical frame of reference** A frame of reference derived from theories in kinetics and kinematics; used with individuals who have deficits in the peripheral nervous, musculoskeletal, integumentary (e.g., skin), or cardiopulmonary system

**Board certification** Certification for the occupational therapist or occupational therapy assistant that incorporates more generalized areas of practice that have an established knowledge base in occupational therapy

**Body functions** Body functions refer to the physiological functioning (such as vision). Body functions include mental functions (such as affective, cognitive and perceptual) as well as higher level cognition, attention, memory, thought, sequencing, emotion and experience of time

**Body structures** Body structures refer to the anatomical structures themselves, such as organs and limbs.

**Brain plasticity**    The phenomenon that the brain is capable of change and that through activity one may get improved neurological synapses, improved dendritic growth, or additional pathways

## C

**Canadian Model of Occupational Performance**    A model of practice that emphasizes client-centered care and spirituality

**Career development**    The process of advancing within the service delivery path or transitioning into a role outside of service delivery

**Centennial Vision [2] [4]**

**Cerebral palsy (CP)**    A disorder caused by an insult to the brain before, during, or soon after birth, which manifests in motor abnormalities

**Certification**    The acknowledgement that an individual has the qualifications to be an entry-level practitioner

**Certified occupational therapy assistant (COTA)**    An individual who completed an associate or bachelors degree from an accredited OT Assistant program and who has passed the NBCOT examination for OT assistants.

**Childhood**    Spans early childhood (1–6 years) and later childhood (6–12 years)

**Civilian Vocational Rehabilitation Act**    Act that provided federal funds to states to provide vocational rehabilitation services to civilians with disabilities

**Clarification**    An active listening technique in which the client's thoughts and feelings are summarized or simplified

**Client**    Person served by occupational therapy in a health facility or training center

**Client-centered approach**    An approach in which the client, family, and significant others are active participants throughout the therapeutic process

**Client factors**    Components of activities consisting of body functions and body structures; used to assess functioning, disability, and health

**Client-related tasks**    Routine tasks in which the aide may interact with the client but not as the primary service provider of occupational therapy

**Client satisfaction**    A measure of the client's perception of the process and the benefits received from occupational therapy services

**Clinical reasoning**    The thought process that therapists use to design and carry out intervention; involves complex cognitive and affective skills

**Close supervision**    The need for direct, daily contact with the supervisee

**Code of ethics**    Professional guidelines for making correct or proper choices and decisions for health-care practice in the field

**Cognitive disability frame of reference**    A frame of reference based on the premise that cognitive disorders in those with mental health disabilities are caused by neurobiologic defects or deficits related to the biologic functioning of the brain

**Competent practitioner**    A level of clinical reasoning skills in which the practitioner is able to see more facts and to determine the importance of these facts and observations, has a broader understanding of the client's problems, and is more likely to individualize treatment; however, flexibility and creativity are still lacking

**Concepts**    Ideas that represent something in the mind of the individual

**Conditional reasoning**    The clinical reasoning strategy in which the occupational therapy practitioner implements intervention and cognitively checks along the way to compare the client's progress in treatment and goals for the future

**Confidentiality**    The expectation that information shared by the client with the occupational therapy practitioner will be kept private and shared only with those directly involved with the intervention

**Consultation**    A type of intervention in which practitioners use their knowledge and expertise to collaborate with the client, caregivers, significant others, or other providers

**Consulting [14]**

**Context**    The setting in which the occupation occurs; includes cultural, physical, social, personal, spiritual, temporal, and virtual conditions within and surrounding the client that influence performance

**Continuing competence**    A process in which the occupational therapy practitioner develops and maintains the knowledge, performance skills, interpersonal abilities, critical reasoning skills, and ethical reasoning skills necessary to perform his or her professional responsibilities

**Continuum of care**    A way of characterizing health-care settings by the level of care required by the client, including the whole spectrum of needs

**Contrived activities**    Made-up activities that may include some of the same skills required to do the occupation

**Cultural competence**    One's ability to be more sensitive to other cultures

**Cultural sensitivity**    The ability to understand the needs and emotions of one's own culture and the culture of others

**Culturally responsive care**    Being aware and knowledgeable of cultures, applying cultural skills to practice

**Culture**    Customs, beliefs, activity patterns, behavioral standards, and expectations accepted by the society of which the client is a member

## D

**Deinstitutionalization**    A national plan to release clients from mental health institutions and into the community—the national **Deinstitutionalization** Plan

**Developmental delays**    The general slowing of skills

**Developmental frame of reference**    A frame of reference that postulates that practice in a skill set will enhance brain development and help the child progress through the stages

**Diagnosis codes**    Billing codes that are based on the client's medical condition or the medical justification for needing services

**Diagnosis-related groups (DRGs)**    Groupings of disease categories that Medicare and other third-party payers use as a basis for hospital payment schedules

**Dignity**    The quality or state of being worthy, honored, or esteemed

**Direct supervision**    The supervising occupational therapist is on site and available to provide immediate assistance to the client or supervisee if needed

**Discharge plan**    The plan developed and implemented to address the resources and supports that may be required upon discontinuation of services

**Distinct value [4]**

**Doctor of Occupational Therapy (OTD)**    Clinical or practice-based doctoral degree; focuses on practice rather than research

**Documentation**    The process of keeping records on all the aspects of service delivery

**Driver rehabilitation specialist**    An occupational therapy practitioner who evaluates and intervenes in physical, social, cognitive, and psychosocial aspects of functioning that affect driving skills

## E

**Education**    The process of gaining knowledge and information

**Education for All Handicapped Children Act of 1975 (PL 94-142)**    Act that established the right of all children to a free and appropriate education, regardless of handicapping condition

**Eleanor Clarke Slagle**    Known as the mother of occupational therapy; developed the area of habit training and organized the first professional school for occupational therapy practitioners

**Emergency procedures**    Actions to follow in case of an injury or accident in the clinic

**Empathy**    The ability of the occupational therapy practitioner to place himself or herself in the client's position and to understand what he or she is experiencing

**Entry-level practitioner**    A practitioner who is still developing his or her skills and is expected to be held responsible for and accountable in professional activities related to the role

**Epistemology**    The part of philosophy that investigates critically the nature, origin, and limits of human knowledge

**Equality**    The treatment of all individuals with an attitude of fairness and impartiality and the respecting of each individual's beliefs, values, and lifestyles

**Ergonomics**    The science of fitting jobs to people

**Ethical dilemma**    A situation in which two or more ethical principles collide with one another, making it difficult to determine the best action

**Ethical distress**    Situations that challenge how a practitioner maintains his or her integrity or the integrity of the profession; involves examining the "right" behaviors or proper choices and decisions

**Ethical element**    The element of clinical reasoning that takes into account the client's perspective and his or her goals for intervention

**Ethics**    The study and philosophy of human conduct

**Evaluation**    The process of obtaining and interpreting data necessary to understand the individual and design appropriate treatment

**Evidence-based practice**    Basing practice on the best available research evidence

**Expert**    A practitioner who has the clinical reasoning skills to recognize and understand rules of practice, use intuition to know what to do next, and use conditional reasoning

## F

**Family-centered care**    Care that involves working with the family members of the child on goals that are considered important to them

**Fidelity**    Faithfulness

**Fieldwork**    Practical experience applying classroom knowledge to a clinical setting; categorized as level I (may be observational) or level II (development of entry-level skills)

**Frame of reference (FOR)**    A system that applies theory and puts principles into practice, providing practitioners with specifics on how to treat specific clients

**Freedom**    An individual's right to exercise choice

**Function**    Action for which a person is fit; the ability to perform

## G

**Gary Kielhofner**    An OT leader who developed the Model of Human Occupation. He conducted research internationally, developed assessments, and published extensively.

**General supervision** At least monthly face-to-face contact with the supervisee

**George Edward Barton** An architect who opened Consolation House for convalescent patients, where occupation was used as a method of treatment

**Goal** End toward which effort is directed

**Grading** Changing the process, environment, tools, or materials of the activity to increase or decrease the performance demands on the client

**Group** More than two people interacting with a common purpose

**Group dynamics** Refers to the interactions among individuals and how they work together

**H**

**Habit training** A reeducation program dedicated to restoring and maintaining health by directing activity to construct new habits and discard ineffective ones

**Handicapped Infants and Toddlers Act of 1986** An amendment to the Education for All Handicapped Children Act; includes children from 3 to 5 years of age and initiates new early intervention programs for children from birth to 3 years of age

**Health** The state of physical, mental, and social well-being

**Herbert Hall** A physician who adapted the arts and crafts movement for medical purposes

**Holistic** An approach deeming that each individual should be seen as a complete and unified whole rather than a series of parts or problems to be managed

**Hospice** Care and services provided to help the client be comfortable during the last stages of a terminal illness

**Humanism** The belief that the client should be treated as a person, not an object

**I**

**Ideal self** What an individual would like to be if free of the demands of mundane reality

**Independence** State or condition of being independent (self-reliant)

**Individualized education plan (IEP)** A plan that charts the problems, goals, and interventions necessary for the child to have success in school

**Individuals with Disabilities Education Act (IDEA) of 1991** Legislation that requires school districts to educate students with disabilities in the least restrictive environment

**Infancy** The period from birth through 1 year of age

**Informed consent** The knowledgeable and voluntary agreement by which a client undergoes intervention that is in accord with his or her values and preferences

**Instrumental activities of daily living (IADLs)** Activities, such as meal preparation, money management, and care of others, that involve interacting with the environment; often complex; may be considered optional

**Interactive reasoning** A strategy used by the occupational therapy practitioner when he or she wants to understand the client as a person

**Interdisciplinary team** A mix of practitioners from different disciplines who maintain their own professional roles and use a cooperative approach that is very interactive and centered on a common problem to solve

**Intermediate-level practitioner** A practitioner who has increased responsibility and typically pursues specialization in a particular area of practice

**Interprofessional education (IPE)** An approach to learning that involves a group of students from multiple professions interacting and providing insight into complex issues.

**Interrater reliability** A measure of the likelihood that test scores will be the same no matter who is the examiner

**Intervention** An approach that involves working with the client through therapy to reach client goals

**Interview** The primary mechanism for gathering information for the occupational profile; achieved by the occupational therapy practitioner asking the client and significant others questions

**J**

**Justice** The need for all occupational therapy practitioners to abide by the laws that govern the practice and the legal rights of the client

**L**

**Later adulthood** The period of development after 65 years of age

**Law** Binding custom or practice of a community; a rule of conduct or action prescribed or formally recognized as binding or enforced by a controlling authority

**Learned helplessness** The phenomenon of less activity and independence in functioning among elderly people that results when older persons are not allowed to engage in activities or when others do everything for them

**Least restrictive environment** The classroom most similar to a regular classroom in which the student can be successful

**Level I fieldwork** An experience completed concurrently with academic coursework; it involves observation and participation in selected aspects of the OT process.

**Level II fieldwork** Hands-on clinical training opportunities designed to provide students with in-depth experience delivering OT services with supervision.

**Licensure** The process by which permission is granted to an individual to engage in a given occupation upon finding that the applicant has attained the minimal degree of competence required to ensure that public health, safety, and welfare will be reasonably protected

**Locus of authority** Situations that require a decision about who should be the primary decision maker

**Long-term care** The level of care needed for clients who are medically stable but have a chronic condition requiring services over time, potentially throughout their lives

**M**

**Mandatory reporting** The requirement that certain professionals, including health-care providers, reported suspected child abuse.

**Mechanistic** The view that sees the human as passive in nature and controlled by the environment in which he or she lives

**Media** The means by which therapeutic effects are transmitted

**Medicare** Enacted in 1965; legislation that provides health-care assistance for individuals 65 years or older or those who are permanently and totally disabled

**Metaphysics** One part of philosophy that addresses questions such as "What is the nature of humankind?"

**Methods** The steps, sequences, and approaches used to activate the therapeutic effect of a medium

**Modality** The media and methods used in occupational therapy intervention

**Model of Human Occupation** A model of practice that views occupation in terms of volition, habituation, performance, and environment

**Model of practice** A way of organizing that takes the philosophical base of the profession and provides terms to describe practice, tools for evaluation, and a guide for intervention

**Moral treatment** A movement grounded in the philosophy that all people, even the most challenged, are entitled to consideration and human compassion

**Morals** A view of right and wrong developed as a result of background, values, religious beliefs, and the society in which a person lives

**Multidisciplinary team** A mix of practitioners from multiple disciplines who work together in a common setting but without an interactive relationship

**N**

**Narrative reasoning** The type of clinical reasoning in which storytelling and story creation are used

**National Board for Certification in Occupational Therapy (NBCOT)** The organization responsible for administering the national certification examination

**National Society for the Promotion of Occupational Therapy** Formed on March 15, 1917; marked the birth of the profession of occupational therapy

**Non–client-related tasks** The preparation of the work area and equipment, clerical tasks, and maintenance activities

**Nonmaleficence** A principle that instructs the practitioner to not inflict harm to the client

**Nonstandardized tests** Tests that do not provide specific guidelines based on a normative sample; do not require standardized procedures

**Nonverbal communication** Communication that includes facial expressions, eye contact, tone of voice, touch, and body language

**Normative data** Information collected from a representative sample that can then be used by the examiner to make comparisons with his or her clients

**Novice** A practitioner who is learning the procedural skills (e.g., assessment, diagnostic, and treatment planning procedures) necessary to practice

**O**

**Observation** The means of gathering information about a person or an environment by watching and noticing

**Occupation** Activity in which one engages that is meaningful and central to one's identity

**Occupation as a means** The use of a specific occupation to bring about a change in the client's performance

**Occupation as an end** The desired outcome or product of intervention

**Occupation-based/occupation-centered activity** The performance of occupation-related activities by the client, including activities of daily living, instrumental activities of daily living, work and school tasks, and play or leisure tasks

**Occupational adaptation** A model of practice that proposes that occupational therapy practitioners examine how they may change the person, environment, or task so the client may engage in occupations

**Occupational justice** The belief that all persons (regardless of ability, age, gender, social class, or economic status) are entitled to have access to participation in everyday occupations.

**Occupational performance** The ability to carry out activities in the areas of occupation

**Occupational profile** An occupational profile is a history of the client's background and functional performance.

**Occupational therapist** An allied health professional who uses occupation, purposeful activity, simulated activities, and preparatory methods to maximize the independence and health of any client who is limited by physical injury or illness, cognitive impairment, psychosocial dysfunction, mental illness, or a developmental or learning disability

**Occupational therapy** A goal-directed activity that promotes independence in function; the practice of using meaningful occupations and purposeful activities to promote function and participation in life activities

**Occupational therapy aide** A person who provides services under the supervision of an occupational therapist to clients and therapists and helps maintain the work space

**Occupational therapy assistant (OTA)** An allied health paraprofessional who, under the direction of an occupational therapist, directs an individual's participation in selected tasks to restore, reinforce, and enhance performance and to promote and maintain health

**Occupational therapy practitioner** Refers to two different levels of clinicians, an occupational therapist or an occupational therapy assistant (OTA)

**Occupational therapy process** The interaction between two active agents involved in the process—the practitioner and the client

**Organismic** The view that a person's behaviors influence the physical and social environment and that, in turn, the person is affected by changes in the environment

**Orthotic device** An apparatus used to support, align, prevent, or correct deformities or to improve the function of movable parts of the body

**Outcome measures** An aspect of program evaluation that evaluates the results of the intervention after the service has been provided

## P

**Participation** Active engagement in one's occupations

**Participatory research** Involves the clinician, client, and faculty member in the research process

**Patient** Person served in a hospital or rehabilitation setting

**Perceived self** The aspect that others see; what they perceive without the benefit of knowing a person's intentions, motivations, and limitations

**Performance patterns** The client's habits, routines, and roles

**Performance skills** Small units of observable action that are linked together in the process of executing a daily life task performance

**Person-Environment-Occupation-Performance** A model of practice that provides definitions and describes the interactive nature of human beings

**Phenomenological** That which is determined by the experience of individuals

**Philippe Pinel** French physician who advocated humane treatment for mentally ill patients in the late 1700s

**Physical agent modalities (PAMs)** Preparatory methods used to bring about a response in soft tissue

**Plain language** Clear, concise wording; language that is understood by those not familiar or educated in health-care environments

**Play** The spontaneous, enjoyable, rule-free, internally motivated activity in which there is no goal or purpose

**Political action committees (PACs)** The legally sanctioned vehicles through which organizations can engage in political action

**Polytrauma [5]**

**Pragmatic reasoning** The type of clinical reasoning that takes into consideration factors in the context of the practice setting and in the personal context of the occupational therapy practitioner that may inhibit or facilitate intervention

**Preparatory activities/methods** Techniques or activities that address the remediation and restoration of problems associated with client factors and body structure, with the long-term purpose of supporting the client's acquisition of performance skills needed to resume his or her roles and daily occupations

**Prevention** Limiting, reducing, slowing down or eliminating disease, trauma, or poor health

**Primary care** Healthcare setting where clients develop a sustained partnership and practice in the context of the family and community

**Principles** Ideas that explain the relationship between two or more concepts

**Private for-profit agencies** Organizations owned and operated by individuals or a group of investors

**Private not-for-profit agencies** Organizations that receive special tax exemptions and typically charge a fee for services and maintain a balanced budget to provide services

**Private funding sources** Businesses that provide funds for medical procedures

**Problem-oriented medical record** A format that provides a structure to documentation

**Procedural reasoning** A clinical reasoning strategy used by the occupational therapy practitioner when he or she focuses on the client's disease or disability and determines what will be the most appropriate modalities to use to improve the functional performance

**Procedure codes** Billing codes that are based on the specific services performed by health-care providers

**Professional association** An organization that exists to protect and promote the profession it represents by (1) providing a communication network and channel for information, (2) regulating itself through the development and enforcement of standards of conduct and performance, and (3) guarding the interests of those within the profession

**Professional development** Organizing and personally managing a cumulative series of work experiences to add to one's knowledge, motivation, perspectives, skills, and job performance

**Professional philosophy** A set of values, beliefs, truths, and principles that guide the practitioner's actions

**Proficient practitioner** A practitioner who views situations as a whole instead of as isolated parts; practical experience allows the proficient practitioner to develop a direction and vision of where the client should be going; able to easily modify the intervention plan if the initial plan does not work

**Program evaluation** Measuring effectiveness by determining which programs are achieving their goals and objectives, then modifying programs accordingly

**Program process** The stages of referral, evaluation, and intervention

**Program structure** The system in which the services are delivered (e.g., staff levels and expertise, equipment, budget and range of services)

**Prudence** The ability to demonstrate sound judgment, care, and discretion

**Psychological sphere** A sphere of practice in which client problems manifest as emotional, cognitive, affective, or personality disorders

**Public agencies** Health-care agencies operated by federal, state, or county governments

**Public funding sources** Agencies at the federal, state, or local level that provide funds for medical procedures

**Purposeful activity** An activity used in treatment that is goal directed; individual is an active voluntary participant; has both inherent and therapeutic goals

## Q

**Quality of life** A relative measurement of what is meaningful and what provides satisfaction to an individual

## R

**Real self** A blending of the internal and external worlds involving intention and action plus environmental awareness

**Reconstruction aides** Civilians who helped rehabilitate soldiers who had been injured in the war so that they could either return to active military duty or be employed in a civilian job

**Reductionistic** View that humankind is reduced to separately functioning parts

**Referral** A request for service for a particular client or a change in the degree and direction of service

**Reflection** A response wherein the purpose is to express in words the feelings and attitudes sensed behind the words of the speaker

**Registered occupational therapist (OTR)** An individual who has completed the requirements for the education of an occupational therapist at an accredited program (masters degree requirement) and passed the NBCOT examination.

**Registration** The listing of qualified individuals by a professional association or government agency

**Regulations** Policies describing the implementation and enforcement of laws

**Rehabilitation Act of 1973** Act that guaranteed certain rights for people with disabilities, emphasized the need for rehabilitation research, and called for priority service for persons with the most severe disabilities

**Rehabilitation movement** The period from 1942 to 1960 in which Veterans Administration hospitals increased in size and number to handle casualties of war and the continued care of veterans

**Relationship** A connection of different roles to one another

**Reliability** A measure of how accurately the scores obtained from the test reflect the true performance of the client

**Restatement** The listener repeats the words of the speaker as they are heard

**Role** A pattern of behavior that involves certain rights and duties that an individual is expected, trained, and encouraged to perform in a particular social situation

**Role competence** The ability to meet the demands of roles

**Routine supervision** Direct contact at least every 2 weeks with interim supervision as needed

## S

**Scientific element** One of the three elements of clinical reasoning that demands careful and accurate assessments, analysis, and recording

**Screening** The process by which the occupational therapy practitioner gathers preliminary information about the client and determines whether further evaluation and occupational therapy intervention are warranted

**Self-awareness** Knowing one's own true nature; the ability to recognize one's own behavior, emotional responses, and effect created on others

**Sensory input** Input that is provided through touch, heat, vibration, or senses (sight, hearing, taste, smell)

**Service competency** A useful mechanism by which it is determined that two people performing the same or equivalent procedures will obtain the same or equivalent results

**Service management functions** Functions that include maintaining a safe and efficient workplace, making daily schedules, documenting treatment, integrating research into practice, billing for services, supervising fieldwork students, handling marketing and public relations, and performing quality assurance activities

**Simulated activity** Activities of which some aspect is "made-up" or involves substituting actual materials or equipment

**SOAP note** The format used for writing the progress note, wherein "S" is subjective information, "O" is objective information, "A" is the assessment, and "P" is the plan

**Social Security Amendments** Changes to social security law which affected the way health-care dollars were dispersed

**Sociological sphere** A sphere of practice wherein clients have problems meeting the expectations of society

**Soldier's Rehabilitation Act** Act that established a program of vocational rehabilitation for soldiers disabled on active duty

**Specialty certification** A credential for occupational therapists and occupational therapy assistants that indicates advanced knowledge in a particular area of practice

**Splint** A device for immobilization, restraint, or support of any part of the body

**Standardized tests** A test that has gone through a rigorous process of scientific inquiry to determine the reliability and validity

**Standards of practice** Guidelines for the delivery of occupational therapy services

**Statutes** Laws that are enacted by the legislative branch of a government

**Structured observation** The means of gathering information about a person by watching the client perform a predetermined activity

**Subacute care** The level in which the client still needs care but does not require an intensive level or specialized service

**Supervision** A cooperative process in which two or more people participate in a joint effort to establish, maintain, and or elevate a level of competence and performance

**Susan Cox Johnson** Demonstrated that occupation could be morally uplifting and could improve the mental and physical state of patients and inmates in public hospitals and almshouses

**Susan Tracy** A nurse involved in the arts and crafts movement and in the training of nurses in the use of occupations

## T

**Task groups basic unit of actions** Groups with specific outcomes and tasks to be completed

**Tasks [1] [3]**

**Technology Related Assistance for Individuals with Disabilities Act of 1988** Act that addressed the availability of assistive technology devices and services to individuals with disabilities

**Test-retest reliability** A measure of the consistency of the results of a given test from one administration to another

**Theory** A set of ideas that help explain things and how they work

**Therapeutic exercise** The scientific supervision of exercise for the purpose of preventing muscular atrophy, restoring joint and muscle function, and improving efficiency of cardiovascular and pulmonary function

**Therapeutic reasoning** The process used to make decisions in occupational therapy practice

**Therapeutic relationship** The interaction between a practitioner and a client in which the occupational therapy practitioner is responsible for facilitating the healing and rehabilitation process

**Therapeutic use of occupations and activity** The selection of activities and occupations that will meet the therapeutic goals

**Therapeutic use of self** The art of relating to clients, which involves being aware of oneself and of the client and being in command of what is communicated

**Therapy** Treatment of an illness or disability

**Thomas Kidner** An architect who was influential in establishing a presence for occupational therapy in vocational rehabilitation and tuberculosis treatment

**Transdisciplinary team** A mix of practitioners from different disciplines in which members cross over professional boundaries and share roles and functions

**Transition services** The coordination or facilitation of services for the purpose of preparing the client for a change

**Truthfulness** The value demonstrated through behavior that is accountable, honest, and accurate and that maintains one's professional competence

## U

**Universal precautions** A set of guidelines designed to prevent the transmission of HIV, hepatitis B virus, and other blood-borne pathogens to health-care providers

**Universal stages of loss** Stages of death and dying first identified by Elisabeth Kübler-Ross, which include denial, anger, bargaining, depression, and acceptance; can also be applied to individuals experiencing loss as a result of a disabling condition

## V

**Validity** The quality of an assessment being a true measure of what it claims to measure

**Veracity** The duty of the health-care professional to tell the truth

**Vision** A statement or ethos of a profession or organization that is developed with the members and constituents over time and that clarifies values, creates a future direction, and focuses the mission

**Volition** One's desire, motivations and interests

## W

**Well-being** Sense of health, quality of life, personal satisfaction

**Wellness** The condition of being in good health

**William Rush Dunton, Jr.** Considered the father of occupational therapy; introduced a regimen of crafts for his patients

**William Tuke** An English Quaker who opened the York Retreat, which pioneered new methods of treatment of mentally ill patients

**World Federation of Occupational Therapists (WFOT)** Organization established in 1952 to help occupational therapy practitioners access international information, engage in international exchange, and promote organizations of occupational therapy in schools in countries where none exists

**World War I** A war fought from 1914 to 1918, in which Great Britain, France, Russia, Belgium, Italy, Japan, the United States, and other allies defeated Germany, Austria-Hungary, Turkey, and Bulgaria. (American Heritage Dictionary)

## Y

**Young adulthood** The ages between 20 and 40 years

# Index

Note: Page numbers followed by *f* indicate figures, *t* indicate tables, and *b* indicate boxes.